Springer Series on Advanced Practice Nursing

Terry T. Fulmer, PhD, C, FAAN, Series Editor
New York University School of Nursing

Mathy Doval Mezey, RN, EdD, FAAN, received her undergraduate and graduate education at Columbia University. She taught at Lehman College of the City University of New York. For 10 years she was a professor at the University of Pennsylvania School of Nursing where she directed the geriatric nurse practitioner program and was Director of the Robert Wood Johnson Foundation Teaching Nursing Home Program, a national initiative to link schools of nursing and nursing homes. Currently, Dr. Mezey is at New York University in the Division of Nursing where she holds a Chair as the Independence Foundation Professor of Nursing Education and directs the Hartford Institute for Geriatric Nursing. The national focus of the Hartford Institute, founded in 1996, is to improve care received by older adults by stimulating best practices in nursing education, clinical care, research and public policy.

Dr. Mezey has authored 5 books and has over 50 publications that focus on nursing care of the elderly and bioethical issues that affect decisions at the end of life. She is Series Editor for the Springer Series in Geriatric Nursing. Her research and writing focus on improving nursing care to older adults, and how best to improve decision making about life-sustaining treatment.

Dr. Mezey is a Fellow in the Gerontological Society of America, and sits on the boards of the Visiting Nurse Service of New York and the American Federation of Aging Research (AFAR).

Diane O'Neill McGivern, RN, PhD, FAAN, began a nursing career after receiving her Bachelor of Science Degree in Nursing from St. John's College in Cleveland, Ohio. During her career, she has worked as a staff nurse, an administrator, and a professor. She earned her MA and PhD from New York University. In 1987 she was appointed Head of the Division of Nursing at New York University. Dr. McGivern has also been a faculty member at Hunter College and at the University of Pennsylvania.

Dr. McGivern has been active in professional nursing and other health organizations and has received honors and awards for her work. She has been a Robert Wood Johnson Health Policy Fellow, elected to the American Academy of Nursing, and is on the board of the Nurses' Educational Fund. She has also produced numerous articles, speeches, and presentations during her prolific career, focusing on professional practice preparation, particularly advanced practice nursing.

Dr. McGivern was elected by the New York State Legislature in 1991 to serve on the Board of Regents, the governing body for education in the state. In March of 1998 she was elected Vice Chancellor of the Board of Regents.

Third Edition

Nurses,
Nurse
Practitioners

Evolution to
Advanced Practice

Mathy D. Mezey, RN, EdD, FAAN
Diane O. McGivern, RN, PhD, FAAN
Editors

 Springer Publishing Company

Springer Publishing Company, Inc.
536 Broadway
New York, NY 10012-3955

Cover design by Janet Joachim
Acquisitions Editor: Ruth Chasek
Production Editor: Helen Song

00 01 02 03/ 5 4 3 2

Library of Congress Cataloging-in-Publication Data

Nurses, nurse practitioners : evolution to advanced practice / edited by
    Mathy D. Mezey and Diane O. McGivern.—third edition
        p. cm.—(Springer series on advanced practice nursing)
    Includes bibliographical references and index.
    ISBN 0-8261-7771-9
    1. Nurse practitioners.   2. Primary care (Medicine)   I. Mezey,
Mathy Doval.   II. McGivern, Diane O'Neill.   III. Series.
    [DNLM: 1. Nurse Practitioners.   2. Primary Health Care.
WY 128N9744 1998]
RT82.8.N884   1998
610.73'06'91   dc21
DNLM/DLC
for Library of Congress   98-26293
                                                                                      CIP

Printed in the United States of America

CONTENTS

CONTRIBUTORS

Ellen D. Baer, RN, PhD, FAAN, Professor Emerita, University of Pennsylvania, School of Nursing; Visiting Professor, New York University, Division of Nursing, New York, New York

Patricia M. Barber, RN, MPA, Coordinator, Clinical Nurse Partnership Managers, Oxford Health Plans of New York, New York, New York

Henry L. Barnett, MD, Senior Consultant, The Children's Aid Society, New York, New York; Distinguished Professor Emeritus, Albert Einstein College of Medicine, Department of Pediatrics, New York, New York

Carol Boland, MSN, RN, Ridgefield Pediatric Associates, Ridgefield, Connecticut

Karen Buhler-Wilkerson, PhD, RN, FAAN, Professor of Community Nursing, University of Pennsylvania, School of Nursing, Philadelphia, Pennsylvania

Bonnie Bullough*, PhD, RN, FAAN, Professor, State University of New York at Buffalo; Dean, School of Nursing, Buffalo, New York

Vern L. Bullough, PhD, RN, Professor, University of Southern California, School of Nursing, Los Angeles, California

---

*deceased

Marina Burke, MSN Candidate, Columbia University, Adult Nurse Practitioner Program, New York, New York; Research Editor, Oxford Health Plans of New York, New York, New York

Winifred Y. Carson, Esq., Nurse Practice Council, American Nurses Association, Washington, DC

Joyce Colling, RN, PhD, FAAN, Professor Emeritus, Gerontological Nursing, Oregon Health Science University, School of Nursing, Portland, Oregon

Lois K. Evans, DNSC, RN, FAAN, Professor and Director; Academic Nursing Practices, Viola MacInnes/Independence Chair in Nursing, University of Pennsylvania, School of Nursing, Philadelphia, Pennsylvania

Claire M. Fagin, PhD, FAAN, Dean, University of Pennsylvania, School of Nursing, Philadelphia, Pennsylvania

Loretta Ford, PhD, RN, FAAN, Professor Emeritus, University of Rochester, School of Nursing, Rochester, New York

Jane A. Fox, EdD, RNCS, PNP, Clinical Associate Professor, New York University, Division of Nursing, New York, New York; Clinical Associate Professor, State University of New York at Stony Brook, School of Nursing, Stony Brook, New York

Cynthia M. Freund, PhD, FAAN, Dean, University of North Carolina at Chapel Hill, School of Nursing, Chapel Hill, North Carolina

Virginia Gillet, MSN, CPNP, Private Practice, Los Angeles, California

Judith B. Igoe, RN, MS, FAAN, Associate Professor, Director, Office of School Health Programs, University of Colorado Health Sciences Center, School of Nursing, Denver, Colorado

Sabrina D. Jarvis, RN, MS, CCRN, SICU Nurse Practitioner, Veteran's Affair Medical Center, Orem, Utah

Melinda Jenkins, PhD, CRNP, Assistant Professor of Primary Care, University of Pennsylvania, School of Nursing, Philadelphia, Pennsylvania

William Kavesh, MD, MPH, Medical Director, Geriatric Primary Care, Philadelphia Veterans Affairs Medical Center; Clinical Assistant Professor of Medicine, University of Pennsylvania, School of Medicine, Philadelphia, Pennsylvania; Adjunct Assistant Professor of Medicine (Health Services), Boston University School of Medicine, Boston, Massachusetts

Susan Leib, MD, Ridgefield Pediatric Associates, Ridgefield, Connecticut

Carolyn Lewis, Executive Director of ANCC, American Nurse Association, Washington, D.C.

Joan E. Lynaugh, RN, PhD, FAAN, Center for the Study of the History of Nursing, University of Pennsylvania, School of Nursing, Philadelphia, Pennsylvania

Betsy Mayberry, MSW, Social Worker and Director of Services, The Children's Aid Society, New York, New York

Connie Mullinix, PhD, MPH, MBA, RN, Flynt Mullinix Health Care Consulting, Chapel Hill, North Carolina

Madeline A. Naegle, RN, PhD, CS, FAAN, Associate Professor, New York University, Division of Nursing, New York, New York

Ann L. O'Sullivan, PhD, CRNP, FAAN, Faculty, University of Pennsylvania School of Medicine, Philadelphia, Pennsylvania; Family and Community Health Section, School of Nursing, University of Pennsylvania, Philadelphia, Pennsylvania; Director, Teen-Baby Program, General Pediatrics Division, The Children's Hospital of Philadelphia, Philadelphia, Pennsylvania

Geraldine S. Paier, PhD, CRNP, Adjunct Professor, University of Arizona, Department of Gerontological Studies, Tucson, Arizona

Frances K. Porcher, EdD, RN, CPNP, Private Pediatric Practice, Bountiful, Utah

Amy Rosenbaum-Welsh, RN, MS, Family Nurse Practitioner, community clinic and school-based teen health center, San Diego, California;

Outstanding Master of Science Student Award, School of Nursing, University of California, San Francisco

Jo Anne Staats, MSN, NP, Bronx-Lebanon Hospital Center, Affiliated with Albert Einstein College of Medicine, Bronx, New York

Ginny Strakosch, PNP, Pediatric Nurse Practitioner, The Children's Aid Society, New York, New York

Neville E. Strumpf, PhD, RN, C, FAAN, Associate Professor and Director, Gerontological Nurse Practitioner Program, University of Pennsylvania, School of Nursing, Philadelphia, Pennsylvania

Eileen M. Sullivan-Marx, PhD, FAAN, Assistant Professor/Program Director Primary Care-Adult Nurse Practitioner Program, University of Pennsylvania, School of Nursing, Philadelphia, Pennsylvania

Joyce E. Thompson, CNM, DrPH, FAAN, FACNM, Professor, University of Pennsylvania, School of Nursing, Philadelphia, Pennsylvania

Jodee Tolomeo, PNP, Pediatric Nurse Practitioner and Clinical Coordinator of The Medical Foster Boarding Home Program, The Children's Aid Society, New York, New York

Rachel Wilson, MS, RN, CS, FNP, Doctoral Candidate, New York University, Division of Nursing, New York, New York; Instructor, Rutgers College of Nursing, Newark, New Jersey

FOREWORD

THIS third edition of *Nurses, Nurse Practitioners: Evolution to Advanced Practice* amply demonstrates that advanced practice nursing (APN) has come of age.

As one of the four most celebrated models of APN, the nurse practitioner (NP), along with nurse-midwives, nurse anesthetists, and clinical nurse specialists, is emerging from a controversial past and is the central theme of this timely publication.

At last, the NP has achieved professional status and indeed has helped to elevate nursing to a new level of professionalism through institutionalization in education, practice, and research. Upon entering the stage of hard intellectual development as an academic discipline, the NPs and other advanced practice nurses are challenged to take their rightful place in the nation's systems of professional education, practice, research, leadership, and policy development. These progressive, important, and historical challenges deserve to be noticed and recorded as they are so cogently in this publication.

This third edition of *Nurses, Nurse Practitioners: Evolution to Advanced Practice* chronicles the progress made since the first edition, adds new dimensions that demonstrate role expansions, the creation of specialties, and delivery system and legislative changes, and addresses the global nature of APN.

New practice paradigms, discussions of specific practice venues, such as acute care and school health, and management of discrete clinical problems like AIDS, pain, incontinence, and others make this a valuable resource for all APNs, students, faculty and their colleagues, and partners in other disciplines. From a historical and philosophical perspective through various practice arenas to policy elements of legislation and financing practice, this new edition provides pathways of understanding, appreciation, and direction as the APN forges ahead into the 21st century.

Loretta C. Ford, RN, EdD, FAAN
Professor and Dean Emeritus
School of Nursing
University of Rochester
Rochester, NY

P A R T **I**

HISTORICAL, EDUCATIONAL, RESEARCH, AND PHILOSOPHICAL PERSPECTIVES

Chapter 1

ADVANCED PRACTICE NURSING: PREPARATION AND CLINICAL PRACTICE

Diane O. McGivern and Mathy D. Mezey

HISTORY AND DEFINITION

B EGINNING in the early 1900s, every decade has provided an additional impetus to support and advance an expanded practice role for nurses. Clinical specialization developed between the 1900s and 1930s through hospital-based courses in anesthesia, operating room, and obstetrical nursing. As post-World War II hospital care became more sophisticated, it required the services of clinical nurse specialists who could provide expert patient care and consultation to less well-prepared nursing staff. The Nurse Training Act, initially enacted in 1964, provided the expanded government funding necessary to support and extend this expert clinician model for inpatient settings (Elder & Bullough, 1990). Functional preparation of nurses for teaching and administration became less a focus through the 1960s and 1970s as clinical training became more important. While graduate programs increased in number and narrowness of specialization, they tended to lack consistency in content or competencies (Kitchens, Piazza, & Ellison, 1989).

The development of the first nurse practitioner program in 1965 by Loretta Ford and Henry Silver was a seminal event in that it was based on a "nursing model focused on the promotion of health in daily living, growth and development for children in families, as well as the prevention of disease and disability" (Ford, 1982, 1986). Ford notes that societal needs and nursing's potential led to the development of nurse practitioners; the primary care physician shortage, which is described as the major contributing factor to the expansion of nurse practitioners in other parts of the country (Elder & Bullough, 1990; McGivern, 1986) is defined by Ford as the *opportunity*, not the reason for the new role (Ford, 1982).

Resistance to the nurse practitioner role initially came from the academic nursing community and some federal agencies, but the idea was born at a time of general concern on the part of consumers for accessible, affordable, and humane care. Bolstered by the supportive governmental and health care environment of the 1960s and 1970s, nurse practitioners created a role that served populations in many settings and became fully integrated into baccalaureate and master's nursing programs. An exhaustive number of studies confirmed the quality, cost effectiveness, productivity, clinical decision-making skills, and job satisfaction of nurse practitioners, making this the most evaluated role in any discipline (Brown & Grimes, 1993, 1995; OTA, 1986).

The evolution of preparatory programs for nurse practitioners, from physician- and nurse-taught certificate programs to well-integrated content in baccalaureate and master's degree programs, was relatively rapid and consistent across the country (McGivern, 1986). The rapid expansion of expert clinicians produced two models of specialization in nursing: the consultative nursing model of clinical nurse specialists and the collaborative model of practitioners, midwives, and anesthetists (Bullough, 1992). These models shared a commitment to research and utilization of knowledge from other disciplines, but differed for several decades in their emphasis on nursing theory, medical content, direct service activities, and practice settings.

More recently, these programs have evolved from separate clinical nurse specialist and nurse practitioner programs to programs that are generally congruent in content and purport to prepare practitioners for a "blended" role providing skills that transcend setting. The most common preparation, family nurse practitioner, would seem to endorse the continued more generalist approach. Common academic program content, practice across fluid practice settings created through vertical systems integration, and legislation that provides for Medicare reimbursement for both nurse practitioners and clinical nurse specialists have further helped to rapidly consolidate these two roles.

Today, advanced practice is defined by the National Council of State Boards of Nursing (NCSBN, 1992) as

> the advanced practice of nursing by nurse practitioners, nurse anesthetists, nurse midwives, and clinical nurse specialists, based on the following: knowledge and skills required in basic nursing education; licensure as a registered nurse; graduate degree and experience in the designated area of practice which includes advanced nursing theory; substantial knowledge of physical and psychosocial assessment; appropriate interventions and management of health care status.
> The skills and abilities essential for the advanced practice role within an identified specialty area include: providing patient/client and community education; promoting stress prevention and management; encouraging self-help; subscribing to caring; advocacy; accountability; accessibility; and collaboration with other health and community professionals.

The Council also noted that "each individual who practices nursing at an advanced level does so with substantial autonomy and independence resulting in a high level of accountability" (NCSBN, p. 4).

Slow but steady growth of preparatory programs and graduation rates for advanced practice nurses have characterized the late 1980s and 90s. This growth has been fueled for reasons similar to those of earlier decades: the continued quest for quality health care, access, and cost containment. In addition, advanced practice nursing is an expression of the autonomy and the health promotion and health maintenance focus of the nursing role. There is a continued search for the right numbers and distribution of health care providers to provide appropriate services increasingly needed by nursing's traditional populations including women and children, urban and rural poor, the chronically ill, the elderly, and patients requiring palliative care and facing end-of-life decisions. More recently, advanced practice nurses are targeting their services to the well, middle class as insurance companies and managed-care organizations include them on panels and practitioners demonstrate greater skills in marketing and financing their services (Winslow, February 7, 1997).

The expansion of master's programs and enrollments in the late 1990s has been fueled also by the loss of nurse-generalist positions in tertiary care settings, expansion of community-based practices, and new reimbursement opportunities. The decrease in the number of nurse-generalists in hospitals and their replacement by less well-prepared, and in some cases unlicensed, personnel has recreated the scenario that first produced the need for specialized nurses earlier in the century. Expert clinicians must once again provide the modeling and direction for less well-prepared workers caring for increasingly more acute and complex patients, and provide the direct care and consultation required of increasingly sophisticated technology-based diagnosis and treatment. Similarly, while the widely publicized unpredictability of the health care delivery systems has tended to depress baccalaureate enrollments, expanded advanced practice programs provide new opportunities to increase overall enrollments by capturing new recruits to nursing, many of whom already have a baccalaureate degree. More recently, the popular media is discussing the "new" nursing shortage and this may stimulate enrollments at both the undergraduate as well as graduate levels (Boivin, 1997; Hawkes, 1998).

MANPOWER PROJECTIONS

Predictions regarding supply and demand for advanced practice nurses are difficult to discuss with precision. Although advanced practice nurses are seen as particularly well prepared for the rapidly evolving health care environment, the advanced practice nursing role is constrained by the relatively limited number of nurses appropriately prepared and credentialed in advanced practice. As of 1996, there were 153,910 advanced practice nurses including nurse practitioners, clinical nurse specialists, certified nurse anesthetists, and nurse-midwives. Of these, approximately 53,799 were clinical nurse specialists, 63,191 nurse practitioners, 30,860 nurse anesthetists, and 6,534 midwives who were recognized by national certification and state board of nursing registration. These practitioners were not necessarily prepared in master's level advanced practice programs (NLN, 1996).

Advanced practice programs have increased in numbers over the last decade with particular emphasis on the primary care areas of family, adult, and pediatrics (Department of Health and Human Services, Division of Nursing, 1994). Currently 274 colleges and universities offer master's and post-master's programs and over 30 schools report the intent to offer advanced practice programs in the near future. Nurse practitioner students make up about 46% of these programs' enrollments and 42% of the graduations (AACN Web site).

Advanced practice nursing, defined by master's degree preparation and certification, is necessarily dependent on sufficient numbers of nurses with the requisite baccalaureate preparation. The current configuration of nursing education programs and numbers of graduates, as described by Aiken and Salmon (1994), is incongruent with health manpower needs for additional advanced practice nurses. While nurses with master's degrees are and will continue to be in great demand, the largest portion of the nursing manpower pool is the community college graduate. It is predicted that shortly there will be a deficit of approximately 428,000 nurses with undergraduate and graduate degrees, severely limiting the number of advanced practice nurses who can be prepared to meet future demand (Aiken, 1995).

Moreover, enrollments are influenced by the limited number of available and appropriate clinical placements; competition with the better-paying service sector for clinician-faculty; and limited institutional budgets that fail to support sufficient faculty. The number of students who graduate annually is further limited by the inability of most students to attend advanced practice programs on a full-time basis.

Demand, on the other hand, is also subject to a variety of factors despite the predictions of need for 91,435–107,689 nurse practitioners (Donaldson, Yordy, Lohr, & Vanselow, 1996) and the goals of the American College of Nurse Midwives for 10,000 providers by 2001. Aiken and Salmon (1994) argue that a number of factors support continued demand for well-prepared nurses: despite hospital downsizing there is continued hospital employment of nurses; expansion is occurring in areas traditionally requiring baccalaureate and higher-degree preparation such as public health, managed care, and home health (AACN Web site); physician capacity to meet the need for primary care services will not be achieved until several decades into the new millennium; and there is a continued demand for the health promotion and maintenance services valued by patients and provided by nurses.

Demand will also be tempered by the perception of standardization of preparation and credentialing. Institutional and organizational employers, insurers, and consumers want assurances that support credibility for practice and reimbursement claims (Aiken & Salmon, 1994; Barber & Burke, 1999, chapter 13). While consistency in preparation and credentialing in master's education is enhanced through criteria promulgated by the National Association of Nurse Practitioner Faculty, the American College of Nurse Midwives and other specialty organizations, and the American

Nurses Credentialing Center, there is strong sentiment for even more standardization which, in turn, will support increased confidence in and utilization of advanced practice nurses.

The future of federal support for the education and reimbursement of advanced practice nursing is the single most powerful determinant of the future growth and utilization of master's-prepared nurses. The use of Medicare monies to support graduate medical education has been the subject of considerable debate in both policy and medical education arenas; this debate extends to support for advanced practice nurses. The argument for redirecting Medicare dollars to graduate nursing preparation is particularly appealing in light of the fact that of the $248 million from Medicare funds that went to support nursing in 1994, two-thirds went to support 124 hospital-based programs that train only 7% of nursing students (National League for Nursing, 1996). Medicare and Medicaid reimbursement of advanced practices nursing services, which is the logical extension of federal support for clinical preparation and training, is also an essential element for continued recruitment of nurses for advanced practice.

Finally, supply of and demand for advanced practice nurses will continue to be strongly influenced by the geographic differences in reorganization of health care systems, managed care organizations' penetration of the market, institutional and regional bias toward physicians or mid-level providers, and states' legal, regulatory, and reimbursement environments (Kovner & Rosenfeld, 1997). The Health Security Act, which provides for direct Medicare reimbursement to nurse practitioners and clinical nurse specialists, will, however, help to create a more uniform reimbursement environment, which in turn should support a more even geographic distribution of advanced practice nurses.

FACTORS SHAPING PRACTICE AND EDUCATION

The volatility of the current health care environment and the relatively slow pace of curricular change in most nursing education programs create a lag in development of appropriate preparatory programs designed to produce new providers and a constriction in the capacity of these institutions to have a greater role in shaping the new care system. Nevertheless, major environmental factors are having an impact on both practice and education. These factors include the corporate health care environment, demands for standardization and credentialing, merging of education and practice efforts, and the demands for financial and professional recognition including reimbursement and practice privileges. Both clinical service and education institutions are attempting to manage unprecedented change and each is responding to forces that until recently touched only one or the other setting. So, for example, colleges and universities are revising academic programs and at the same time attempting to negotiate with the combined clinical-fiscal organizations that exercise control over clinical practice of faculty and students, opportunities for field-based research, and employment opportunities for graduates.

Health Care Environment

Few if any predictions about the eventual shape of the health care delivery system can be offered with confidence. However, common themes do describe the current environment and may give some hint as to its future condition. These themes include managed care, continued vertical integration of delivery systems, growth of the proprietary sector, evolution of occupational and professional roles, more limited access for the underinsured and uninsured, and lack of flexibility in academic health centers to move toward new curricular and delivery models (Donaldson et al., 1996).

The market penetration of managed care varies geographically and between the public and private sectors. Managed care is characterized by selective lists of providers; mechanisms for influencing the nature, amount, and site of services provided; limited access to specialists; and a decline in the distinction between insuring, financing, and clinical decisions affecting the availability of services. The move from discounted services to capitation, and the fact that some large purchasers are negotiating directly with providers for services as is already occurring in some states, offer opportunities for full integration of health services. These characteristics will continue to evolve over time as a result of corporate policy, legal action, and/or government policy (Freudenheim, 1997). Corporate policy of private sector large business groups and large managed care organizations will effect changes in public sector policy and practice.

The continued development of vertically integrated systems that combine acute care, rehabilitation, chronic care, special services, mental health, substance abuse, health maintenance, and other primary care services is prompted by the desire to protect market share and, within the system, to increase efficiency (Donaldson et al., 1996). System survival depends on increased volume of routine care, much of which could be provided by nurses (Aiken & Salmon, 1994).

It would seem advantageous to large provider groups to understand this along with the fact that most nurses, accustomed to working in large organizations (Kovner & Rosenfeld, 1997), find such organizational settings less stressful than other clinicians whose tradition has been free-standing private practice. Health care organizations are consolidating in order to create larger, more powerful organizations to secure more capital, marketing advantage, and economies of scale in infrastructure. Consolidation may lead to increased cost-effectiveness and access to capital, but it is also raises questions about quality of care and economic viability. For patients, concerns about personal attention, quality and comprehensiveness of services, and overall responsiveness are triggered by health care organizational mergers and restructuring.

The economic imperatives of the evolving system are accelerating the natural evolution of the health professions' practices. Primary care is achieving greater monetary and hierarchial status, mid-level providers are assuming a more central role, and interdisciplinary teamwork is again being valued. While incremental changes in scope and site of practice for traditional and new providers are generally expected and accepted, there is less acceptance when the evolution speeds up and is directly linked with potential economic competition (Kovner & Rosenfeld, 1997). Up until recently, professions have attempted to control their educational preparation, their relationship with patients and other professionals, and the payment they receive for their services. There is now the potential for managed-care companies and others to substantially influence education by creating their own training programs, lobbying legislative bodies to modify scopes of practice to their benefit, and mandating levels of provider mix and models for collaboration.

Access to care for the urban poor and people living in rural areas is not addressed in the new health environment. Rural hospitals have been more susceptible to closure and primary care services are more difficult to sustain in less populated areas. Urban providers who treat uninsured or underinsured clients are threatened by the loss of cross-subsidies and the erosion of federal programs that help to defray the losses (Donaldson et al., 1996). Nurses could be key to providing these services if they had greater access to capital, fewer barriers to practice, and greater access to consultation. Nurses have traditionally served these populations successfully and would continue to do so if the economic and legal obstacles were removed, including the link to physicians who are not well distributed geographically (Aiken & Salmon, 1994). The extent to which technology, such as telemedicine or telehealthcare, could change the access to services and the improved utilization of advanced practice nurses will depend on the national investment in the technology and the resolution of jurisdictional issues related to cross-state or country boundaries.

Academic health centers, which prepare large numbers of professionals from a variety of health-related disciplines, are viewed as lacking the ability to train more primary care providers, but will be called on to train fewer medical specialists and fewer physicians overall. Teaching hospitals could develop the cadres of highly qualified and technically skilled professional nurses to staff acute-care units and could collaborate with their schools of nursing in the development of primary care services in their ambulatory settings, home care services, and related enterprises (Aiken & Salmon, 1994; Donaldson et al., 1996). They also, by definition, could provide the setting for interdisciplinary training and practice that could ultimately produce cost-savings by having the most appropriate team member be responsible for interventions thus improving quality of care and reducing mortality and morbidity (Aiken, Smith, & Lake, 1994; Frank & Della Penna, 1998; Knaus, Draper, Wagner, & Zimmerman, 1986; Siegler, Hyer, Fulmer, & Mezey, 1999). To date, however, academic health centers appear to lack both the ability and the will to make nursing excellence a key component to outpatient and inpatient quality.

Thus the major common elements in the transition to the new health care system, including managed care, consolidation and vertical integration, decreased access for the rural and urban poor populations, maintaining the viability and relevance of the academic health science centers, are ripe for nursing to play a vitalizing role with appropriate opportunities for nursing education and nursing generalist and advanced clinical practice (Aiken, 1995).

Education Program Expansion and Standardization

Despite some growth in master's programs and the potential for increased utilization of advanced practice nurses across a wide range of settings, operant factors effecting program development make it difficult to predict the future of education of advanced practice nurses.

Enrollment

The immediate response of many academic institutions to the perceived need for and interest in advanced practice nursing is reflected in the increased numbers of institutions offering such programs at the master's level. As of 1996, there were 274 colleges and universities offering advanced practice nursing programs. Programs in order of prevalence of specialty practice preparation include family nurse practitioners (49%), adult primary care (19%), pediatrics (10.5%), geriatrics (4.7%), women's health care (4%), and mental health (2%) (AACN Web site).

Despite the interest in master's programs preparing advanced practice nurses, there are significant factors that mitigate against expanding programs and enrollments. These forces include intensified corporate emphasis on clinicians' productivity and cost-containment; the identified costs of students in the clinical setting in a corporate culture that does not necessarily value teaching and research; new competition with medical students and residents for primary care placements and preceptors; competition for clinically skilled faculty; and the expanded and prolonged risk management and legal reviews of institutional and agency placement contracts.

These factors limit clinical placements for students in advanced practice nursing programs and create significant difficulties in coordination for faculty and administrators. Academic programs are accommodating to these pressures and their own budgetary constraints in a variety of ways including limiting enrollments, attempting to create nursing centers and other clinical settings over which they have greater control, requiring students to seek their own clinical practice placements, paying agencies for student placements, reducing the number of required clinical hours, and reducing faculty field supervision.

The general uncertainty about the future of the health care system reduces the impetus for students, academic institutions, and clinical service providers to aggressively plan for the advanced practice model in other than incremental steps. Students are predominantly part-time, and in many regions where downsizing and reorganizing of health care institutions create uncertainty, students are preparing for advanced practice while staying in their current roles and institutions without specific plans to move into new practice opportunities.

Curriculum

Curricular content is increasingly prescribed by specialty organizations, credentialing bodies, state education departments, and boards of nursing, a movement with many repercussions on program development and consumer confidence. Content generally includes advanced nursing theory; research and statistics; professional and systems issues; advanced assessment; sciences including pharmacology and prescriptive authority knowledge and skills, pathophysiology, psycho-immunology, epidemiology and/ or others depending on the specialty focus; clinical content; and 600 to 800 hours of precepted clinical experiences congruent with the objectives of the program are now the norm.

The didactic content requirements of the programs are generally understood by students. However, the less tangible expectations of the advanced practice programs do catch students unaware even though they are described in program materials and are part of the conversation with faculty. Students who enroll in advanced practice programs often do not appreciate the difference in role expectations between their current practice and the demands of advanced practice until they are far along in the program. Accountability, autonomy, continuous responsibility, and new collaborative relationships with physicians and others are behaviors that some students have not necessarily developed in their generalist nursing practice and ultimately find difficult or are unable to cultivate in their new role.

Advanced practice programs are attempting to create a balance between general and specialized content and focus. The argument for more general preparation is linked to flexibility and ability to take advantage of employment opportunities. It also is used to counteract the criticism that nursing is mimicking medical specialization. The argument for greater specialty preparation includes the fact that many generalist skills have been incorporated into baccalaureate preparation, expectations for more autonomous practice and more complex care required of patients regardless of settings require greater depth, and advanced practice nurses work with distinct populations, diseases, and/or in defined settings. The balance of generalist and specialist knowledge and skills in programs also varies with the generally accepted role of the graduate in that region, the anticipated number and type of practice opportunities, the faculty's curricular and clinical expertise, and outside funding which drives program development.

The issue of nurse practitioner versus clinical nurse specialist preparation was blurred by the findings that curricular preparation and practice were increasingly similar (Elder & Bullough, 1990; Forbes, Rafson, Spross, & Kozlowski, 1990). The debate over the parallel or fused roles of clinical nurse specialists and nurse practitioners has become even more muted due to the significant shifts in practice opportunities: reduction of nurses with master's preparation in tertiary care facilities; Medicare reimbursement legislation that recognizes nurse practitioners and clinical specialists; the rapid movement of patients across settings; and registration of many programs which entitle graduates to take either or both certification examinations. The roles that all advanced practice nurses are expected to engage in: provider, consultant, patient educator, and researcher continue to be addressed in both nurse practitioner and clinical specialist curricula. On the other hand, as is discussed further below, clinicians often lack the pedagogical skills needed to assume faculty positions (Kovner & Rosenfeld, 1997).

The extended time it takes for most colleges and universities to respond to environmental changes and develop new courses and programs presents opportunities for nonacademic institutions to meet their own needs and the interests of their employees. Health care institutions and now, managed-care companies, are demanding new workers with different skills and, where they have the capacity to offer the knowledge and skills corporately valued, compete with academic institutions and professional organizations for control of training and credentialing (Frank & Della Penna, 1998; Yordy, 1996). Academic program faculty need to take the initiative and work collaboratively with employers, consumers, and payers to develop academic degree programs and certificate and continuing education offerings that meet current needs. The latter programs are more easily offered in a timely way and can assist alumni in maintaining their edge in the marketplace.

Faculty

Securing appropriately prepared faculty to teach in the advanced practice programs is a major ongoing issue in light of the increased competition from the increased number of programs, the lower salary structure in the academic setting, limited cadre of experienced and credentialed clinicians, and the varying degrees of flexibility in academic institutions to combine teaching responsibilities with clinical practice opportunities outside of student practica in order to maintain clinical expertise.

Once appointed, however, faculty clinicians are presented with other challenges, including their lack of traditional preparation in teaching, course and curriculum development, and assessment and evaluation; their lack of awareness of the academic cultural expectations; and the obligations thus shifted to other faculty. Programs, such as the one offered to clinicians by the University of Pennsylvania School of Nursing, address these requirements and demonstrate a need for other comparable formal and informal programs to prepare clinicians as knowledgeable teachers. Clinicians often come to the academic setting anticipating that it is less consuming and less stressful work than that of the practice setting. They are unprepared for the diversity of demands and the stress of being responsive to students, patients, clinical agency administrators, and academic colleagues and administrators. These clinicians bring to the program their network of clinicians and their good working relationships with physicians and others which infuses a practice paradigm into the educational program and improves access to new preceptors and new agencies. Students obviously benefit from working with experts who have, in addition to clinical skills, the skills gained from experience in handling ethical, legal, fiscal, and interpersonal practice issues. Clinical agencies are more cooperative and comfortable in dealing with expert clinician faculty, and the preceptors in the agencies view these faculty as knowledgeable colleagues.

Nursing faculty are supplemented by other scientists with credentials appropriate to pharmacology, pathophysiology, and other program requirements, by researchers with a variety of backgrounds, and by experts in legal, ethical, organizational, and fiscal aspects of practice. Physicians continue to serve as faculty in the didactic portions of programs as well as preceptors in clinical practica. While the need for medical expertise may have lessened with the relative increase in prepared advanced practice faculty, there continue to be advantages to the ongoing physician involvement in preparatory programs. Physicians provide clinical expertise and the perspective of the collaborating professional. In the process, they become more informed and conversant with the advanced practice role and confident in the knowledge and skills of students and graduates. Students gain experience in dealing with physicians in new capacities thereby facilitating future collaboration and interdisciplinary practice.

Funding

As practice shifts from structured acute-care settings to ambulatory, home, and community-based settings, the need for better educated, more autonomous practitioners is escalating. Acute-care settings are also changing with fewer medical residents in specialty training, opening of attending physician and nurse practitioner-managed units, and the overall downsizing of nursing staff including the loss of senior clinicians and supervisory staff. But funding for nursing education and clinical training by all levels of government is at odds with the anticipated consumer needs and provider skill mix. While baccalaureate nursing programs received $10 million in 1994 in federal funding and advanced practice programs more than $50 million in Title VIII funding, a disproportionate amount of support still flows to a small number of hospital-based diploma programs. Moreover, community college programs, which are supported by county and state governments, and prepare graduates for the shrinking inhospital positions, are not cost-effective or efficient since graduates eventually seek baccalaureate preparation at additional cost in time and money.

Medicare support of physician training, at $6 billion in 1995, dwarfs the amounts targeted to nursing and the inequity continues through clinical training and service. Hospitals receive an average of $125,000 annually for each resident they train, of which only approximately $30,000 to $40,000 goes to pay the resident's salary, whereas Professional Nurse Traineeship money is extremely limited and primarily used for tuition; stipends, when available, only approximate the costs of texts and supplies. Schools of nursing are heavily dependent on tuition revenue and lack the other revenue streams that typically support medical schools. As noted in Table 1.1, tuition is a negligible part of medical school support in contrast to colleges and universities that house schools and departments of nursing. Employer costs for nursing education are carried through tuition benefits. These benefits vary, may have little relation to local tuition costs, and frequently are the target of budget reductions and bargaining unit negotiations.

There are other costs associated with the preparation of the current inappropriate mix of nurses, advanced practice nurses, and physicians. Advanced practice nurses typically cost $20,000 per year for two years (Alliance for Health Care Reform, 1996), while medical training costs $70,000 per year for three to six years. It is estimated that the cost of not utilizing nurse practitioners approaches $18.75 billion (Nichols, 1992).

The capacity of advanced practice nursing programs could be easily expanded by utilizing existing levels of funding redirected to appropriate levels of education and preparation of clinicians, including those prepared to teach in academic programs. Thus, funding for advanced practice nursing preparation should be aligned with anticipated need and coordinated by all levels of government. Appropriate government support that makes education more available would address a range of issues including the need for greater diversity, the need to recruit a younger workforce, and the need to enhance baccalaureate and master's graduation rates through increased full-time study.

**TABLE 1.1   How Medical School and Other Higher
Education Is Financed**

Distribution of total revenues of institutions of higher education[*] compared with medical schools (by percents)

	Tuition	State/ Local Government	Federal Research	Services Hospital[**]	Other[***]	Other
Medical Schools	4	12	19	12	36	17
Institutions of Higher Education						
Public Universities	17	37	12	13	14	8
Public 2-Year Colleges	20	64	5	0	7	4
Private Universities	40	3	16	11	13	18

[*]Not specific to nursing schools.

[**]Medicare education revenues are included under the hospital category.

[***]Other services for medical schools are primarily practice plan revenues; for institutions of higher education, other services include educational activities and auxiliary enterprises. Totals may exceed 100% because of rounding.

Source: Alliance for Health Reform, *The Twenty-First Century Nurse*, Feb. 1997, Washington, D.C. Table reprinted by permission.

Credentialing

Credentialing is a process common to education and practice encompassing a variety of mechanisms that share a set of common goals: to assure quality, competency, and accountability, and to achieve recognition for funding or reimbursement (Porcher, 1999, chapter 23). These goals take on greater immediacy and broader utility in the fluctuating health care environment, since they define uniform quality and competency which are of increasing importance to payers, consumers, employers, and nurses and other health care professionals. The meaning of each of the current credentialing mechanisms should be widely disseminated to the constituencies requiring the information in order that they may select and pay for programs and services knowledgeably.

Credentialing targets individuals, academic institutions, and health care organizations through various mechanisms. Individual practitioners are credentialed through registration, licensure, and certification. Registration, the earliest form of credentialing, lists the qualified individuals who have met the minimum qualification. Licensure is the state government's permission to practice the profession, and it is the protection of title which prohibits use of such designation by those not appropriately prepared or tested. Certification is carried out by nongovernmental bodies recognized by the profession, and the process attests that a licensed professional has met certain standards including preparation, experience, and successful testing.

Certification still lacks the clarity and consistency of standards since it recognizes both generalist and specialist practice, a range of educational preparation, and other variable criteria. To be useful to advanced practice nursing, certification should uniformly require advanced practice preparation embedded in master's degree programs and represent a uniform level of expertise. Certification, however, should also be continually redefined in keeping with the development of new technologies, expanding knowledge base, and the natural evolution of scope of practice.

In the case of individual provider certification, practitioners who meet specific criteria apply as individuals to a credentialing body, and a certificate is conferred upon review of eligibility or successful completion of an examination. Examples of such certification mechanisms include the American Nurses Credentialing Center (ANCC) certification examination for primary care practice as an adult, pediatric, and geriatric nurse practitioner (ANA, 1991) and specialty organization certification, such as National Association of Pediatric Nurse Associates and Practitioners (NAP-NAP). In contrast to individual certification, some states and professional organizations certify educational programs following review of curricula and faculty credentials. Certification in such instances is automatically conferred on graduates who successfully complete the certified program.

Institutional credentialing includes accreditation of academic institutions and programs and review of hospitals and community health care agencies. Accreditation is the process by which nongovernmental agencies and organizations made up of member institutions review and grant accreditation status to institutions and programs according to stated criteria. Officially designated accrediting bodies are, in turn, reviewed and recognized by national accrediting bodies. In addition to the Joint Commission, The Community Health Accreditation Program (CHAP) reviews and accredits community and home health care agencies. Agencies meeting CHAP standards also meet conditions of participation in Medicare and Medicaid programs set by the federal government.

The American College of Nurse Midwifery maintains the dual function of specifying curriculum requirements and certification requirements; such credentialing has served to create a standard minimum curriculum that assures comparability of preparation. In contrast to nurse-midwifery, the lack of comparability in credentialing in most other practice areas lends itself to unevenness in advanced practice master's programs and different levels of graduates' proficiency.

For advanced practice nurses, more consistent and explicit credentialing is needed to assure payers, consumers, and employers that they are contracting for an expected level of competence and expertise. To date, certification requirements do not provide that assurance, nor is program accreditation sufficiently outcome based to support confidence in comparability of providers.

All states have some mechanism for credentialing nurse practitioners and nurse midwives. However, the mechanisms for achieving certification vary by state and include the national certification exam, state board of medicine and/or nursing approval, state examination, an academic degree, or some combination of these (Bullough, 1999, chapter 21). These state variations are confusing to all constituent groups and limit practitioner mobility. The national recognition practice model being discussed by the National Council of State Boards of Nursing would be based on an interstate contract that would allow generalist nurses to hold licensure in one state and practice in others consistent with each state's laws. In the face of distance learning and telemedicine the model may eventually address advanced practice nursing issues (National Council of State Boards of Nursing, www.ncsbn.org).

LINKING EDUCATION AND PRACTICE

The links between educational programs and clinical practice began in the 1960s when nursing leaders at the University of Florida (Smith, 1965) and Case Western Reserve University (MacPhail, 1972) published accounts of their projects. For many years university schools of nursing such as the University of Rochester and Rush University have been centrally involved in the administration and delivery of nursing services in their affiliated teaching hospitals (Christman & Grace, 1981; Ford, 1981). There have been a variety of other affiliation models with nursing homes, home care agencies, and dedicated units within hospitals.

The drive to reduce medical specialty practice preparation and, therefore, the number of available residents for inpatient care, the desire to manage cases in a more holistic way, and recognition of the cost-effective, mid-level provider care appropriate to some hospital-based populations has stimulated further interest in collaboration between schools of nursing and other diverse providers. The result of these collaborations is greater access for students' clinical placements, access to subjects for clinical research, and opportunities to shape clinical care. The provider organizations gain linkages to academic institutions and quality of care is improved through the participation of skilled faculty and students from the academic programs.

In a continued effort to capture the benefits of our earlier practice-based education, nursing programs and hospital departments of nursing are attempting to integrate the education, research, and clinical practice elements. Schools of nursing are collaborating with clinical service institutions and/or developing independent practice arrangements. Faculty practice represents points on a continuum: faculty with clinical practice positions outside of their faculty appointments to formally organized practices managed by faculty-providers which may or may not accommodate students (Evans, Jenkins, & Buhler-Wilkerson, 1999, chapter 19). Schools of nursing are investing in practice arrangements for a variety of reasons including the need to offer clinicians a clinical component to their faculty appointments, creating the opportunity for faculty and students to learn the complex clinical, resource, fiscal, and risk aspects of the role being taught, and in some cases, to create a revenue stream that will support the school of nursing in ways similar to medical school faculty practice. Nursing faculty also desire to influence the style and quality of practice in ambulatory, acute-, and long-term care settings.

Several examples of community-based practice include management of adult primary care practices (Winslow, February, 1997), school-based health clinics (McClowry, 1996), university health care services (Shortridge & McLain, 1983), home care, and nursing homes (Mitty, Bottrell, & Mezey, 1997). The Teaching Nursing Home Program, cosponsored by the Robert Wood Johnson Foundation and the American Academy of Nursing, was a joint practice-education model that linked schools of nursing in affiliations with nursing homes in order to pool personnel, physical, and financial resources. These affiliations focused on innovations in patient-resident health care, reality-based health professions education, and new understandings of care needs through clinical research (Garrad, Kane, Ratner, & Buchanon, 1991; Mezey & Lynaugh, 1989; Mitty, Bottrell, & Mezey, 1997). Such projects have demonstrated that collaborative relationships can improve patient care and provide important clinical learning opportunities for students (Mitty, Bottrell, & Mezey, 1997; Shaughnessey, Kramer, Hittle, & Steiner, 1996). In addition, faculty practice arrangements provide faculty and students with the opportunity to shape clinical practice consistent with the values and standards of the profession of nursing and the standards of specialty practice groups.

FINANCIAL AND PROFESSIONAL RECOGNITION OF ADVANCED PRACTICE NURSING

Recognition of advanced practice nursing's central role in health care is directly linked to compensation, credentialing, and prescriptive, admitting, and other privileges and remains high on nursing's legislative and policy agenda.

As is addressed at length in several chapters in this text (Boland & Leib, chapter 7; Evans, Jenkins, Buhler-Wilkerson, 1999, chapter 19; Sullivan-Marx & Mullinix, 1999, chapter 20), recognition of a professional group's authority to practice is payment; barrier to payment is a code for the other professional recognition issues. Ironically, many nurses are unaware of how practice revenue is generated. In a 1994 survey of nurses, including 46% advanced practice nurses, conducted by the American Nurses Association and the National Organizational Liaison Forum, most nurses were not knowledgeable of the sources of revenue that supported their practice sites (American Nurses Association, 1994). Moreover, while most advanced practice nurses have prescriptive privileges, many extending to controlled substances, many fewer have admitting privileges. In a recent New York State survey of approximately 1300 community-based nurse practitioners, 70% did not have hospital privileges; 8.8% could see inpatients but were split about entering progress notes; 16.3% could also write orders; and 44.9% could admit patients (Kovner & Rosenfeld, 1997).

While advanced practice nurses are generally unaware of sources of payment, probably because they are largely salaried, certain professional associations and lobbyists have generated support for third-party payment for advanced practice nursing services, from Medicaid, managed-care organizations, and, most recently, Medicare. "The Primary Care Health Practitioner Incentive Act of 1997" provides for direct Medicare reimbursement at 85% of the physician fee schedule for legally authorized services regardless of setting or physician association. The estimates of extending Medicare Part B to nurse practitioners and physician assistants amounts to less than one-half of 1% of Part B expenditures which is comparable to what is anticipated to be expended on the increased bonuses paid to physicians practicing in shortage areas (Aiken & Salmon, 1994). Nevertheless, consistent reimbursement policies under Medicare will encourage payment by other insurance providers, enhance the geographic distribution of advanced practice nursing, improve consumer choice, and broaden the practice opportunities for nurses.

THE FUTURE OF ADVANCED PRACTICE NURSING

Despite the uncertainty, the future of advanced practice nursing and the profession of nursing is potentially in the most exciting and momentous period in our profession's history. The current state of education and practice suggests that nursing can play a central role in a new, more effective health care delivery system. Positioning for nursing's opportunity to make health care accessible, humane, and efficacious depends on assurances that education and clinical training and standards for individual and institutional credentialing are rigorous and consistent. This is necessary to convey clear information and expectations to consumers and payers. The expansion, more even distribution, access to, and utilization of advanced practice nurses depends on more uniform reimbursement policies and practice privileges that meet consumer and patient needs consistent with high quality, cost-effective care.

In the face of this range of opportunities for advanced practice nursing, what will be the most important areas for the focused attention of educators, practitioners, and policy makers?

Practice Opportunities

A kaleidoscope of institutional and community-based practices will continue to offer new practice opportunities to academically and clinically prepared and credentialed providers. In order to anticipate and produce change, or simply take advantage of existing opportunities advantageous to their consumers, advanced practice nurses need preparation as experts, socialization as autonomous, accountable, and ethical providers, and grounding in the fiscal, technologic, legal, and political requirements of health care delivery.

Primary care practice will continue to occupy the majority of nurse practitioners and nurse-midwives. However, the potential for acute-care practice will be realized in the next five years as the reduction in specialty medical training programs creates needs for skilled inpatient management. The development of additional free-standing group practices, following the pattern set by nurse-midwives and some nurse practitioners, and the expansion of advanced practice nurses into home care and nursing homes will continue as direct payment for services becomes more available and as advanced practice nurses gain access to capital and legal, fiscal, and risk management expertise.

Research on the effectiveness of advanced practice nursing services will continue and broaden to focus on the new specialties and settings such as acute care and home care, and on the nature of advanced practice in relation to specific patient outcomes (Brown & Grimes, 1995). As advanced practice nurses are reimbursed and become visible parts of large databases, their interventions will be available to examine in relation to patient care outcomes.

Continued Standardization through Credentialing

The call for consistency in program content started years ago, reinforced by the articulate voice of Rozella Scholdtfeldt and others. Professional associations and accrediting bodies, informed by their members, have much to do to generate consensus and create mechanisms that ensure quality, consistency, and accountability in the preparation and monitoring of professional competence. Credentialing that is well understood by nurses, consumers, and payers, raises standards, keeps pace with practice demands, and supports practice in the broader jurisdictions requires more aggressive dialog and implementation. It is therefore imperative that nurses and credentialing bodies recognize that this effort is key to successful expansion and institutionalization of advanced practice nursing.

Collaboration and Interdisciplinary Practice

Preparation for collaboration and interdisciplinary practice is expensive in both time and human resources. Unlike the 1970s when available funding made training possible, with a few notable exceptions (Tsukuda, 1998) the current call for interdisciplinary practice is based only on recognized need but no additional support. With a few exceptions (Siegler, Hyer, Fulmer, & Mezey, 1998), the national funding that often persuades academic and training institutions to create training programs is largely missing.

In the past, the drive to collaboration and interdisciplinary practice often came from groups regarded as secondary to medicine who used it as a way to gain recognition. Collaboration is an activity that has been a staple in nursing but is neither well taught nor practiced. As advanced practice nursing becomes more central and less dependent on medicine for authority and status, it is not clear what the impetus will be to promote interdisciplinary practice. Beyond rhetoric, it will be interesting to see what nursing does to continue its stated commitment to interdisciplinary practice and whether the corporate values associated with teamwork will prevail.

Increasing Diversity and Cultural Competence

The 1992 national survey of 4,000 nurse practitioners and clinical specialists projected that the then 30,000 practitioners in the United States were predominantly White (91%), married (70%), females (96%), over the age of 35 (88%). A more recent survey conducted by the New York State Department of Health of the state's 3,800 nurse practitioners reveals similar characteristics. Of the almost 2,500 respondents, the median age was 44 years, 89.5% were White, and 96% were female (Kovner & Rosenfeld, 1997). The national data, confirmed by survey data in one state, reveal the picture of a provider group considerably less diverse than the population served. Nursing has long expressed commitment to educational mobility, equal access, and career mobility. However, the lack of diversity among advanced practice nurses suggests the need for much more aggressive recruitment efforts by academic programs and more creative systems of engaging nurses working in local communities.

While successful federal funding for advanced practice programs is linked to projected numbers of students and graduates from underrepresented groups, other funding incentives need to be targeted to individual students and institutions. *Healthy People 2000* (1991) speaks eloquently to the need for broader representation in the ranks of health care professionals. Clearly the solutions to underrepresentation are complex and include improved elementary and secondary education consistent with preparation for higher education, commitment of resources for effective career information, and recruitment, and financial aid including scholarships to make career preparation possible. Ensuring cultural competence of advanced practice nurses is another important goal. Understanding clients'/patients' culturally determined health values and health-seeking behaviors continues to be an essential element in providing appropriate care.

Other Emerging Issues

Several important and interesting issues will continue to develop over the next few years that will directly impact on the practice and influence of advanced practice nurses. These include the continued corporate development of health care and perhaps education, expansion of telemedicine, and the extension internationally of expanded roles for nursing and advanced practice nursing particularly.

Continued Corporatization

The health care reform initiated by the federal government but monopolized by the corporate sector has produced changes with unprecedented speed and with little or no regard for the traditional assumptions about access, quality, and control. Corporate practice of health care does not address "public good" issues such as public or consumer protection, support for education and research, maintenance of distinct scopes of practice while fostering flexibility and collaboration, or providing for continued professional competency.

Health care institutions and organizations are increasingly making or influencing clinical decisions in the name of cost-effectiveness and control of resources. There is discussion at state levels to determine how to maintain licensure requirements in an environment in which corporations increasingly bring out-of-state personnel to facilities where one or more licensed groups are striking. States are also examining the need to make health maintenance organizations, like individual practitioners, liable under professional malpractice laws.

Ironically, in the era of less governmental regulation and limited budgets, it is government that may need to take on these public-good issues. State governments are increasingly being asked to provide user-friendly information which reflects statutory and regulatory language about professional practice and public protection, to conduct and publish more research about professional competency, to investigate and prosecute instances of illegal practice; provide outcome data related to providers' services; and to review complaints as part of a system of due process. It is not clear how government will accommodate these needs and make provider organizations and practitioners more accountable. State governments have traditionally controlled scope of practice and the disciplinary process as well as determinations about requirements for continued professional development and peer review. Practice across jurisdictional boundaries raises the question about the feasibility of exclusive state control. All levels of government will be asked to meet the funding needs for education and research, though the historic uncertainty of government support for these functions remains an issue (New York State Education Department, 1997).

The swing to health care regulation by free market forces may be reversing itself, prompted by consumers who are no longer persuaded that their best interests are being served and providers who are unwilling to lose any more clinical or fiscal control. The flux between government regulation and free market forces is being pushed by the improved economy, lower unemployment rates, and, therefore, more secure employees, a recognition of the impact of the current system on the uninsured and underinsured, and growing questions as to the values of for-profit care (Passell, December 7, 1997).

Telemedicine/Telehealthcare

Telemedicine or telehealthcare is the provision of medical services over geographical distances by means of modern telecommunications and computer systems. It has existed since the 1970s and is already well developed and practiced despite significant variation among states regarding policy development and regulation. The opportunities for consultation, direct examination, diagnosis, and treatment are unlimited. The potential of telemedicine for advanced practice nursing includes better distribution of practitioners using distance consultation, increased practice opportunities and broader availability of services, more available research-based information, improved clinical education, and opportunities for interdisciplinary collaboration.

Concerns associated with technology-based practice include the desirability of the extension of the mutual recognition practice model to advanced practice nursing, issues of confidentiality of electronic information as part of patients' records, unlicensed practice, fraud and abuse, and practice exemptions. These issues will need to be resolved in the near future if this technology is to achieve its full potential to improve health care. Telehealthcare will also have economic implications for nursing practice and education that as yet are not totally predictable.

International Extension of Advanced Nursing Practice

The United States experience with advanced practice nursing is being examined by governments and institutions in many other countries for reasons similar to those that stimulated the development and growth of advanced practice here over the last thirty years. The opportunities to develop the nurse practitioner role grew out of nurses' being well prepared but underutilized and the limited number of primary care physicians in the face of dramatically increased demand. These factors, evident in European, African, and Asian countries, may have different causes but seem strikingly familiar: nurses' current skills are underutilized; changing demographics reflecting greater needs among the elderly and people with chronic illness; and heightened demand for services, coupled with limited manpower or inefficient provider mix. For example, the current interest in the nurse practitioner role in the Netherlands relates to nurses being underutilized in comparison to their preparation and physicians and others seeking a shorter work week, thereby creating a need for additional providers. Similarly, in the United Kingdom, as patients face delays in signing onto generalist physicians' panels, nurse practitioners are potentially an option to improve access to primary care.

Despite the thirty years of experience and research, other countries may not necessarily avoid the same developmental problems or leapfrog over the implementation issues based on our experience. The Netherlands has recently established a hospital-based certificate program for nurse practitioners, with the training and instruction provided by the physicians in the specialty areas to which the students are assigned.

CONCLUSION

Advanced practice nursing is on the cusp of exciting new developments. The openness of the health care system to change provides opportunities for broader professional recognition, more innovative practices, adequate compensation and organizational support, and greater autonomy. At the same time, system flux creates demands on individual practitioners, professional associations, academic institutions, and fiscal-clinical entities to anticipate the knowledge and skills necessary to provide expert clinical care and to hold fast to values that assure public access to quality health care.

REFERENCES

Aiken, L. (1995). Transformation of the nursing workforce. *Nursing Outlook, 43,* 201–209.

Aiken, L., & Mullinex, C. (1987). The nursing shortage—myth or reality. *New England Journal of Medicine, 317*(1), 641.

Aiken, L., & Salmon, M. (1994). Healthcare workforce priorities: What nursing should do now. *Inquiry, 31,* 318–329.

Aiken, L., Smith, H.L., & Lake, E.T. (1994). Lower medicare mortality among a set of hospitals known for good nursing care. *Medical Care, 32,* 781–787.

Alliance for Health Reform. (1996). *The twenty-first century nurse.* Washington, DC: Author.

American Association of Colleges of Nursing. (1998). (Web site www: aacn.nch.edu).

American Association of Colleges of Nursing. (1995). 1994–95 Special Report on Master's and Post-Master's Nurse Practitioner Programs, Faculty Clinical Practice. Washington, DC: Author.

American Nurses Association. (1991). *Certification for advanced practice.* Washington, DC: Author.

American Nurses Association. (1994). American Nurses Association/Nursing Organization Liaison Forum. *Current Procedural Terminology Utilization Survey.* Washington, DC: Author.

Barber, P. M., & Burke, M. (1998). Advanced practice nursing in managed care. In M. Mezey, & D. McGivern (Eds.), *Nurse, nurse practitioners: Evolution to advanced practice* (pp. 203–218). New York: Springer.

Boivin, L. (1997). The nursing shortage: It's back. *The Nursing Spectrum, 9*(24), 3.

Boland, C., & Leib, S. (1998). Collaborative physician and nurse practitioner's practice. In M. Mezey & D. McGivern (Eds.), *Nurses, nurse practitioners: Evolution to advanced practice nursing* (pp.133–141). New York: Springer.

Brown, S. A., & Grimes, D. E. (1995). A meta-analysis of nurse practitioners and nurse midwives in primary care. *Nursing Research, 44*(6), 332–339.

Brown, S. A., & Grimes, D. E. (1993). *A meta-analysis of process of care, clinical outcomes, and cost-effectiveness of nurses in primary care roles: Nurse practitioners and certified nurse-midwives.* Washington, DC: American Nurses Association, Division of Health Policy.

Bullough B., Gillett, V., & Bullough, B. (1998). State nurse practice acts. In M. Mezey & D. McGivern (Eds.), *Nurses, nurse practitioners: Evolution to advanced practice.* New York: Springer.

Bullough, B. (1992). Alternative models for specialty practice. *Nursing and Health Care, 13,* 254–259.

Christman, L., & Grace, H. (1981). Unification, reunification: Reconciliation or collaboration. *Modes for Collaboration.* Fall Conference Proceeding, Midwest Alliance in Nursing, September 1980–81. Unpublished.

Department of Health and Human Services. (1990). *Healthy People 2000: National Health Promotion and Disease Prevention Objectives,* Publication No 91-50212. Washington, DC: Author.

Department of Health and Human Services, Division of Nursing. (February 2, 1994). *Survey of Certified Nurse Practitioners and Clinical Nurse Specialists: December 1992—Final Report.* Publication No 240-91-0055. Washington, DC: U.S. Department of Health and Human Services.

Department of Health and Human Services, Division of Nursing. (March, 1996). *The Registered Nurse population: Findings from the National Sample Survey of Registered Nurses.* Washington, DC: Author.

Donaldson, M. S., Yordy, K., Lohr, K., & Vanselow, N. (1996). The delivery of primary care. In M. S. Donaldson, K. Yordy, K. Lohr, & N. Vanselow (Eds.), *Primary care: America's health in a new era* (pp. 104–147). Washington, DC: National Academy Press.

Elder, R., & Bullough, B. (1990). Nurse practitioners and clinical nurse specialists: Are the roles merging? *Clinical Nurse Specialist, 4,* 78–84.

Evans, L., Jenkins, M., & Buhler-Wilkerson, K. (1998). Power nursing for the 21st century: The role of academic practice. In M. Mezey & D. McGivern (Eds.), *Nurses, nurse practitioners: Evolution to advanced practice nursing.* New York: Springer.

Forbes, K., Rafson, J., Spross, J., & Kozlowski, D. (1990). The clinical nurse specialist and nurse practitioner: Core curriculum survey results. *Clinical Nurse Specialist, 4,* 63–66.

Ford, L. (1986). Nurse, nurse practitioners: The evolution of primary care. Review. *Image: Journal of Nursing Scholarship, 18,* 177–178.

Ford, L. (1982). Nurse practitioner: History of a new idea and predictions for the future (pp. 231–247). In L. H. Aiken & S. R. Gortner (Eds.), *Nursing in the 1980's: Crises, opportunities, challenges.* Philadelphia: Lippincott.

Ford, L. (1981). Creating a center of excellence in nursing. In L. Aiken (Ed.), *Health Policy and Nursing Practice* (pp. 430–451). New York: McGraw-Hill.

Frank, J. C., & Della Penna, R. (1998). Geriatric team training in managed care organizations. In E. Seigler, K. Hyer, T. Fulmer, & M. Mezey (Eds.), *Geriatric interdisciplinary team training.* New York: Springer.

Freudenheim, M. (1997, Oct. 10). HMO switches to flat fee for treatment by specialists. *New York Times,* A1 and D4.

Garrard, J., Kane, R., Ratner, E., & Buchanon, J. (1991). The impact of nurse practitioners on the care of nursing home residents. In P. Katz, R. Kane, & M. Mezey (Eds.), *Advances in long-term care: Vol 1.* New York: Springer.

Hawkes, M. (1998). Needed by 2005: More (good) nurses. *The Nursing Spectrum, 10*(2), 4–5.

Herman, C., & Krall, K. (1983). University-sponsored home care agency as a clinical site. Paper presented at Clinical Experience Today and Tomorrow: A Conference for Baccalaureate Nurse Educators, St. Paul, Minnesota.

Kitchens, E., Piazza, D., & Ellison, K. (1989). Specialization in adult health/medical surgical nursing: What does it mean? *Journal of Nursing Education, 28,* 221–226.

Knaus, W., Draper, E., Wagner, D., & Zimmerman, J. (1986). An evaluation of outcome from intensive care in a major medical center. *Annals of Internal Medicine, 104,* 410–418.

Kovner, C., & Rosenfeld, P. (1997). Practice and employment trends among nurse practitioners in New York State. *Journal of the New York State Nurses Association, 28*(4), 4–8.

MacPhail, J. (1972). *An experiment in nursing: Planning, implementing and assessing in planned change.* Cleveland: Case Western Reserve University Press.

McClowry, S. (1996). A comprehensive school-based clinic: University and community partnership. *Journal of the Society of Pediatric Nurses, 1*(1), 19–26.

McGivern, D. (1986). The evolution of primary care nursing. In M. Mezey & D. McGivern (Eds.), *Nurses, nurse practitioners: The evolution of primary care* (pp. 3–14). Boston: Little, Brown.

Mezey, M. (1992). Nursing homes: Resident's needs, nursing's response. In L. Aiken & C. Fagin (Eds.), *Charting nursing's future: Agenda for the 1990s* (pp. 198–215). Philadelphia: J. B. Lippincott.

Mezey, M., & Lynaugh, J. (1989). The teaching nursing home program: Outcomes of care. *Nursing Clinics of North America, 24*(3), 130–141.

Mitty, E., Bottrell, M., & Mezey, M. (1997). The teaching nursing home program: Enduring educational outcomes. *Nursing Outlook, 45,* 133–140.

National Council of State Boards of Nursing (1998). (Web site www.ncsbn.org).

National Council of State Boards of Nursing. (1992). Position paper on the licensure of advanced practice nursing. Unpublished manuscript, pp. 1–8.

National League for Nursing (1996). *Nursing Data Review.* New York: Author.

New York State Education Department Conference on the Professions. (1997, October). New York City.

Nichols, L. M. (1992). Estimating costs of underusing advanced practice nurses. *Nursing Economics, 10,* 343–351.

Passell, P. (1997, December 7). In medicine, government rises again. *New York Times,* pp. 1, 4.

Porcher, F. K. (1996). Licensure, certification and credentialing. In J. V. Hickey (Ed.), *Advanced practice nursing.* Philadelphia: Lippincott-Raven Publishers.

Shaughnessey, P., Kramer, A., Hittle, D., & Steiner, J. (1995). Quality of care in teaching nursing homes: Finding and implications. *Health Care Financing Review, 16*(4), 55–83.

Shortridge, L. M., & MacLain, B. R. (1983). Levels of intervention for a coexistence model. *Nurse Practitioner, 8,* 74–80.

Siegler, J., Hyer, K., Fulmer, T., & Mezey, M., (Eds.). (1998). *Geriatric Interdisciplinary Team Training.* New York: Springer Publishing Company.

Smith, D. M. (1965). Education and service under one administration. *Nursing Outlook, 13,* 54–58.

Sullivan-Marx, E., & Mullinix, C. (1999). Payment for advanced practice nurses: Economic structures and systems. In M. Mezey & D. McGivern (Eds.), *Nurses, nurse practitioners: Evolution to advanced practice nursing.* New York: Springer.

Tsukuda, R. A. (1998). A perspective on health care teams and team training. In E. Seigler, K. Hyer, T. Fulmer, & M. Mezey (Eds.), *Geriatric Interdisciplinary Team Training.* New York: Springer.

U.S. Congress, Office of Technology Assessment. (1986). *Nurse practitioners, physician assistants, and certified nurse-midwives: A policy analysis.* (Health Technology Case Study 37, OTA-HCS-37). Washington, DC: U.S. Government Printing Office.

U.S. Department of Health and Human Services. (1991). *Health People 2000: National Health Promotion and Disease Prevention.* Rockville, MD: Public Health Service.

U.S. Department of Health and Human Services. (1992). *The registered nurse population.* Washington, DC: Author.

U.S. Department of Health and Human Services, Office of the Assistant Secretary of Health. (1995). *Registered Nurse Chart Book.* Washington, DC: Author.

Winslow, R. (1997, February 7). Nurses to take doctors duties, Oxford says. *The Wall Street Journal*, A3.

Yordy, K. (1996). The nursing workforce in a time of change. In M. Osterweis, J. McLaughlin, H. Manasse, & C. Hopper (Eds.), *The US Health Workforce* (pp. 141–152). Washington, DC: Association of Academic Health Centers.

Chapter 2

RESEARCH IN SUPPORT OF NURSE PRACTITIONERS

Cynthia M. Freund and Jane A. Fox

THE political context that influenced nurse practitioner practice in the 1980s and 1990s differed considerably from that in earlier years. During the 1960s and 1970s, practitioners, researchers, and policy makers involved in the nurse practitioner movement were excited about its potential; many saw it as a reform movement, or even a revolution. While the movement was in its formative stages, some supporters saw it as a way to enhance nurses' stature within the health care community and with patients and consumers; others saw nurse practitioners as a quick solution to the physician shortage and the lack of primary care services, particularly in rural and other underserved areas.

The purpose of this chapter is not to provide an exhaustive review of the literature. Several comprehensive review articles, by Edmunds (1978), Prescott and Driscoll (1979, 1980), Goodwin (1981), Abdellah (1982), Yankauer and Sullivan (1982), Shamansky (1984), Molde and Diers (1985), Crosby, Ventura, and Feldman (1987), Feldman, Ventura, and Crosby (1987), LaRochelle (1987), Stanford (1987), Donley (1995), Brush and Capezuti (1996), and Dunn (1997) provide extensive discussions of the research. Their work will not be repeated here.

The authors of report after report have concluded that nurse practitioners are successful and effective, no matter what measure is used or what question is addressed—access, availability, acceptance, satisfaction, cost, or clinical outcomes. There are studies that could be more methodologically rigorous, but more recent studies are both methodologically and conceptually sound. True, there are some reports whose findings are not favorable to nurse practitioners, but the overwhelming majority of findings support their effectiveness.

The purposes here are, first, to highlight the significant historical and new findings from research in the 1980s and 1990s that give us new knowledge about nurse practitioners, their practice, and their effectiveness; and, second, to examine these findings in the context of the policy issues of the time.

POLITICAL CONTEXT: HISTORICAL AND CURRENT

From the beginning of the nurse practitioner movement there was both wide support for and resistance to nurse practitioners. Thus the research of the 1960s and 1970s was motivated not only by scientific objectives, but also by the need for evidence to support the claims of the advocates of nurse practitioners, or to refute the claims of those opposed to them.

Early research primarily addressed nurse practitioners' impact in four areas: (1) access and availability of services; (2) consumer and employee acceptance; (3) productivity, profitability, and cost of care; and (4) quality of care (Freund, 1986). In general, this research yielded positive findings in all four areas. The majority of nurse practitioners distributed themselves in underserved areas (Sultz, Henry, & Carroll, 1977; Weston, 1980). They increased the availability of primary care services (Mendenhall, Repicky, & Neville, 1980; Morris & Smith, 1977). Patients (Alonzi et al., 1979; Charney & Kitzman, 1973; Day, Egli, & Silver, 1970; Levine, Orr, Sheatsley, Lohr, & Brodie, 1978; Lewis & Resnick, 1967; Morris & Smith, 1977; Pender & Pender, 1980; Physician Extender Work Group, 1977; Schulman & Wood, 1972; Storms & Fox, 1979; Sultz, Henry, & Carroll, 1977) and physicians (Alonzi et al., 1979; Congressional Budget Office, 1979; Connelly & Connelly, 1979; Lawrence et al., 1977; Schiff, Fraser, & Walter, 1969) were satisfied with nurse practitioner care. The care provided by nurse practitioners was found to cost less than the same care provided by physicians (Freund, 1981; Record, McCally, Schweitzer, Bloomquist, & Berger, 1980; Schneider & Foley, 1977). And the quality of care provided by nurse practitioners was found to cost less than the same care provided by physicians (Freund, 1981; Record, McNally, Schweitzer, Bloomquist, & Berger, 1980; Schneider & Foley, 1977). And the quality of care provided by nurse practitioners equaled and, in some instances, exceeded that provided by physicians (Bessman, 1974; Freund, 1986; Lewis, Resnik, Schmidt, & Waxman, 1969; Merenstein & Rogers, 1974; Perrin & Goodman, 1978; Runyan, 1976; Sox, 1979; Spector, McGrath, Alpert, Cohen, & Aikens, 1975).

Recent studies also concluded that nurse practitioners, when compared to physicians, deliver the same or better quality care at a lower cost with high patient satisfaction (Avorn, 1991; Brown & Grimes, 1993; Brush & Capezuti, 1996; Hall et al., 1990; Safriet, 1992; Salkever, 1992; U.S. Congress OTA, 1986).

These conclusions could not be drawn without qualifications. Many earlier studies were case examples, with small samples of nurse practitioners, physicians, and patients; random assignment was rarely used; control over variables such as patient acuity, practice type, provider-training, and experience was not exercised; and definitions and measurements varied, making cross-study comparability difficult. Nevertheless, by the end of the 1970s, many asserted that several questions about nurse practitioner practice had been answered satisfactorily. The policy initiatives of the decade had been to provide increased quality primary care services at reasonable cost; nurse practitioners had contributed to that end.

The same factors that motivated research on nurse practitioner practice in the 1970s (access, acceptance, productivity, cost, and quality) continued into the 1980s. During the 1980s, however, the conditions that had provided a fertile environment for the development of the nurse practitioner movement changed. The physician shortage of the previous decades became a physician glut: physicians who once could not be enticed to rural and underserved areas now sought them out. Community and state agencies established to help rural communities develop primary health care services had embraced nurse practitioners in the 1960s and 1970s; in the 1980s, they abandoned them in favor of physicians seeking new practice options. Further, the availability and accessibility of primary care services lost favor as a national health policy issue, in part because of the physician surplus. In the eyes of those who viewed them merely as physician substitutes, there was no further need for nurse practitioners.

Although the physician shortage was easing into a surplus, escalating health care expenditures were modifying the nation's goal of quality health care as a right for all. Quality health care at reasonable cost became the new health policy goal, and throughout the 1980s, a variety of cost-containment measures were studied and implemented. Policies aimed at stimulating a market economy in the health care sector were introduced, and competition among health care providers began. Although procompetition policies were directed primarily at institutional providers, because of the increase in their numbers, physicians found themselves competing with each other, and with nurse practitioners. Issues of encroachment and territoriality became prominent, and the earlier emphasis on collaboration and collegiality faded. The 1990s have brought increased competition in the health care marketplace among health care providers (Safran, Tarlov, & Rogers, 1994; Sekscenski, Sansom, Bazell, Salmon, & Mullan, 1994).

Another noteworthy change in the sociopolitical environment during the 1980s was the growing influence of business and industry on health policy. As health care costs continued to rise, corporations, as underwriters of these costs, began to work for the development of policies to contain costs. Insurers, feeling the pressure from both business and government, instituted their own cost-containment strategies. The 1990s have seen the growth of managed care as an attempt at cost containment.

Although a variety of cost-containment strategies were introduced, those that limited access to services and the volume of services had the greatest impact on nurse practitioners. On the assumption that nurse practitioner services represented an increase in the quantity of services provided (and thus an increase in overall costs), legal barriers and restrictive reimbursement policies were established; these limited patients' access to nurse practitioners, provided a disincentive for employers of nurse practitioners, and, in some instances, actually prohibited nurse practitioners from engaging in their trade. These restrictive policies designated the physician as the gatekeeper for health care services, assuming that the physician would limit the volume, and hence the costs, of the services provided (an assumption not founded, however, on fact). Thus, not only did procompetition policies put nurse practitioners in competition with physicians, but policies of cost containment put nurse practitioners at physicians' mercy.

Although many policy makers saw nurse practitioners purely as physician substitutes, the nursing profession never viewed them in that way. On the contrary, the profession took advantage of the physician shortage, the lack of access to and availability of primary care services, and the maldistribution of providers in the 1960s to introduce an innovation that not only met the pressing needs of the time, but went beyond them. Nurse practitioners could safely and effectively provide the bulk of primary care needed by most people and thus could substitute for and replace physicians; and nurse practitioners would and did practice in underserved areas. But in the profession's view, nurse practitioners would do more than that: they would change the nature of primary care services. With their focus on the traditional nursing values of health promotion and prevention, teaching and counseling, and family involvement, nurse practitioners would improve both the quality of services provided and patient outcomes. Unfortunately, policy makers did not agree.

As has been noted, research during the early period of the nurse practitioner movement addressed questions dictated by political realities and policy considerations, and as a result did not focus on the "added" advantages of nurse practitioners, that is, those aspects of the nurse practitioner's performance that go beyond traditional medical services. However, toward the end of the 1970s, research initiatives began to address more encompassing questions related to nurse practitioner practice, and this broader focus has continued.

Given the political climate of the 1980s and the restrictions on further expansion of the nurse practitioner innovation during that period, the question might be asked: what purpose have these new research initiatives served? If the time frame is limited to the 1980s, then the new initiatives appear to have advanced the nurse practitioner movement very little. However, as we moved into the decade of the 1990s, there were already signs of change. For certain programs and under certain conditions, direct reimbursement is now provided to nurse practitioners for services rendered. Legal barriers to nurse practitioner practice have been tested in courts, and the courts have ruled that nurse practitioners engage in legal practice. Further, there are indications that the role of the nurse practitioner as originally conceived by the nursing profession is beginning to be understood, accepted, and endorsed by policy makers, business and community leaders, and consumers.

The research of the 1980s, like that of previous decades, provides testimony to the effectiveness of nurse practitioners. Many of the research initiatives begun earlier continued (for example, emphasis on availability, acceptance, economic impact, and quality of care). A move both toward greater scientific rigor and toward a broader conception of primary care and the nurse practitioner role began toward the end of the 1970s (Diers & Molde, 1979; Sullivan & Dachelet, 1979; Williams, 1975); much of the research of the 1980s was characterized by this broader focus. This research has also added to the already large accumulation of evidence about nurse practitioners—evidence vital in deciding the policy questions of the 1990s. Thus, even though the political climate for nurse practitioners was not overwhelmingly positive during the 1980s, the research of the period has served well the nurse practitioner movement in the 1990s.

Nurse practitioners are constantly required to justify their existence. Facts and figures are needed to support nurse practitioner practice before lawmakers, bureaucrats, and business people. This has been especially important in the 1990s with cost containment and managed care. Physician groups, when confronted with favorable data regarding the effectiveness of nurse practitioners, have criticized the rigor upon which the analyses are based. Three recent studies (Avorn, 1991; Hall et al., 1990; Salkever, 1992), conducted by non-nurse researchers, seem to withstand the criticism about study design and the impartiality of the investigator. These studies compared nurse practitioner and physician practice and found the nurse practitioner to be the better practitioner. Brown and Grimes (1993) reached similar conclusions: " . . . NPs and CNMs had patient outcomes equivalent to or slightly better than those of physicians . . . it can be concluded that nurse practitioners in advanced practice roles are cost-effective providers of primary care" (p. 31). Hall and colleagues (1990) found nurse practitioner performance to be equal to or superior on seven of eight tasks studied on the 426 audited charts of physicians and nurse practitioners in sixteen ambulatory care practices. Avorn (1991) asked 799 physicians and nurse practitioners to answer two questions based on a case study. Nurse practitioners were found to be far more likely to gather additional historical data and far less likely to recommend a prescription drug than the physician. Salkever (1992) compared the cost and effectiveness of nurse practitioners' and physicians' care for otitis media and sore throat. Nurse practitioners were found to be 20% less costly in the care they offered and at least as effective as physicians in resolving problems.

RESEARCH INITIATIVES

Access and Availability

Access and availability of primary care services were no longer predominant concerns in the 1980s. The physician shortage had abated, and the physician surplus that was predicted for 1990 had actually occurred early in the mid-1980s. In five years, from 1975 to 1980, the number of primary care physicians nearly doubled (Graduate Medical Education National Advisory Committee, 1978). Not only were more physicians providing primary care services, but some even went to rural underserved areas and replaced nurse practitioners (Brooks, Bernstein, DeFriese, & Graham, 1981; Brooks & Johnson, 1986). As early as 1981, it was suggested that if nurse practitioners were viewed as physician substitutes, " . . . they may serve their purpose only temporarily before their usefulness expires and before they are displaced by physicians" (Brooks et al., 1981, p. 254). Thus, from the perspective of many policy makers, the basic rationale for nurse practitioners—to increase access to and availability of primary care services—no longer existed.

The issues driving the debate on adequate access to services and physician availability has changed in the 1990s. In the United States less than 30% of physicians are generalists and the number continues to decline. Less than 15% of 1992 medical school graduates in the United States plan to become generalists (Schroeder, 1993). This shrinking pool of primary care physicians has forced hospitals to utilize the nurse practitioner, midwives, and nurse anesthetists on the inpatient unit (Mezey, Dougherty, Wade, & Mersmann, 1994).

Cost-containment strategies that began in the 1980s have accelerated in the 1990s and have further contributed to diminished concern over access and availability. Controlled utilization became a policy goal, replacing access and availability. With the increase in the number of physicians, it was argued that an increase in the number of nurse practitioners would only lead to increased utilization and consequent increases in costs. Nevertheless, a study of nurse practitioner-staffed clinics across the country over a 10-year period found that when nurse practitioners were replaced by physicians or physicians were added to the staff, the clinics experienced greater patient utilization, charged more for office visits, had larger budgets, and generated more of their budgets from fees for services (Brooks & Johnson, 1986). Thus, it is doubtful whether the physician surplus that drove physicians to rural underserved areas to replace nurse practitioners actually resulted in cost savings or even cost neutrality.

The debate in the 1980s as to whether nurse practitioners should continue to be supported also involved their distribution in rural and underserved areas. The factors that influence choice of practice location for nurse practitioners do not differ from those that influence physicians and dentists (Beck & Gernert, 1971; Bible, 1970; Cooper, Heald, Samuels, &

Coleman, 1975). Nurse practitioner location in rural areas is affected by clinical training experiences in rural areas (Hafferty & Goldberg, 1986), the rural background of the nurse practitioners, and the rural background of their spouses and families (Moscovice & Nestegard, 1980). Also, salaries of nurse practitioners in rural areas are 38% lower than those of their counterparts in nonrural areas—another factor affecting practice location choice (Roos & Crooker, 1983). Nevertheless, nurse practitioners do locate in rural and inner-city areas at a higher rate than do physicians (Weiner, Steinwachs, & Williamson, 1986), even though the actual percentage in these areas is low. In one state, the number of nurse practitioners in rural areas was found to be 9.2%, compared to 7.1% for primary care physicians (Salmon & Stein, 1986).

Some policy makers expected that a still greater proportion of nurse practitioners would choose practice locations that physicians found undesirable, that is, rural and inner-city locations. Weston (1980), however, noted that the ratio of nurse practitioners to the rural population is higher in states with more liberal legal sanctions and reimbursement policies, suggesting that nurse practitioners do not avoid underserved areas; rather, they are excluded from underserved areas by legal prohibitions and restrictive reimbursement policies. Further, it is unlikely that these legal sanctions and reimbursement policies will change in order to stimulate nurse practitioner practice in underserved areas, as nurse practitioner acceptance is no longer related to access and availability, but to the increasing number of physicians competing for similar opportunities (Weiner et al., 1986).

Career Patterns and the Acute-Care Nurse Practitioner

Even though access and availability were not policy concerns of the 1980s, questions about nurse practitioner distribution and career patterns remained. With increasing competition from physicians for similar opportunities, were nurse practitioners practicing in primary care settings? Were they in underserved locations? Was the scope of their practice fully realized, or was it constrained? Did master's degree and certificate degree program graduates differ? Were nurse practitioners, a predominantly female group, fully employed? Though these questions had less relevance for policy considerations in the 1980s, they continued to be relevant for the profession.

Nurse practitioners are continuing to expand their roles and are now providing care in inpatient as well as outpatient settings. The changing health care environment of the 1990s has caused the recent expansion of the role of the tertiary nurse practitioner and the acute-care nurse practitioner (ACNP)—a title used to describe the role of the nurse with advanced degrees and credentials engaged in the delivery of care to complex, acutely or chronically ill patients (Davitt & Jensen, 1981; Ford & Knight, 1990; Keane & Richmond, 1993; Parrinello, 1995). Nurse practitioners are moving into the acute-care setting in large numbers. Recent changes in the delivery of health care, a steady decrease in the size and number of medical residency training programs (Cohen, 1993; Foster & Seltzer, 1991), and the need to contain health care costs while maintaining quality of care have created opportunities for nurse practitioners to practice in more specialized roles and settings (Brundige, 1997; Gaedeke & Blount, 1995; Iglehart, 1994).

It is important to recognize that the role of the ACNP has been in existence since the 1970s (Davitt & Jensen, 1981); it was the neonatal nurse practitioner (NNP) who initiated the new acute-care and tertiary-care practitioner roles. NNPs practice collaboratively with physicians utilizing highly complex technical skills and clinical decision making. McGee (1995) describes a similar role for perinatal nurse practitioners (PNNPs) in a hospital in Colorado. Hospitals are employing nurse practitioners and midwives on general and specialty units (Knaus, Felten, Burton, Fobes, & Davis, 1997) in areas such as intensive care (Keane, Richmond, & Kaiser, 1994; Snyder et al., 1994), pediatrics (Gaedeke & Blount, 1995), surgery (Davitt & Jensen, 1981; Nemes & Barnaby, 1992; Callahan, 1996), trauma (Spisso, O'Callaghan, McKennan, & Holcroft, 1990), and neonatal intensive care units (Clancy & Maguire, 1995).

As acute-care practice has expanded, many nurse practitioners have shifted their role from generalist to that of specialist. Some nurse practitioners are specializing in specific areas of patient care, particular areas of practice such as adult cardiac care and surgery (Callahan, 1996; Giacalone, Mullaney, DeJoseph, & Cosma, 1995), oncology (Kinney, Hawkins, & Hudmon, 1997), mental health (Cornwell & Chiverton, 1997), critical care/emergency/trauma care (Buchanan & Powers, 1997; Cole & Ramirez, 1997; Keough, Jennrich, Holm, & Marshall, 1996), and vascular surgery (Knaus, Davis, Burton, Fellen, & Fobes, 1996) or have focused on the care of certain groups of patients such as those with HIV infection (Aiken et al., 1993).

By the end of the 1980s nurse practitioners were differentiated by a number of specialties beyond pediatrics and family nurse practitioner, for example, adult, geriatric, occupational health, women's health, school health, and psych/mental health. They were employed in a variety of settings: rural clinics and physician offices as well as health departments, hospitals (in ambulatory care, emergency departments, and inpatient units), industry and business, schools, nursing homes, and home health agencies (Bellet & Leeper, 1982; Bennett, 1984; Brooks & Johnson, 1986; Cruikshank & Lakin, 1986; Glascock, Webster-Stratton, & McCarthy, 1985; Hayden, Davies, & Clore, 1982; Martin & Davis, 1989; Scharon & Bernacki, 1984; Sobolewski, 1981; Weston, 1980; Wilbur, Zoeller, Talashek, & Sullivan, 1990; Zimmer, Groth-Juncker, & McCusker, 1985).

With the expansion of the role of the ACNP the practice settings have also expanded to include hospital-based specialties (Spisso et al., 1990), unit-based areas (Rudisill, 1995), and urgent care centers (Buchanan & Powers, 1997). This differentiation and broadening of the scope of practice of nurse practitioners clearly points to the fact that the nurse practitioner role is an advanced practice role in nursing, not merely a physician substitute role. Nemes (1994) agrees and describes the ACNP role in the hospital setting as one which strengthens and promotes a multidisciplinary approach to patient care and offers an opportunity to improve the delivery of health care. Martin and Coniglio (1996) report that the collaborative practice model, implemented on a Head and Neck Surgical Oncology unit, between an ACNP and a physician, is effective and impacts positively on patient care. Knaus et al. (1996) had similar findings on a vascular acute-care service. Ingersoll (1995) found, in interviews she conducted with ACNPs, that they described their role as complementary to the physician's. This disputes findings in other studies which describe the nurse practitioner as a physician substitute or physician extender (Poirier-Elliott, 1984; Spisso et al., 1990). Ingersoll (1995) supported findings concluded in other studies of primary care nurse practitioners which also reported a strong nursing orientation in their roles (Thibodeau & Hawkins, 1994).

Several investigators have surveyed graduates of nurse practitioner training programs. Others have studied nurse practitioners in a particular state or region to explore employment opportunities and career patterns (Bullough, 1984; Cruikshank & Lakin, 1986; Cruikshank, Clow, & Lakin, 1986; Hayden et al., 1982; Pulcini & Fitzgerald, 1997; Radosevich et al., 1990; Roos, 1979; Sirles, Leeper, Northrup, & O'Rear, 1986). These investigators report unemployment among nurse practitioners in the range of 2% to 22%. Reasons given for unemployment are similar to those for all nurses: pregnancy, childrearing, family responsibilities, and family relocation. However, barriers to practice as a nurse practitioner are also cited as reasons for unemployment.

The most comprehensive recent survey of nurse practitioners was conducted by the American Academy of Nurse Practitioners in 1989; 12,000 nurse practitioners were sent questionnaires, and close to 59% responded (Towers, 1989a, 1989b, 1990a, 1990b). Respondents represented all nurse practitioner specialties; 47% held master's degrees, and most were in primary care practices. Of those in rural areas and small communities, 37% held a master's or higher degree. Of those in urban areas, 53% held a master's or higher degree, and close to half (45%) worked in inner-city locations (Towers, 1990a).

Only 30% of the respondents had a physician on site 100% of the time, but most had access to a physician by phone; nevertheless, 70% reported asking physicians to see fewer than 20% of their patients (Towers, 1990b). A similar rate of physician consultation has been found by others (Cruikshank et al., 1986; Record et al., 1980), and these findings support the claim by Steinwachs et al. (1986) that the need for primary care physicians cited by the Graduate Medical Education National Advisory Committee was overestimated, whereas the need for nurse practitioners was underestimated.

Similar practice characteristics were also reported as part of the 1992 National Survey of Certified Nurse Practitioners and Clinical Nurse Specialists. Pan, Geller, Gullicks, Muus, and Larson (1997) compared similarities and differences between primary care nurse practitioners and physician assistants. The nurse practitioner data were collected as part of the 1992 national survey.

Charges for nurse practitioner services have been reported to be considerably less than charges for comparable physician services: first-visit charges ranged from 12% to 45% less than first-visit charges for a physician, and regular visit charges ranged from 7% to 40% less. The variability in the nurse practitioner-physician difference in charges is a factor of the particular specialty, with the least difference noted between pediatric nurse practitioners and physicians and the greatest difference noted between psych/mental health nurse practitioners and physicians (Towers, 1989a). Medicare reimbursement has recently changed. On August 5, 1997 President Clinton signed the Budget Reconciliation Act of 1997. This bill includes legislation that allows nurse practitioners to be reimbursed, at 80% of the actual charge or 85% of the Medicare fee schedule, for services provided to Medicare patients regardless of setting. This legislation became effective January 1, 1998.

The national survey of nurse practitioners found that they were managing pharmacologic therapeutics in all 50 states, across all specialties and in all locales—rural areas, small communities, and urban areas. Most used written protocols to guide their prescriptive activity, the extent of which was governed by state laws. In rural areas and small communities, 58% and 55%, respectively, of nurse practitioner respondents wrote prescriptions under their own name, whereas 43% of the urban nurse practitioner respondents did so. The advanced practice nurse (APN) currently has some prescriptive authority in all but one state (Pearson, 1997).

Fewer than 1% of APNs had been primary defendants in malpractice claims (Towers, 1989b). Pearson and Birkholz (1995) concluded from their survey that APNs, specifically readers of the *Nurse Practitioner*, are at low risk for malpractice allegations and claims. Birkholz (1995) studied data from a 17 1/2-month period provided by the National Practitioner Data Bank (NPDB). The NPDB is a computer depository of health care providers' malpractice payments by insurers and adverse actions taken by hospitals, licensing boards, or professional organizations accumulated since September 1, 1990. The NPDB is checked by a hospital when granting clinical privileges and then every 2 years. It can be accessed only by specified agencies and individuals. The collected data show nurses have less than 3% of the reported malpractice payments while physicians have 97%. APNs, when separated from RNs, have even fewer malpractice reports. Malpractice payment reports of APNs vary from 0.6% to 7.6%. These data have several flaws. Malpractice reports of APNs and RNs may be underreported, as clients may attempt to collect money from the deepest pockets, the hospital and/or physician. Claims may be five to eight years old which does not reflect the APNs' increased malpractice exposure from expanded scope of practice including prescriptive privileges.

Most nurse practitioners reported being responsible for taking histories, performing physical exams, ordering and evaluating lab tests, and prescribing medications—traditional medical services. All the nurse practitioners also reported nursing activities such as patient teaching, family counseling, and group education for health promotion and disease prevention. The ACNP is expected to assess complex, acutely ill patients, think critically, utilize diagnostic reasoning, perform case management and advanced therapeutic interventions (Clochesy, Daly, Idemotu, Steel, & Fitzpatrick, 1993).

Thus, during the 1990s, the comprehensive nature of nurse practitioner practice has become more apparent, and nurse practitioners are more clearly demonstrating an advanced practice nursing role. They are providing a broad range of services in underserved areas and doing so at less cost than physicians. The 1990s have seen new roles for nurse practitioners evolve as managed care has impacted every aspect of the health care delivery system.

Acceptance

Patient Acceptance

Studies of patient acceptance of nurse practitioners conducted in the mid-1980s and 1990s confirmed the findings of previous studies: patients are accepting of and satisfied with nurse practitioner services, and their acceptance increases after they have had experiences with nurse practitioners. For example, in a study of nurse practitioners and patients in the Army health care system, Southby (1980) found that patients who had experience with nurse practitioners were more accepting of them than were patients who had not had such experience. Furthermore, patients who had previous experience with nurse practitioners had higher expectations of them than did patients with no experience. Matas, Brown, and Holman (1996) noted that all the parents in their study reported having a positive visit at the nursing center and 30% stated they preferred nurse practitioners as primary health care providers. Buchanan and Powers (1997) studied staffing a fast track or minor emergency area with nurse practitioners. Their on-site analysis of nurse practitioner effectiveness indicated that patients were satisfied with their care. Larrabee, Ferri, and Hartig (1997) also found high patient satisfaction.

Investigators also began to examine factors associated with this acceptance, to determine which patients were more accepting of nurse practitioners. Some investigators found that women (Smith & Shamansky, 1983) and others found that men were more accepting (Enggist & Hatcher, 1983); still others noted no difference between men and women (Shamansky, Schilling, & Holbrook, 1985). Findings on the relationship between income level and nurse practitioner acceptance were also inconsistent (Enggist & Hatcher, 1983; Hogan & Hogan, 1982; Shamansky, Schilling, & Holbrook, 1985; Smith & Shamansky, 1983). However, findings on the relation of educational level and age to nurse practitioner acceptance were more consistent. Generally, patients with more education were more accepting of nurse practitioners (Brands, 1983; Fox & Storms, 1980; Pender & Pender, 1980; Schilling, Shamansky, & Swerz, 1985), and younger people were more likely to accept nurse practitioners than older persons (Enggist & Hatcher, 1983; Hogan & Hogan, 1982; Smith & Shamansky, 1983).

Higher educational level, younger age, and previous knowledge of or experience with nurse practitioners are likely to be interrelated. This interrelationship was noted by Fox and Storms (1980), who found that persons age 65 and older were less likely to have heard about nurse practitioners than were younger persons. Whether or not older persons had heard of nurse practitioners, after the services provided by nurse practitioners were described, 68% said they would accept their care; however, the percentage who would accept care by nurse practitioners was significantly higher among those who had heard of nurse practitioners than among those who had not. Fox and Storms found that more younger people would accept care by nurse practitioners (76%), but more younger people had heard of nurse practitioners prior to the study. Brands (1983) noted that among older persons, those with formal education beyond high school were more accepting of nurse practitioners than those with less formal education. These findings reflect the fact that exposure to and acceptance of innovations (such as nurse practitioners) is more likely to occur among younger persons and those with higher educational levels.

Some of the studies of patient acceptance provide additional insights into why and under what conditions patients are accepting of nurse practitioners. Brands (1983), for example, who studied patient acceptance of nurse practitioners among older persons, differentiated patient acceptance between traditional, transitional (health maintenance and promotion), and nontraditional (physical assessment and management of health problems) nursing activities. Most of the older persons surveyed would accept nurse practitioners for traditional activities; three-quarters preferred nurse practitioners for transitional activities; and proportions ranging from 15% to 63% (depending on the specific activity) would accept nurse practitioners for nontraditional activities.

A study by Molde and Baker (1985) provides further evidence of the type of services patients desire from nurse practitioners. These authors studied 128 patients in a primary care center to determine whether their visit was motivated primarily by their "chief complaint" or whether they had hidden agendas. They found that 30% of the patients had hidden agendas, but did not verbalize these hidden agendas unless sanctioned to do so; the hidden agendas—often the real reason for the visit—were related to their need for nursing care. These findings suggest that patients may need the services of nurse practitioners more than the services of physicians, even if they do not recognize this. Further, if patients do recognize their need for nursing services, to seek such services outright is not sanctioned, and thus they must mask their real need, making appointments for visits under the guise of having traditional medical problems.

A series of studies of potential nurse practitioner consumers in New Haven, Connecticut, identified the characteristics of services most likely to predict intent to use nurse practitioners among consumers of all ages (Shamansky et al., 1985). Although fewer than 33% of the survey respondents had heard of nurse practitioners and fewer than 10% had actual experience with them, 62% said they would use nurse practitioner services, while 24% were unsure and 13% would not. Prior knowledge or experience was not a significant predictor of intent to use nurse practitioner services. The strongest predictor was dissatisfaction with present care, and the most frequently expressed areas of dissatisfaction were availability and cost of care.

Holbrook and Shamansky (1985) examined the market for nurse practitioner services among women 18 to 40 years of age, a subsample of the consumers surveyed in the larger Connecticut study. Eighty percent of the women said they would use nurse practitioner services if they were covered by insurance. Shamansky and St. Germain (1987) also studied acceptance of nurse practitioners by the elderly; they found that although 73% had no prior knowledge of nurse practitioners, 51% thought there were no differences between physician and nurse practitioner services and were accepting of nurse practitioners.

These investigators also found that cost of care and health insurance coverage were significant predictors of intent to use nurse practitioner services. Prior knowledge of nurse practitioner services and perceived differences between physician and nurse practitioner care were not significant predictors. Shamansky and St. German (1987) conclude that patient acceptance and utilization of nurse practitioner services may not depend on prior knowledge or preference of provider, but on characteristics of the service which meet the particular needs of a population group, such as time spent during a visit, cost of care, convenience, and whether the services were covered by insurance.

The studies by Brands (1983), Molde and Baker (1985), and Shamansky et al. (1985) all suggest that health care consumers are discerning. They not only evaluate providers in determining their choice of services; they also evaluate the cost of the care provided, insurance coverage, accessibility and convenience of services, and inclusion of services beyond those traditionally provided. The question of patient acceptance of nurse practitioners is thus a marketing question—what kinds of services, at what cost and convenience, are the determining factors. The question involves the benefits sought by consumers and the relative advantage of nurse practitioners and the services they provide over and above other alternative forms of health service.

Physician Acceptance

Physicians tended to be accepting of nurse practitioners in the early 1970s when there was a shortage of physicians and they were overly worked. However, toward the late 1970s, nurse practitioners began to be viewed as a threat. Today, competition in the health care market among health care providers has been described as fierce and is expected to increase (Safran, Tarlov, & Rogers, 1994; Sekscenski et al., 1994). Competition exists between physician generalists and specialists as well as between nurse practitioners and physician generalists, and physician assistants. The current disagreement between organized medicine and nursing focuses on the independent practice of the nurse practitioner or practice without physician control (DeAngelis, 1994; Mundinger, 1994). Several authors have suggested a collaborative practice arrangement with physicians (DeAngelis, 1994). A collaborative practice arrangement may be appropriate for the ACNP (Britton, 1997; Genet et al., 1995; Martin & Coniglio, 1996), but restrictive to the nurse practitioner in primary care.

As with patient acceptance, physician acceptance is thought to be related to prior experience with nurse practitioners. Several studies support this view (Pierce, Quattlebaum, & Corley, 1985; Sharpe & Banahan, 1982; Weinberger, Greene, & Mamlin, 1980). Two studies that examined the effect of working with nurse practitioners during residency training on physicians' acceptance of nurse practitioners found that house staff acceptance and expectations of these practitioners increased during the residency period; further, these physicians indicated a willingness to employ nurse practitioners (Sharpe & Banahan, 1982; Weinberger et al., 1980). However, despite these findings, there are few reports in the literature of nurse practitioner involvement in residency training programs.

It has been suggested that physician acceptance is also related to traditional hierarchical structures, particularly gender hierarchy, which limits physicians' ability to view nurse practitioners as colleagues (Campbell-Heider & Pollock, 1987); at the same time, gender bias leads physicians to see nurse practitioners as less of a threat than physician assistants (Johnson & Freeborn, 1986). Both Weinberger et al. (1980) and Sharpe and Banahan (1982) have noted that physician acceptance of nurse practitioners is influenced by the effect of nurse practitioners on physician income and by issues of licensing, legal status, and reimbursement for services. More than likely, gender is and will remain a factor in physicians' acceptance of nurse practitioners. However, during the 1980s, with the physician surplus and various efforts at cost containment, the question of physician acceptance became clouded by issues of encroachment, territoriality, and competition. Cairo (1996) examined the attitudes of a group of emergency physicians toward collaborative practice with emergency nurse practitioners and found that the physicians supported the role of the emergency nurse practitioner provided that they were supervised in the traditional fashion by the physician.

Economic Impact

By the early 1980s, there was conclusive evidence that nurse practitioners were cost-effective. However, questions continued to be raised about their economic impact: Were nurse practitioners as productive as physicians? Were there true cost savings associated with nurse practitioners? Some argued, for example, that nurse practitioners were not economically viable because in many remote (and nonremote) settings, they " . . . fail to meet expenses or produce only minimal profits" (Mendenhall, Repicky, & Neville, 1980, p. 621). In this argument, however, the primary criterion used to assess economic effectiveness was income (and profit) generation; reimbursement policies were not acknowledged as a major influencing variable.

Throughout the 1980s, the question remained: what is the *potential* economic impact of nurse practitioners—for restrictive reimbursement policies prohibited coverage of many nurse practitioner services. Investigators had to conclude from the evidence available that cost savings could result from the use of nurse practitioners if nurse practitioner services were reimbursed by third-party payers. For example, in a study of nurse practitioners in one state with very restrictive reimbursement policies, investigators noted that in most settings, nurse practitioners could, if reimbursed, generate at least two to four times their salary and benefits; however, they could not realize this income because of restrictive reimbursement policies (Sirles et al., 1986).

Several studies conducted during the 1980s in settings not dependent on third-party reimbursement demonstrated actual cost savings associated with nurse practitioner services. Over a 4-year period, Dellinger, Zentner, McDowell, and Annas (1986), for example, reported a net savings of $273,986 a year when nurse practitioners were used to provide primary care and prevention services to company employees. They also noted that dependents who had the benefit of nurse practitioner services had lower insurance claims than did other dependents. The company is now considering extending nurse practitioner services to dependents, with the prospect of further cost savings. Since in industry many companies are self-insured and, for others, insurance rates are determined by the actual claims made by employees, any program that reduces health care expenditures and insurance claims results in cost savings.

Savings similar to those reported by Dellinger et al. have also been reported by others. At Tenneco, Inc., nurse practitioners provide a comprehensive program of services to 3,622 employees, On an annual basis, their services cost $469,562, compared to $978,057 for equivalent services provided by community physicians (Scharon & Bernacki, 1984; Scharon, Tsai, & Bernacki, 1987). Caward (1981) reported a net savings of $43,452 for a company of only 165 employees. Touger and Butts (1989) showed a substantial reduction in employer health care costs with a nurse practitioner primary care clinic at the worksite—from $120 per month per employee to $87 per month per employee between 1984 and 1987. It is important to note that during this same period, on average, employer health care costs rose as much as 20% to 30%. Lawler and Bernhardt (1986) argue convincingly that the marginal benefit (extra benefit realized for each added dollar spent, taking into account marginal productivity and cost) of nurse practitioners in occupational settings is substantial.

More recently, Lugo (1997) demonstrate how nurse practitioner services in a nurse-managed wellness center reduced a corporation's medical costs by $100,000 during the first six months of operation. Cost savings were realized while fostering employee satisfaction and addressing the health needs of the 1,000 employees. McGrath (1990) reported the overall financial savings of employing a nurse practitioner rather than a physician to be about 24%. Hooker (1993) noted that nonphysician providers are employed at about one-half of physician costs (including salary and benefits); combined with the "hands on" attention nurse practitioners provide patients, utilizing nurse practitioners in managed care is beneficial. Avron (1991) and Salkever (1992) also showed nurse practitioners to be cost-effective.

Studies have also been conducted in other settings not dependent (or not solely dependent) on third-party reimbursement for financial viability. Yeater (1985) noted that a 1980 CHAMPUS evaluation found that reimbursed expenses to nurse practitioners were 31% less than those for physicians. Brodie, Bancroft, Rowell, and Wolf (1982) compared care provided by nurse practitioners and physicians in a military pediatric outpatient clinic and found no differences except that the mean nurse practitioner cost per visit was 38% less than the mean physician cost per visit. A study of the costs of care for services in a jail compared program costs before and after the inclusion of nurse practitioners on the staff. Volume of care doubled, while the average cost per visit was reduced by one-third and various measures of quality improved (Hastings et al., 1980). And in HMOs per-episode costs for pediatric patients with nurse practitioners as the initial provider were 20% less than with physicians as the initial provider; general examination costs for women ages 40 to 55 were 52% less for nurse practitioners than for physicians (Salkever, Skinner, Steinwachs, & Katz, 1982).

All of these studies demonstrate that when reimbursement from third-party payers is not an issue, the use of nurse practitioners results in cost savings, as well as other added benefits. Yet while most of the studies to date provide evidence of nurse practitioner cost-effectiveness, they are limited in one respect. Except for those conducted in industrial settings, most have measured cost-effectiveness on a per-visit episode of illness or total-program basis, without considering costs incurred in other health care sectors, such as for hospitalization. In one study, however, both the costs for primary care services and the costs for hospitalization were examined for patients with congestive heart failure. The study compared costs at a Veterans Administration Center before and after the institution of a nurse practitioner clinic. Even though outpatient costs increased from $5,518 to $16,555, inpatient costs decreased from $153,450 to $22,275, resulting in a net savings of $120,138. These savings were largely attributed to a 60% reduction in the number of hospitalizations and an 85% reduction in the mean number of hospitalized days of nurse practitioner patients (Cintron, Bigas, Linares, Aranda, & Hernandez, 1983).

In the Veterans Administration study, the sample was small and patients were not randomly assigned to the nurse practitioner clinic. However, several other studies have reported similar results. In two studies of geriatric nurse practitioners in nursing homes, fewer hospital transfers from the nursing home were noted after the employment of a geriatric nurse practitioner (Garrard et al., 1990; Wieland, Rubinstein, Ouslander, & Martin, 1986). A 48% reduction in hospital transfers resulted in a reduction of 250 acute bed-days (Wieland et al., 1986). Also, in a randomized controlled trial of a home health care team using nurse practitioners, average daily costs were significantly less for patients cared for by the team with a nurse practitioner, due to the lower hospital utilization rates for these patients (Zimmer, Groth-Juncker, & McCusker, 1985).

Several recent studies suggest that cost savings associated with nurse practitioners increase if expensive institutionalization costs are considered. The findings also suggest that more comprehensive studies of nurse practitioner cost-effectiveness may show that the true cost-savings may have been underestimated. Naylor, Brooten, Jones, Lavizzo-Mourey, Mezey, and Pauly (1994) studied how a comprehensive discharge plan designed for the elderly and implemented by a gerontologic nurse specialist improved patient outcomes and decreased the cost of care by delaying or preventing rehospitalization. Parsons and McMurtry (1997) conducted a pilot study to review patient characteristics and outcomes of emergency room and hospital readmission rates for chronically ill elderly patients receiving primary care and discharge planning by a nurse practitioner. These studies suggest that primary care and discharge planning provided by nurse practitioners can reduce emergency room use and possibly decrease the number of hospital readmissions.

Few studies have examined the cost-effectiveness of inpatient nurse practitioners. Spisso et al. (1990) found that with the utilization of the nurse practitioner on a trauma service in a teaching hospital costs decreased and quality of care increased. Genet et al. (1995) looked at the implementation of the nurse practitioner role on a medical patient care division of a university hospital and offered suggestions for evaluating the cost benefits of nurse practitioner services. Rudisill (1995) described how an advanced practice nurse based on an inhospital unit can demonstrate improved outcomes, decreased costs, and patient satisfaction. Bissinger, Allred, Arford, and Bellig (1997) concluded that both the medical house staff and the neonatal nurse practitioner provide above-average care in the neonatal intensive care unit but that the nurse practitioner is more cost-effective and offers an acceptable alternative to house staff in the neonatal care unit studied. Nichols (1992) documented a model that predicts the costs of underusing advanced practice nurses. The results of underutilization may cost the nation $8.75 billion annually resulting from scope-of-practice restrictions and denied access for consumers.

In perhaps the most rigorous and conclusive study of nurse practitioner cost-effectiveness (Record et al., 1980), one full-time nurse practitioner was shown to provide the same care as a .63 full-time equivalent (FT) physician at one-third the cost. When the training cost differential between nurse practitioners and physicians is added in, the savings are staggering.

In 1986, the U.S. Congress Office of Technology Assessment (1986) published its report on nurse practitioner and certified nurse midwife cost and quality. The policy analysis was directed by a 20-member interdisciplinary advisory committee and was based on an extensive review of the research. The report repeatedly affirmed the cost-effectiveness of nurse practitioners for society, and stressed the effects of prohibitive legal constraints and restrictive reimbursement policies in limiting the true cost savings of nurse practitioners.

Sweet (1986) and Jacox (1987) thus suggest that the challenge is to change laws and reimbursement policies. Despite enabling federal legislation for nurse practitioner reimbursement, in 1990 only 26 states had mandatory benefit laws to reimburse nurse practitioners, and even in those states implementation of the laws was stalled and reimbursement limited (Scott & Harrison, 1990). State licensing laws meant to protect the public are actually serving to limit competition (Jacox, 1987). Licensing laws limit nurse practitioner practice by prohibiting certain activities, or by making their performance dependent on physician supervision—both of which protect the physicians' monopoly and direct the reimbursement to the physician. Further, these laws result in a double charge to society, which Jacox (1987) illustrates:

> For example, an NP working in a hospital may perform an admission history and physical on a newly admitted patient who has a private attending physician. The hospital pays the nurse's salary; the attending physician "validates" the history and physical exam and collects a fee, so that consumers or payers pay twice for a single service, hence raising the total cost of care. (p. 266)

Thus, for 30 years, study results have for the most part provided evidence in favor of nurse practitioners. Yet barriers continue to restrict their full contribution to the health care system in this country.

Quality of Care

The quality of care provided by nurse practitioners continued to be studied extensively during the 1980s and the 1990s. "From the beginning, the quality of services delivered by the new health professionals was a source of concern, receiving far more attention than the quality of services delivered by physicians had ever received" (Yankauer & Sullivan, 1982, p. 263). Many studies continued to use physician care as the standard for quality (Goldberg, Jolly, Hosek, & Chu, 1981; Hall et al., 1990; Hickman, Sox, & Sox, 1985; McDowell, Martin, Snustad, & Flynn, 1986; Palmer et al., 1985; Powers, Jalowiec, & Reichelt, 1984; Ramsay, McKenzie, & Fish, 1982; Thompson, Basden, & Howell, 1982; Watkins & Wagner, 1982). In other words, if nurse practitioner care, in terms of process or outcome or both, was equivalent to physician care, it was considered safe, competent quality care (Prescott and Driscoll [1979] provide an excellent review of earlier studies).

In the comparison studies of the 1980s, subtle and important differences between nurse practitioners and physicians were noted. For example, nurse practitioners had fewer missed appointments and higher return rates for follow-up visits (Becker, Fournier, & Garner, 1982; Bibb, 1982; Fosarelli, DeAngelis, Kaszuba, & Hafferty, 1985), and they prescribed fewer medications (Rosenaur, Stanford, Morgan, & Curtin, 1984). In a study comparing physician and nurse practitioner care for hypertensive patients, nurse practitioners had more success in managing obesity: nurse practitioner patients tended to lose weight, while physician patients tended to gain weight. In addition, nurse practitioner patients had better control of their hypertension (Ramsay, McKenzie, & Fish, 1982). The investigators concluded that successful outcomes were contingent on more than technical skills.

Hall et al. (1990) asked whether some of the more favorable outcomes associated with nurse practitioners were attributable to gender, since in most studies nurse practitioners were female and physicians were male. In a randomized controlled clinical trial of 16 ambulatory clinics, they compared the practices of female physicians and nurse practitioners.

"Comparable or superior performance for nonphysicians was found for all tasks but one [cancer screening in women]" (Hall et al., 1990, p. 489).

In comparing nurse practitioners to physicians, investigators have also noted differences in caseloads between nurse practitioners and physicians (Barkauskas, Chen, Chen, & Ohlson, 1981; Chen, Barkauskas, Ohlson, Chen, & DeStefano, 1983; Diers, Hamman, & Molde, 1986; Dunn & Higgins, 1986). In some studies, caseload differences were by design— nurse practitioners were assigned "well" visits (Sackett, Spitzer, Gent, & Roberts, 1974); or, in contrast, they were assigned patients with multiple chronic conditions (Runyan, 1976). In other studies, however, more nurse practitioner patients had problems not included in the ICD-9 codes (Barkauskas et al., 1981; Chen et al., 1983; Diers et al., 1986). Other research found that the caseloads of nurse practitioners included individuals whose overall health status was poorer than that of those seen by physicians (Aiken et al., 1993). Also, fewer nurse practitioner patients had private insurance, and 84% of the nurse practitioners' patients received public assistance, as compared to 62% of physicians' (Diers et al., 1986).

In some of these studies, investigators looked at differences in style or pattern of practice between physicians and nurse practitioners, rather than focusing solely on medical variables. Chen et al. (1983), for example, noted that pediatric nurse practitioners emphasized wellness more than their pediatrician counterparts. Diers et al. (1986) noted that nurse practitioners attended more to symptoms of nonpathological conditions, comfort, and comprehensiveness of care than did physicians. Campbell, Neikirk, and Hosokawa (1990) noted that nurse practitioners exhibited more concern with psychosocial issues than did physicians. However, in this study, when the type of visit (acute-care, chronic-care, well-care, and follow-up) was controlled, differences between nurse practitioners and physicians were not significant (Campbell, Mauksch, Neikirk, & Hosokawa, 1990; Campbell, Neikirk, & Hosokawa, 1990). Nonetheless, in many studies, differences have been apparent in nurse practitioner and physician style, emphasis, and pattern of practice. Brown and Grimes (1993) found nurse practitioners to spend more time, 24.9 minutes, with their patients as compared to the physician's 16.5 minutes. Courtney and Rice (1997) found in their study that the typical primary care visit lasted 18 minutes with history taking and teaching being the predominant activities.

Since the late 1960s, nurse practitioners have claimed that their style or pattern of practice is different from that of physicians, and that they are more than physician substitutes. Several studies have supported this view (Ingersoll, 1995; Thibodeau & Hawkins, 1994). However, results from one study suggest that this assertion requires questioning. In a study of nurse practitioner-patient interactions during well-child visits, taped interactions were analyzed. Pediatric nurse practitioners conducted comprehensive assessments and gave mothers a wealth of educational information. "However, the process of assessing and intervening was dominated by PNP questions, commands, and opinions" (Webster-Stratton, Glascock, & McCarthy, 1986, p. 249).

In a review of the Webster-Stratton et al. study, Lynn (1987) says:

> One of the early arguments for the creation of the nurse practitioner was that nurses would bring to the diagnosis and management of common health problems a more holistic approach to the patient. A preponderance of closed questioning of patients, the lack of patient input into the "nurse patient" interaction, the lack of description of or rationale for interventions suggested, and the nonrecognition of the patient by name or actions would seem to bring this holistic orientation into question. (p. 270)

Webster-Stratton et al. attribute their findings to the educational preparation of nurse practitioners, suggesting that nurse practitioners are knowledgeable about and committed to holistic care, but have less skill in the areas of counseling and teaching.

Results from many studies over the last three decades have produced evidence of the high quality of care provided by nurse practitioners, particularly when physician care is used as the standard. More recent studies have begun to identify the differences in both process and outcome between nurse practitioners and physicians (Mezey & Lynaugh, 1989). In an editorial in the *American Journal of Public Health*, Sullivan (1982) noted: "Nurse practitioners continue to show an uncanny ability not only to provide primary care equivalent to that of physicians, but also to offer something special that increases adherence . . . " (p. 8) and results in fewer prescribed medications and hospital days, decreased symptoms, and improved nutritional changes. Identification of practice style differences between physicians and nurse practitioners, and examination of their effects on patient outcomes and satisfaction, are clearly research priorities for the future. As Diers et al. (1986) suggest, these are important questions, because policy decisions about substitution and reimbursement rest on the answers. Safriet (1992) discusses the importance of obtaining an adequate history and patient counseling. The additional time spent in these two activities results in higher quality and more cost-effective patient care.

In 1979, Diers and Molde (1979) called for more conceptual and methodological rigor in nurse practitioner research and suggested that more attention be paid to sampling, measurement of chronically ill and well populations, definition of comparison groups, and consideration of new sources of data and more relevant standards of care. Stanford (1987) and Sullivan (1982) called for studies of process related to outcome and studies of the nursing component of nurse practitioner practice. While much of the research in the 1980s was conceptually sound and addressed these methodological issues, major gaps in the literature still exist. Although Courtney and Rice (1997) investigated the practice of the nurse practitioner and described the process of nurse practitioner primary care, several authors have suggested that research studies must focus more on processes of care, cost-effectiveness analyses, and outcomes of care to better understand the practice of the nurse practitioner (Crosby, Ventura, & Feldman, 1987).

Crosby et al. (1987) conducted a synthesis of the literature on nurse practitioner effectiveness, and noted that studies to identify current conditions that either enhance or impede nurse practitioner practice were needed. These researchers noted that studies addressing barriers to nurse practitioner practice were reported in the early 1970s, but "a reassessment of this issue in view of the changes that have occurred would contribute to an awareness of current factors having an impact on nurse practitioners" (p. 79). As one of the expert reviewers in the study concluded, the research agenda is the policy agenda.

SUMMARY AND CONCLUSIONS

In 1998, significant barriers to independent practice remain. Direct reimbursement (Nichols, 1992; Scott & Harrison, 1990); prescriptive authority (Mahoney, 1995); physician opposition; and gender issues all contribute to the underutilization of the nurse practitioner. Martin and Hutchinson (1997) explored the practice of nurse practitioners from their perspective. The nurse practitioners in the study describe establishing their roles from a marginalized, or discounted, position. Nurse practitioners, despite hundreds of studies which prove their effectiveness, still must convince the public that they are highly skilled and able to provide high-quality care. The public must believe in the nurse practitioner's superior skills and seek out their care. In the media physicians are portrayed as God-like while nurse practitioners are invisible (Martin & Hutchinson, 1997).

In 1986, in an examination of the factors influencing the workplace encroachment experienced by nurse practitioners, Ostwald and Abanobi (1986) wrote: "After 20 years of nurse practitioners' participation in the delivery of primary care services, the questions asked are no longer about their cost-effectiveness, the quality of services, or, for that matter, their viability" (p. 154). Researchers had made the same assertion 5 years earlier and many continue to make the same assertion today. The review in this chapter and the reviews by others note that there is ample evidence of the quality of services provided by nurse practitioners in all types of settings, as well as their cost-effectiveness and their acceptance by consumers. However, the full potential of nurse practitioners has never been accepted, according to Yankauer and Sullivan (1982) because it is too threatening.

Despite the evidence, Ostwald and Abanobi (1986) note:

> stupendous growth in the supply of primary health care providers in the face of declining utilization raises serious questions about the professional autonomy of nurse practitioners and about practice domains between nurse practitioners and physicians. Although nurse practitioners have won social acceptance from consumers, resistance from conservative policy makers, physicians, and health-care administrators, as well as restrictive reimbursement systems, continue to pose serious barriers to optimal utilization of nurse practitioner services, favoring more costly alternatives instead. (p. 154)

Early in the history of the nurse practitioner movement, resistance was attributed to reluctance to try a new, innovative role because questions of quality, cost, and patient acceptance were unanswered. These were legitimate questions. Today, 30 years later, the questions have been answered, but the resistance continues.

That resistance has recently been described as "encroachment" or as "restraint of trade." In one state, 38% of the nurse practitioners have experienced job encroachment (Ostwald & Abanobi, 1987). Another study of nurse practitioners in emergency rooms found that 57% left for practice in other settings because of resistance to their roles by physicians and hospital administrators (Hayden, Davies, & Clore, 1982). Bullough (1984), in an examination of major legal actions against nurse practitioners over a period of 10 years, found that of 17 major legal actions, only 2 were malpractice claims. The remainder were actions brought by medical societies and medical boards in an attempt to restrict nurse practitioner practice. Bullough concluded that most of the actions "look like harassment of nursing" (p. 441).

Kelly (1985) recommends that nurse practitioners turn to the judicial system to challenge restraints on their practice. She cites four major obstacles to the practice of nurse practitioners—or, in other words, restrictions that restrain their trade: (1) licensing restrictions; (2) denial or restrictions of third-party reimbursement; (3) denial of access to medical facilities; and (4) restrictions on access to physician backup services. The Sherman Act has great potential for correcting abuses in the marketplace, and antitrust actions can now be brought against licensing boards, third-party payers, health care organizations, and physicians. Success in any such antitrust action, however, is dependent on a new kind of evidence.

Evidence supporting nurse practitioner competence and safety, and the quality and cost-effectiveness of their services, will not withstand judicial scrutiny under the antitrust doctrine. In any judicial challenge, evidence must be case-specific. In addition, evidence is needed to support the demand for nurse practitioner services and limitations on consumers' free choice. In her review of restraint of trade challenges in the health care industry with relevance to nurse practitioners, Kelly (1985) describes several arguments that can be made by nurse practitioners in support of restraint of trade claims. Evidence to support such claims is being accumulated (note particularly the studies reviewed in the Patient Acceptance section), though more is needed.

During the 1980s, a great deal of research did address the essence of this practice, focusing on both its process and its outcome. The findings confirm that nurse practitioners, in all types of settings, and with various patient populations, provide care and services that lead to positive patient outcomes; in many instances, when compared to physicians, nurse practitioner outcomes are better.

Despite the findings, more research is still needed. What nurse practitioners do that results in better patient outcomes is an important question. They do it for less cost, or at least they have the potential of providing services at less cost, which could be fulfilled if system barriers were removed so that savings could be passed on to consumers and society. Furthermore, it is unlikely there will ever be enough nurse practitioners to meet societal needs. Consequently, if what nurse practitioners do that leads to positive patient outcomes can be identified, this knowledge can be transferred to other health care providers who, along with nurse practitioners, will make up the constellation of health care professionals working to meet society's needs.

After reviewing the literature from 1980 to 1990, it is apparent that encroachment and restraint of trade are real issues that inhibit the full use of nurse practitioners. Although the questions are slightly different from those of the late 1960s and 1970s, questions derived from political considerations are perhaps even more important today than previously. Evidence to support claims of encroachment and restraint of trade is crucial if nurse practitioners are to realize their full potential.

A challenge facing nurse practitioners today is the need to provide quality care and improved patient outcomes in less time at lower cost (Jones, 1993). Matas, Brown, and Holman (1996) conducted a study to measure qualitative and quantitative outcomes and the effectiveness and quality of health care provided by nurse practitioners. Research should focus on the actual process of care provided by nurse practitioners. It is essential to know what processes produce what outcomes. Nurse practitioners must be able to describe what they do with clients and relate these interventions to particular clinical outcomes (Courtney & Rice, 1997). This information is essential if the nurse practitioner is to meet the challenges of the next millennium. Mundinger (1997) writes in an editorial that well-designed and rigorously conducted studies on cost, quality, and outcomes of APNs are critically needed. Patients need to know what they are choosing when they choose a nurse practitioner as their health care provider. Policy makers and APNs need to know exactly what they are reimbursing.

REFERENCES AND BIBLIOGRAPHY

Abdellah, F. (1982). The nurse practitioner 17 years later: Present and emerging issues. *Inquiry, 19*(2), 105–116.

Ackerman, M. H., Norsen, L., Martin, B., Wiedrich, & Kitzman, H. J. (1996). Development of a model of advanced practice. *American Journal of Critical Care, 5*(1), 68–73.

Aiken, L. H., Lake, E. T., Semaan, S., Lehman, H. P., O'Hare, P. A., Cole, C. S., Dunbar, D., & Frank, I. (1993). Nurse practitioner managed care for persons with HIV infection. *Image, 25*(3), 172–177.

Alonzi, S., Geolot, D., Richter, L., Mapstone, S., Edgerton, M., & Edlich, R. R. (1979). Physician and patient acceptance of emergency nurse practitioners. *Journal of the American College of Emergency Physicians, 8,* 357–359.

American Nurses Association and American Association of Critical Care Nurses. (1995). *Standards of clinical practice and scope of practice for the acute care nurse practitioner.* Washington, DC: American Nurses Publishing.

Avorn, J. (1991). The neglected medical history and therapeutic choices for abdominal pain: A nationwide study of 799 physicians and nurses. *Archives of Internal Medicine, 151,* 694–698.

Barkauskas, V., Chen, S., Chen, E., & Ohlson, V. (1981). Health problems encountered by nurse-practitioners and physicians in obstetric-gynecologic ambulatory care clinics. *American Journal of Obstetrics and Gynecology, 140*(4), 393–400.

Beal, J. A., Steven, K., & Quinn, M. (1997). Neonatal nurse practitioner role satisfaction. *Journal of Perinatal Neonatal Nursing, 11*(1), 65–76.

Beck, J., & Gernert, E. (1971). Attitudes and background values and predictors of urban-rural practice location. *Journal of Dental Education, 35*(9), 45–53.

Becker, D., Fournier, A., & Garner, L. (1982). A description of a means of improving ambulatory care in a large municipal hospital: A new role for nurse practitioners. *Medical Care, 20*(10), 1046–1050.

Bellet, P., & Leeper, J. (1982). Effectiveness of the pediatric nurse practitioner well-baby clinics in West Alabama. *The Alabama Journal of Medical Sciences, 19*(2), 126–128.

Bennett, M. L. (1984). The rural family nurse practitioner: The quest for role identity. *Journal of Advanced Nursing, 9*(2), 145–155.

Bessman, A. (1974). Comparison of medical care in nurse clinician and physician clinics in medical school affiliated hospitals. *Journal of Chronic Disease, 27,* 115–125.

Bibb, B. N. (1982). Comparing nurse practitioners and physicians: A simulation study on processes of care. *Evaluation of Health Professions, 5*(1), 29–42.

Bible, B. L. (1970). Physicians' view of medical practice in nonmetropolitan communities. *Public Health Reports, 85*(1), 11–17.

Birkholz, G. (1995). Malpractice data from the national practitioner data bank. *Nurse Practitioner, 20*(3), 32–35.

Bissinger, R. L., Allred, C. A., Arford, P. H., & Bellig, L. L. (1997). A cost-effectiveness analysis of neonatal nurse practitioners. *Nursing Economics, 15*(2), 92–99.

Brands, R. (1983). Acceptance of nurses as primary-care providers by retired people. *Advances in Nursing Science, 5*(3), 37–49.

Brodie, B., Bancroft, B., Rowell, P., & Wolf, W. (1982). A comparison of nurse practitioner and physician costs in a military out-patient facility. *Military Medicine, 147*(12), 1051–1053.

Brooks, E. F., Bernstein, J. D., DeFriese, G. H., & Graham, R. M. (1981). New health practitioners in rural satellite health centers: The past and future. *Journal of Community Health, 6*(4), 246–256.

Brooks, E. F., & Johnson, S. L. (1986). Nurse practitioner and physician assistant satellite health centers: The pending demise of an organizational form? *Medical Care, 24*(10), 881–890.

Brown, S. A., & Grimes, D. E. (1993). *A meta-analysis of process of care, clinical outcomes, and cost-effectiveness of nurses in primary care roles: Nurse practitioners and certified nurse-midwives.* Washington, DC: American Nurses' Association, Division of Health Policy.

Brundige, K. J. (1997). Preparing pediatric nurse practitioners for roles in specialty practice. *Journal of Pediatric Health Care, 11*(4), 198–200.

Brush, B. L., & Capezuti, E. A. (1996). Revisiting "A nurse for all settings": The nurse practitioner movement, 1965–1995. *Journal of the American Academy of Nurse Practitioners, 8*(1), 5–11.

Buchanan, L. (1996). The acute care nurse practitioner in collaborative practice. *Journal of the American Academy of Nurse Practitioners, 8*(1), 13–20.

Buchanan, L., & Powers, R. D., (1997). Establishing an NP-staffed minor emergency area. *Nurse Practitioner, 22*(4), 175–187.

Bullough, B. (1984). Legal restrictions as a barrier to nurse practitioner role development. *Pediatric Nursing, 10*(6), 439–442.

Bullough, B., Sultz, H., Henry, O. M., & Fiedler, R. (1984). Trends in pediatric nurse practitioner education and employment. *Pediatric Nursing, 10*(3), 193–196.

Buppert, C. K. (1995). Justifying nurse practitioner existence: Hard facts to hard figures. *Nurse Practitioner, 20*(8), 43–48.

Cairo, M. J. (1996). Emergency physician's attitudes toward the emergency nurse practitioner role: Validation versus rejection. *Journal of the American Academy of Nurse Practitioners, 8*(9), 411–417.

Callahan, M. (1996). The advanced practice nurse in an acute care setting: The nurse practitioner in adult cardiac surgery care. *Nursing Clinics of North America, 31*(3), 487–493.

Campbell, J. D., Mauksch, H. O., Neikirk, H. J., & Hosokawa, M. C. (1990). Collaborative practice and provider styles of delivering health care. *Social Science Medicine, 30*(12), 1359–1385.

Campbell, J. D., Neikirk, H. J., & Hosokawa, M. C. (1990). Development of a psychosocial concern index from videotaped interviews of nurse practitioners and family physicians. *Journal of Family Practice, 30*(3), 321–326.

Campbell-Heider, N., & Pollock, O. (1987). Barriers to physician-nurse collegiality: An anthropological perspective. *Social Science and Medicine, 25*(5), 421–425.

Capan, P., Beard, M., & Mashburn, M. (1993). Nurse-managed clinics provide access and improved health care. *Nurse Practitioner, 18*(5), 50–55.

Caward, J. (1981). Economics of the nurse practitioner role in an industrial setting. *Nurse Practitioner, 6*(6), 17–18.

Charney, E., & Kitzman, H. (1973). The child health nurse (pediatric nurse practitioner) in private practice: A controlled trial. *New England Journal of Medicine, 108*, 998–1003.

Chen, S., Barkauskas, V., Ohlson, V., Chen, E., & DeStefano, L. (1983). Health problems encountered by pediatric nurse practitioners and pediatricians in ambulatory care clinics. *Medical Care, 21*(2), 168–179.

Cintron, G., Bigas, C., Linares, E., Aranda, J., & Hernandez, E. (1983). Nurse practitioner role in a chronic congestive heart failure clinic: In-hospital time costs, and patient satisfaction. *Heart and Lung, 12*(3), 237–240.

Clancy, G. T., & Maguire, D. (1995). Advanced practice nursing in the neonatal intensive care unit. *Critical Care Nursing Clinics of North America, 7*(1), 71–76.

Clochesy, J. M., Daly, B. J., Idemoto, B. K., Steel, J., & Fitzpatrick, J. J. (1994). Preparing advanced practice nurses for acute care. *American Journal of Critical Care, 3*(4), 255–259.

Cohen, J. (1993). Transforming the size and composition of the physician workforce to meet the demands of health care reform. *New England Journal of Medicine, 329*, 1810.

Cole, F. L., & Ramirez, E. (1997). The emergency nurse practitioner: An educational model. *Journal of Emergency Nursing, 23*(2), 112–115.

Congressional Budget Office. (1979) *Physician extenders: Their current and future role in medical care delivery.* Washington, DC: U.S. Government Printing Office.

Connelly, S. V., & Connelley, P. A. (1979). Physician's patient referrals to a nurse practitioner in a primary medical clinic. *American Journal of Public Health, 69*, 73–75.

Cooper, R. A. (1997). The growing independence of nonphysician clinicians in clinical practice. *JAMA - Journal of the American Medical Association, 277*(13), 1092–1093.

Cooper, J., Heald, K., Samuels, M., & Coleman, S. (1975). Rural or urban: Factors influencing the location decision of primary care physicians. *Inquiry, 12*(1), 18–25.

Cornwell, C., & Chiverton, P. (1997). The psychiatric advanced practice nurse with prescriptive authority: Role development, practice issues, and outcomes measurement. *Archives of Psychiatric Nursing, 11*(2), 57–65.

Courtney, R., & Rice, C. (1997). Investigation of nurse practitioner-patient interactions: Using the nurse practitioner rating form. *Nurse Practitioner, 22*(2), 46–65.

Crosby, F., Ventura, M., & Feldman, M. J. (1987). Future research recommendations for establishing NP effectiveness. *Nurse Practitioner, 12*(1), 75–79.

Cruikshank, B. M., Clow, T. J., & Lakin, J. A. (1986). Use of physician consultation by nurse practitioners in community health and ambulatory clinic settings. *Journal of Community Health Nursing, 3*(4), 211–223.

Cruikshank, B. M., & Lakin, J. A. (1986). Professional and employment characteristics of NPs with master's and non-master's preparation. *Nurse Practitioner, 11*(11), 45–52.

Daly, B. J. (1997). Acute-care nurse practitioners: 'Strangers in a strange land.' *AACN Clinical Issues, 8*(1), 93–100.

Davitt, P., & Jensen, L. (1981). The role of the acute care nurse practitioner in cardiac surgery. *Nursing Administration Quarterly, 6,* 16–19.

Day, L., Egli, R., & Silver, H. (1970). Acceptance of pediatric nurse practitioners. *American Journal of Disease of Children, 119,* 204–208.

DeAngelis, C. D. (1994). Nurse practitioner redux. *Journal of the American Medical Association, 271,* 868–871.

Dellinger, C. J., Zentner, J. L., & Annas, W. (1984). A report on the use of a family nurse practitioner to reduce industrial health care costs. *North Carolina Medical Journal, 45*(12), 800–802.

Dellinger, C. J., Zentner, J. P., McDowell, P. H., & Annas, A. W. (1986). The family nurse practitioner in industry. *American Association of Occupational Health Nursing Journals, 34*(7), 323–325.

Diers, D., Hamman, A., & Molde, S. (1986). Complexity of ambulatory care: Nurse practitioner and physician caseloads. *Nursing Research, 35*(5), 310–314.

Diers, D., & Molde, S. (1979). Some conceptual and methodological issues in nurse practitioner research. *Research in Nursing and Health, 2*(2), 73–84.

Donley, R. (1995). Advanced practice nursing after health care reform. *Nursing Economics, 13*(2), 84–88, 98.

Dunn, E. V., & Higgins, C. A. (1986). Health problems encountered by three levels of providers in a remote setting. *American Journal of Public Health, 76*(2), 154–159.

Dunn, L. (1997). A literature review of advanced clinical nursing practice in the United States of America. *Journal of Advanced Nursing, 25*(4), 814–819.

Edmunds, M. W. (1978). Evaluation of nurse practitioner effectiveness: An overview of the literature. *Evaluation and the Health Professions, 1*(1), 69–82.

Edmunds, M. W., & Ruth, M. W. (1991). NPs who replace physicians: Role expansion or exploitation? *Nurse Practitioner, 16*(9), 46–49.

Enggist, R. E., & Hatcher, M. E. (1983). Factors influencing consumer receptivity to the nurse practitioner. *Journal of Medical Systems, 7*(6), 495–512.

Feldman, M., Ventura, M., & Crosby, F. (1987). Studies of nurse practitioner effectiveness. *Nursing Research, 36*(5), 303–308.

Finerfrock, W., & Havens, D. H. (1997). Coverage and reimbursement issues for nurse practitioners. *Journal of Pediatric Health Care, 11*(3), 139–143.

Finocchio, L. J., Dower, C. M., McMahon, T., & Gragnola, C. M., The taskforce on Health Care Workforce Regulation. (1995). *Reforming Health Care workforce regulation: Policy considerations for the 21st century.* San Francisco, CA: Pew Health Professions Commission.

Fitzgerald, S. M., & Wood, S. H. (!997). Advanced practice nursing: Back to the future. *JOGNN - Journal of Obstetric, Gynecologic, & Neonatal Nursing, 26*(1), 101–107.

Ford, L., & Knight, R. (1990). Advanced nursing practice. *Today's OR Nurse, 12,* 22.

Fosarelli, P., DeAngelis, C., Kaszuba, A., & Hafferty, F. (1985). Compliance with follow-up appointments generated in a pediatric emergency room. *American Journal of Preventative Medicine, 1*(3), 23–29.

Foster, H., & Seltzer, V. (1991). Accommodating to restrictions on residents' working hours. *Academic Medicine, 66,* 94.

Fox, J. G., & Storms, D. (1980). New health professionals and older persons. *Journal of Community Health, 5*(4), 254–260.

Freund, C. M. (1981). Unpublished doctoral dissertation, The University of Alabama at Birmingham.

Freund, C. (1986). Nurse practitioners in primary care. In M. Mezey & D. McGivern (Eds.), *Nurses, nurse practitioners: The evolution of primary care* (pp. 305–333). Boston: Little, Brown.

Gaedeke, M. K., & Blount, K. (1995). Advanced practice nursing in pediatric acute care. *Critical Care Nursing Clinics of North America, 7*(1), 61–70.

Garrard, J., Kane, R. L., Radosevich, D. M., Skay, C. L., Arnold, S., Kepferle, L., McDermott, S., & Buchanan, J. L. (1990). Impact of geriatric nurse practitioners on nursing-home residents' functional status, satisfaction, and discharge outcomes. *Medical Care, 28*(3), 271–283.

Genet, C. A., Brennan, P. F., Ibbotson-Wolff, S., Phelps, C., Rosenthal, G., Landefeld, C. S., & Daly, B. (1995). Nurse practitioners in a teaching hospital. *Nurse Practitioner, 20*(9), 47–54.

Giacalone, M. B., Mullaney, D., DeJoseph, D. A., & Cosma, M. (1995). Development of a nurse-managed unit and the advanced practitioner role. *Critical Care Nursing Clinics of North America, 7*(1), 35–41.

Glascock, J., Webster-Stratton, C., & McCarthy, A. M. (1985). Infant and preschool well-child care: Master's- and nonmaster's-prepared pediatric nurse practitioners. *Nursing Research, 34*(1), 39–43.

Goldberg, G., Jolly, D., Hosek, S., & Chu, D. (1981). Physician's extenders' performance in Air Force clinics. *Medical Care, 19*(9), 951–964.

Goodwin, L. (1981). The effectiveness of school nurse practitioners: A review of the literature. *The Journal of School Health, 51*(11), 623–624.

Graduate Medical Education National Advisory Committee. (1978). *Supply and distribution of physicians and physician extenders* (DHEW Publication No. HRA 78-11). Washington, DC: Government Printing Office.

Greenberg, E. M. (1996). Violence and the older adult: The role of the acute care nurse practitioner. *Critical Care Nursing Quarterly, 19*(2), 76–84.

Hafferty, F. W., & Goldberg, H. I. (1986). Educational strategies for targeted retention of nonphysician health care providers. *Health Services Research, 21*(1), 107–125.

Hall, J. A., Palmer, R. H., Orav, E. J., Hargraves, J. L., Wright, E. A., & Louis, I. A. (1990). Performance quality, gender, and professional role: A study of physicians and nonphysicians in 16 ambulatory care practices. *Medical Care, 28*(6), 489–501.

Hardy-Havens, D. M., & Evans, E. C. (1995). A future for nurse practitioners in managed care. *Journal of Pediatric Health Care, 9*(2), 88–91.

Hastings, G., Vick, L., Lee, G., Sasmor, L., Natiello, T., & Sanders, J. (1980). Nurse practitioners in a jailhouse clinic. *Medical Care, 18*(7), 731–744.

Hayden, M. L., Davies, L., & Clore, E. (1982). Facilitators and inhibitors of the emergency nurse practitioner role. *Nursing Research, 31*(5), 294–299.

Hickman, D., Sox, H., & Sox, C. (1985). Systematic bias in recording the history in patients with chest pain. *Journal of Chronic Disease, 38*(1), 91–100.

Hogan, K., & Hogan, R. (1982). Assessment of the consumer's potential response to the nurse practitioner model. *Journal of Nursing Education, 21*(9), 4–12.

Holbrook, T., & Shamansky, S. (1985). The market for nurse practitioner services among women 18 to 40 years of age. *Health Care for Women International, 6*(5), 309–325.

Hooker, R. S. (1993). The roles of physician assistants and nurse practitioners in a managed care organization. In D. K. Clawson & M. Osterweis (Eds.), *The Role of Physician Assistants and Nurse Practitioners in Primary Care* (pp. 51–67). Washington, DC: Association of Academic Health Centers.

Hravnak, M., Kobert, S. N., Risco, K. G., Balsisseri, M., Hoffman, L. A., Clochesy, J. M., Rudy, E. B., & Snyder, J. V. (1995). Acute care nurse practitioner curriculum: Content and development process. *American Journal of Critical Care, 3,* 179–188.

Iglehart, J. K. (1994). Health care reform and graduate medical education. *New England Journal of Medicine, 330,* 1167–1171.

Ingersoll, G. L. (1995). *Critical Care Nursing Clinics of North America, 7*(1), 25–33.

Jacox, A. (1987). The OTA report: A policy analysis. *Nursing Outlook, 35*(6), 262–267.

Johnson, R., & Freeborn, D. (1986). Comparing HMO physicians' attitudes toward NPs and PAs. *Nurse Practitioner, 11*(1), 39, 43–46, 49.

Jones, K. R. (1993). Outcomes analysis methods and issues. *Nursing Economics, 11*(3), 145–152.

Keane, A., & Richmond, T. (1993). Tertiary nurse practitioners. *Image, 25,* 281.

Keane, A., Richmond, T., & Kaiser, L. (1994). Critical care nurse practitioners: Evolution of the advanced practice nursing role. *American Journal of Critical Care, 3,* 232–237.

Kelly, K. (1985). Nurse practitioner challenges to the orthodox structure of health care delivery: Regulation and restraints of trade. *American Journal of Law and Medicine, 11*(2), 195–225.

Keough, V., Jennrich, J., Holm, K., & Marshall, W. (1996). A collaborative program for advanced practice in trauma/critical care nursing. *Critical Care Nurse, 16*(2), 120–127.

King, K., & Ackerman, M. (1995). An educational model for the acute care nurse practitioner. *Critical Care Nursing Clinics of North America, 7,* 1–7.

Kinney, A. Y., Hawkins, R., & Hudmon, K. S. (1997). A descriptive study of the role of the oncology nurse practitioner. *Oncology Nursing Forum, 24*(5), 811–820.

Kleinpell, R. M. (1997). Acute care nurse practitioners: Roles and practice profiles. *AACN Clinical Issues, 8*(1), 156–162.

Knaus, V. L., Davis, K., Burton, S., Felten, S., & Fobes, P. (1996). Vascular nurse practitioner: A collaborative practice role in the acute care setting. *Journal of Vascular Nursing, 14*(2), 40–44.

Knaus, V. L., Felten, S., Burton, S., Fobes, & Davis, K. (1997). The use of nurse practitioners in the acute care setting. *Journal of Nursing Administration, 27*(2), 20–27.

LaRochelle, D. (1987). Research studies on nurse practitioners in ambulatory health care: A review, 1980–1985. *Journal of Ambulatory Care Management, 10*(3), 65–75.

Larrabee, J. H., Ferri, J. A., & Hartig, M. T. (1997). Patient satisfaction with nurse practitioner care in primary care. *Journal of Nursing Care Quality, 11*(5), 9–14.

Lawler, T., & Bernhardt, J. (1986). Nurse practitioners and HMOs in occupational health. *AAOHN - American Association of Occupational Health Nursing, 34*(7), 333–336.

Lawrence, R. S., DeFriese, G. H., Putnam, S. M., Pickard, Cyr, A. B., & Whiteside, S. W. (1977). Physician receptivity to nurse practitioners: A study of the correlates of the delegation of clinical responsibility. *Medical Care, 15,* 298–310.

Levine, J. I., Orr, S. T., Sheatsley, D. W., Lohr, J. A., & Brodie, B. M. (1978). The nurse practitioner: Role, physician utilization, and patient acceptance. *Nursing Research, 27,* 245–254.

Lewis, C. E., & Resnik, B. (1967). Nurse clinics and progressive ambulatory patient care. *New England Journal of Medicine, 277,* 1236–1241.

Lewis, C. E., Resnick, B., Schmidt, G., & Waxman, D. (1969). Activities, events and outcomes in ambulatory patient care. *New England Journal of Medicine, 280,* 645–649.

Lugo, N. R. (1997). Nurse-managed corporate employee wellness centers. *Nurse Practitioner, 22*(4), 104–113.

Lynn, M. (1987). Pediatric nurse practitioner-patient interactions: A study of the process. *Journal of Pediatric Nursing, 2*(4), 268–271.

Mahoney, D. F. (1995). Employer resistance to state authorized prescriptive authority for NPs: Results of a Pilot Study. *Nurse Practitioner, 20*(1), 58–61.

Martin, A., & Davis, L. (1989). Mental health problems in primary care: A study of nurse practitioners practice. *Nurse Practitioner, 14*(10), 50–56.

Martin, B., & Coniglio, J. U. (1996). The acute care nurse in collaborative practice. *AACN Clinical Issues, 7*(2), 309–314.

Martin, P. D., & Hutchinson, S. A. (1997). Negotiating symbolic space: Strategies to increase NP status and value. *Nurse Practitioner, 22*(1), 89–102.

Martin, S. R. (1995). Caring advanced nursing practice. *Nurse Practitioner, 20,* 16, 21.

Master, R., Feltin, M., Jainchill, J., Mark, R., Kavesh, W., Rabkin, H., Turner, B., Bachrach, S., & Lennox, S. (1980). A continuum of care for the inner city. *New England Journal of Medicine, 302*(26), 2622–2627.

Matas, K. E., Brown, N. C., & Holman, E. J. (1996). Measuring outcomes in nursing centers: Otts media as a sample case. *Nurse Practitioner, 21*(6), 116–125.

McDowell, B., Martin, D., Snustad, D., & Flynn, W. (1986). Comparison of the clinical practice of a geriatric nurse practitioner and two internists. *Public Health Nursing, 3*(3), 140–146.

McGee, D. C. (1995). The perinatal nurse practitioner: An innovative model of advanced practice. *JOGNN - Journal of Obstetric, Gynecologic, and Neonatal Nursing, 24,* 602–606.

McGrath, S. (1990). The cost-effectiveness of nurse practitioners. *Nurse Practitioner, 15*(7), 40–42.

Mendenhall, R., Repicky, P., & Neville, R. (1980). Assessing the utilization and productivity of nurse practitioners and physicians assistants: Methodology and findings on productivity. *Medical Care, 18*(6), 609–623.

Merenstein, J. H., & Rogers, K. D. (1974). Streptococcal pharyngitis: Early treatment and management by nurse practitioners. *Journal of the American Medical Association, 227,* 1278–1282.

Mezey, M., Dougherty, M., Wade, P., & Mersmann, C. (1994). Nurse practitioners, certified nurse midwives, and nurse anesthetists: Changing care in acute care hospitals in New York City. *Journal of the New York State Nurses Association, 25*(4), 13–17.

Mezey, M., & Lynaugh, J. (1984). The teaching Nursing Home program: Outcomes of care. *Nursing Clinics of North America, 24*(3), 769–780.

Molde, S., & Baker, D. (1985). Explaining primary care visits. *Image, 17*(3), 72–76.

Molde, S., & Diers, D. (1985). Nurse practitioner research: Selected literature review and research agenda. *Nursing Research, 34*(6), 362–367.

Morris, S. B., & Smith, D. B. (1977). The distribution of physician extenders. *Medical Care, 15,* 1045–1057.

Moscovice, I., & Nestegard, M. (1980). The influence of values and background on the location decision of nurse practitioners. *Journal of Community Health, 5*(4), 244–253.

Mundinger, M. O. (1994). Advanced practice nursing—good medicine for physicians. *New England Journal of Medicine, 330,* 211.

Mundinger, M. O. (1997). Editorial: New medicare access for advanced practice nurses: Good medicine for elders? *APNSCAN*(17), 1–2.

Naylor, M., Brooten, D., Jones, R., Lavizzo-Mourey, Mezey, M., & Pauly, M. (1994). Comprehensive discharge planning for the hospitalized elderly. *Annals of Internal Medicine, 120*(12), 999–1006.

Nemes, J. (1994). Nurse practitioners in acute care units. *Nursing Standard, 9*(8), 37–40.

Nemes, J., & Barnaby, K. (1992). The pediatric nurse practitioner in a surgical inpatient setting. *Nurse Management, 23,* 44.

Nichols, L. (1992). Estimating costs of underusing advanced practice nurses. *Nursing Economics, 10*(5), 343–351.

Nugent, K. E., & Lambert, V. A. (1996). The advanced practice nurse in collaborative practice. *Nursing Connections, 9,* 5–14.

Nugent, K. E., & Lambert, V. A. (1997). Evaluating the performance of the APN. *Nursing Management, 28*(2), 29–32.

Ostwald, S., & Abanobi, 0. (1986). Nurse practitioners in a crowded marketplace: 1965–1985. *Journal of Community Health Nursing, 3*(3), 145–156.

Ostwald, S., & Abanobi, 0. (1987). Strategies used by nurse practitioners to adjust to workplace encroachment. *Pediatric Nursing, 13*(3), 189–190.

Palmer, R., Louis, T., Hsu, L-N, Peterson, H., Rothrock, J., Strain, R., Thompson, M., & Wright, E. (1985). A randomized controlled trial of quality assurance in sixteen ambulatory care practices. *Medical Care, 23*(6), 751–770.

Pan, S., Geller, J. M., Gullicks, J. N., Muus, K. J., & Larson, A. C. (1997). A comparative analysis of primary care nurse practitioners and physician assistants. *The Nurse Practitioner, 22*(1), 14–17.

Parrinello, K. M. (1995). Advanced practice nursing: An administrative perspective. *Critical Care Nursing Clinics of North America, 7*(1), 9–16.

Parsons, P. L., & McMurtry, C. T. (1997). NP care/discharge planning saves money. *The Nurse Practitioner, 22*(3), 238–240.

Parrinello, K. M. (1995). Advanced practice nursing: An administrative perspective. *Advanced Practice Nursing, 7*(1), 9–16.

Pearson, L. J. (1996). The annual update of how each state stands on legislative issues affecting advanced nursing practice. *Nurse Practitioner, 21*(1), 10–70.

Pearson, L. J. (1997). Annual update of how each state stands on legislative issues affecting advanced nursing practice. *Nurse Practitioner, 22*(1), 18–86.

Pearson, L. J., & Birkholz, G. (1995). Report on the 1994 readership survey on NP experiences with malpractice issues. *Nurse Practitioner, 20*(3), 18–29.

Pender, N., & Pender, A. (1980). Illness prevention and health promotion services provided by nurse practitioners: Predicting potential consumers. *American Journal of Public Health, 70*(8), 798–803.

Perrin, E., & Goodman, H. (1978). Telephone management of acute pediatric illness. *New England Journal of Medicine, 298,* 130–135.

Pew Health Professions Commission. (1995, November). *Reforming health care workforce regulation: Policy considerations for the 21st century.* San Francisco, CA: Author.

Physician Extender Work Group. (1977). *Report of the Physician Extender WorkGroup.* (No. 017-022-00555-6) Hyattsville, MD: U.S. Government Printing Office.

Piano, M. R., Kleinpell, R., & Johnson, J. A. (1996). The acute care nurse practitioner and management of common health problems: A proposal. *American Journal of Critical Care, 5*(4), 289–292.

Pierce, M., Quattlebaum, T. G., & Corley, J. (1985). Significant attitude changes among residents associated with a pediatric nurse practitioner. *Journal of Medical Education, 60*(9), 712–718.

Poirier-Elliott, E. (1984). Cost-effectiveness of non-physician health care professionals. *Nurse Practitioner, 9,* 54.

Powers, M., Jalowiec, A., & Reichelt, P. (1984). Nurse practitioner and physician care compared for nonurgent emergency room patients. *Nurse Practitioner 9*(2), 39–52.

Prescott, P., & Driscoll, L. (1979). Nurse practitioner effectiveness: A review of physician-nurse comparison studies. *Evaluation and the Health Professions, 2*(4), 387–411.

Prescott, P., & Driscoll, L. (1980). Evaluating nurse practitioner performance: The nurse practitioner. *American Journal of Primary Health Care, 28*(4), 32–53.

Pulcini, J., & Fitzgerald, M. A. (1997). NPACE nurse practitioner practice characteristics, salary, and benefits survey: Eastern United States. *Clinical Excellence for Nurse Practitioners, 1*(3), 185–190.

Radosevich, D., Kane, R., Garrard, J., Skay, C., McDermott, S., Kepferle, L., Buchanan, J., & Arnold, S. (1990). Career paths of geriatric nurse practitioners employed in nursing homes. *Public Health Report, 105*(1), 65–71.

Ramsay, J., McKenzie, J., & Fish, D. (1982). Physicians and nurse practitioners: Do they provide equivalent health care? *American Journal of Public Health, 72*(1), 55–57.

Record, J., McCally, M., Schweitzer, S., Blomquist, R., & Berger, B. (1980). New health professions after a decade and a half: Delegation, productivity and costs in primary care. *Journal of Health Politics, Policy and Law, 5*(3), 470–497.

Roos, P. (1979). Nurse practitioner employment, unemployment, reemployment. *Nursing Research, 28*(6), 348–353.

Roos, P., & Crooker, M. (1983). Variables affecting nurse practitioner salaries. *Nurse Practitioner, 8*(5), 36–44.

Rosenaur, J., Stanford, S., Morgan, W., & Curtin, B. (1984). Prescribing behaviors of primary care nurse practitioners. *American Journal of Public Health, 74*(1), 10–13.

Rudisill, P. T. (1995). Unit-based advanced practice nurse in critical care. *Critical Care Nursing Clinics of North America, 7*(1), 53–59.

Runyan, J. W. (1976). The Memphis chronic disease program: Comparisons in outcome and the nurse's extended role. *Nurse Practitioner, 1*(5), 27–30.

Sabo, C. E., & Louis, M. (1996). Nurse practitioners: Reevaluation of the need for and willingness to hire by nurse administrators, nurse practitioners, and physicians. *Journal of the American Academy of Nurse Practitioners, 8*(8), 375–381.

Sackett, D. L., Spitzer, W. O., Gent, M., & Roberts, R. S. (1974). The Burlington randomized trial of the nurse practitioner: Health outcomes of patients. *Annals of Internal Medicine, 80,* 137–142.

Safran, D. G., Tarlov, A. R., & Rogers, W. H. (1994). Primary care performance in fee-for-service and prepaid health care systems. *Journal of the American Medical Association, 271,* 1579–1586.

Safriet, B. J. (1992). Health care dollars and regulatory sense: The role of advanced practice nursing. *Yale Journal of Regulation, 9*(2), 417–488.

Salkever, D., Skinner, E., Steinwachs, D., & Katz, H. (1982). Episode-based efficiency comparisons for physicians and nurse practitioners. *Medical Care, 20*(2), 143–153.

Salmon, M. A., & Stein, J. (1986). Distribution of nurse practitioners and physician assistants: Are they meeting the need for primary care? *North Carolina Medical Journal, 47*(3), 147–148.

Scharon, G. M., & Bernacki, E. J. (1984). A corporate role for nurse practitioners. *Business and Health, 1*(9), 26–27.

Scharon, G., Tsai, S., & Bernacki, E. (1987). Nurse practitioners in an occupational setting: Utilizing patterns for the delivery of primary care. *American Association of Occupational Health Nurses Journal, 35*(6), 280–284.

Schiff, D. W., Fraser, C. H., & Walter, H. L. (1969). The pediatric nurse practitioner in the office of pediatricians in private practice. *Pediatrics, 44,* 62–68.

Schilling, L., Shamansky, S., & Swerz, M. (1985). Profiles of the consumer and nonconsumer of pediatric nurse practitioner services: New Haven, Connecticut. *Journal of Community Health Nursing, 2*(2), 79–92.

Schneider, D. P., & Foley, W. J. (1977). A systems analysis of the impact of physician extenders on medical cost and manpower requirements. *Medical Care, 15,* 277–297.

Schroeder, S. A. (1993). The U.S. physician supply: Generalism in retreat. *Bulletin of the New York Academy of Medicine,* Winter, 103–117.

Schulman, J., & Wood, C. (1972). Experience of a nurse practitioner in a general medical clinic. *Journal of the American Medical Association, 219,* 1453–1461.

Scott, C., & Harrison, 0. A. (1990). Direct reimbursement of nurse practitioners in health insurance plans of research universities. *Journal of Professional Nursing, 6*(1), 21–32.

Sekscenski, E. S., Sansom, S., Bazell, C., Salmon, M. E., & Mullan, F. (1994). State practice environments and the supply of physician assistants, nurse practitioners, and certified nurse-midwives. *The New England Journal of Medicine, 331,* 1266–1271.

Shah, H. S., Bruttomesso, K. A., Sullivan, D. T., & Lattanzio, J. (1997). An evaluation of the role and practices of the acute-care nurse practitioner. *AACN Clinical Issues, 8*(1), 147–155.

Shamansky, S. (1984). Nurse practitioners and primary care research: Promises and pitfalls. *Annual Review of Nursing Research, 3,* 107–125.

Shamansky, S., Schilling, L., & Holbrook, T. (1985). Determining the market for nurse practitioner services: The New Haven experience. *Nursing Research, 34*(4), 242–247.

Shamansky, S., & St. Germain, L. (1987). The elderly market for nurse practitioner services. *Western Journal of Nursing Research, 9*(1), 87–106.

Sharpe, T., & Banahan, B. (1982). Evaluation of the use of rural health clinics: Attitudes and behaviors of primary care physicians in service areas of nurse practitioner clinics. *Public Health Reports, 97*(6), 566–571.

Sharp, N. (1996). Nurse practitioner reimbursement: History and politics. *Nurse Practitioner, 21*(3), 100–104.

Sharp, N. (1997). Medicare reimbursement: For NPs, CNSs, MDs, and telehealth. *Nurse Practitioner, 22*(8), 143–146.

Shay, L. E., Goldstein, J. T., Matthews, D., Trail, L. L., & Edmunds, M. W. (1996). Guidelines for developing a nurse practitioner practice. *Nurse Practitioner, 21*(1), 72–81.

Sinclair, B. P. (1997). Advanced practice nurses in integrated health care systems. *JOGNN - Journal of Obstetric, Gynecologic, and Neonatal Nursing, 26*(2), 217–223.

Sirles, A., Leeper, J., Northrup, R., & O'Rear, M. (1986). The education, employment situations and practice activities of nurse practitioners in Alabama. *The Alabama Journal of Medical Sciences, 23*(4), 379–384.

Smith, D., & Shamansky, S. (1983). Determining the market for family nurse practitioner services: The Seattle experience. *Nursing Research, 32*(5), 301–305.

Snyder, J. V., Sirio, C. A., Angus, D. C., Hravnak, M. T., Kobert, S. N., Sinz, E. H., & Rudy, E. B. (1994). Trial of nurse practitioners in intensive care. *New Horizons, 2*(3), 296–304.

Sobolewski, S. (1981). Cost-effective school nurse practitioner services. *The Journal of School Health, 51*(9), 585–588.

Southby, J. (1980). Primary care nurse practitioners within the Army health care system: Expectations and perceptions of the role. *Military Medicine, 145*(10), 659–665.

Sox, H. C. (1979). Quality of patient care by nurse practitioners and physicians' assistants: A ten-year perspective. *Annals of Internal Medicine, 91,* 459–468.

Spector, R., McGrath, P., Alpert, J., Cohen, P., & Aikens, H. (1975). Medical care by nurses in an internal medicine clinic. *Journal of the American Medical Association, 232,* 1234–1237.

Spisso, J., O'Callaghan, C., McKennan, M., & Holcroft, J. W. (1990). Improved quality of care and reduction of housestaff workload using trauma nurse practitioners. *Journal of Trauma, 30*(6), 660–665.

Stanford, D. (1987). Nurse Practitioner research: Issues in practice and theory. *Nurse Practitioner, 12*(1), 64–74.

Steinwachs, D., Weiner, J., Shapiro, S., Bataldon, P., Coltin, K., & Wasserman, F. (1986). A comparison of the requirements for primary care physicians in HMOs with projections made by the GMENAC. *New England Journal of Medicine, 314*(4), 217–222.

Storms, D. M., & Fox, J. G. (1979). The public's view of physicians' assistants and nurse practitioners. *Medical Care, 17,* 526–535.

Strickland, W. J., & Hanson, C. M. (1995). Practice characteristics and satisfaction of contemporary nonphysician providers. *Family & Community Health, 18*(3), 78–88.

Sullivan, J. A., & Dachelet, C. Z. (1979). Evaluative research and the nurse practitioner: Where we've been, where we are and what's ahead. In H. Sultz, O. M. Henry, & J. A. Sullivan (Eds.), *Nurse practitioners: USA* (pp. 187–197). Lexington, MA: Lexington Books.

Sullivan, J. (1982). Research on nurse practitioners: Process behind the outcome? *American Journal of Public Health, 72*(1), 8–9.

Sultz, H., Henry, 0. M., & Carroll, H. (1977). Nurse practitioners: An overview of nurses in the expanded role. In A. Bliss & E. Cohen (Eds.), *The health professionals* (pp. 41–76). Germantown, MD: Aspen Systems.

Sweet, J. B. (1986). The cost-effectiveness of nurse practitioners. *Nurse Economics, 4*(4), 190–193.

Thibodeau, J. A., & Hawkins, J. W. (1994). Moving toward a nursing model in advanced practice. *Western Journal of Nursing Research, 16,* 205.

Thompson, R., Basden, P., & Howell, L. (1982). Evaluation of initial implementation of an organized adult health program employing family nurse practitioners. *Medical Care, 20*(11), 1109–1127.

Touger, G. N., & Butts, J. K. (1989). The workplace: An innovative and cost-effective practice site. *Nurse Practitioner, 14*(1), 35–42.

Towers, J. (1989a). Part 1: Report of the American Academy of Nurse Practitioners national nurse practitioner survey. *Journal of the American Academy of Nurse Practitioners, 1*(3), 91–94.

Towers, J. (1989b). Report of the national survey of the American Academy of Nurse Practitioners, part 11: Pharmacologic management practices. *Journal of the American Academy of Nurse Practitioners, 1*(4), 137–142.

Towers, J. (1990a). Report of the national survey of the American Academy of Nurse Practitioners, part III: Comparison of nurse practitioner characteristics according to education. *Journal of the American Academy of Nurse Practitioners, 2*(3), 121–124.

Towers, J. (1990b). Report of the national survey of the American Academy of Nurse Practitioners, part IV: Practice characteristics and marketing activities of nurse practitioners. *Journal of American Academy of Nurse Practitioners, 2*(4), 164–167.

U.S. Congress, Office of Technology Assessment. (1986). *Nurse practitioners, physician assistants, and certified nurse midwives: A policy analysis.* Washington, DC: U.S. Government Printing Office.

Watkins, L., & Wagner, E. (1982). Nurse practitioner and physician adherence to standing orders criteria for consultation or referral. *American Journal of Public Health, 72*(1), 22–29.

Watson, L. J. (1996). A national profile of nursing centers. *Nurse Practitioner, 21*(3), 72–81.

Webster-Stratton, C., Glascock, J., & McCarthy, A. M. (1986). Nurse practitioner-patient interactional analyses during well-child visits. *Nursing Research, 35*(4), 247–249.

Weinberger, M., Greene, J., & Mamlin, J. (1980). Changing house staff attitudes toward nurse practitioners during their residency training. *American Journal of Public Health, 70*(11), 1204–1206.

Weiner, J., Steinwachs, D., & Williamson, J. (1986). Nurse practitioner and physician assistant practices in three HMOs: Implications for future U. S. health power needs. *American Journal of Public Health, 76*(5), 507–511,

Weston, J. L. (1980). Distribution of nurse practitioners and physician assistants: Implications of legal constraints and reimbursement. *Public Health Reports, 95*(3), 253–258.

Wieland, D., Rubenstein, L., Ouslander, J., & Martin, S. (1986). Organizing an academic nursing home. *Journal of American Medical Association, 255*(19), 2622–2627.

Wilbur, J., Zoeller, L., Talashek, M., & Sullivan, J. (1990). Career trends of master's prepared family nurse practitioners. *Journal of American Academy of Nurse Practitioners, 2*(2), 69–78.

Williams, C. A. (1975). Nurse practitioner research: Some neglected issues. *Nursing Outlook, 23*(3), 172–177.

Yankauer, A., & Sullivan, J. (1982). The new health professionals: Three examples. *Annual Review of Public Health, 3,* 249–276.

Yeater, D. (1985). 1985 health care cost management update. *Occupational Health Nursing, 31*(12), 594–599.

Zimmer, J. G., Groth-Juncker, A., & McCusker, J. (1985). Randomized controlled study of a home health care team. *American Journal of Public Health, 75*(2), 134–141.

Chapter 3

PHILOSOPHICAL AND HISTORICAL BASES OF ADVANCED PRACTICE NURSING ROLES

Ellen D. Baer

SINCE almost the inception of modern nursing in America toward the end of the 19th century, certain nurses practiced in ways considered more independent and advanced than the usual nursing activities. Drawn to such practice by their own inclinations, inspired by progressive ideals, and paid by society to acculturate its newest and neediest members, public health and visiting nurses tended to the sick, the poor, the young, the old, in their homes. In addition to providing physical ministrations, these nurses introduced immigrant mothers to illness prevention techniques, taught them sanitary ideals, and encouraged their use of nutritious foods. For the most part, such independent nursing practices developed in fields not yet noticed by physicians, such as midwifery and anesthesia, or outside of mainstream settings, such as among the rural populations served by the Frontier Nursing Service.

By the middle of the 20th century, America's success in World War II had changed the way Americans viewed the world. All things seemed possible, even the eradication of disease. Advances in technology, chemistry, atomic energy, transportation, manufacturing, and a host of other fields developed to assist the war effort, were turned to civilian uses. Health care was a major beneficiary of these new discoveries. Nurses shared in the expansive view of health care possibilities as both providers of many new, expanded services and as beneficiaries of its largesse. Nurses left World War II with officer rank, some federal funding for nursing educational programs, and access to free university education through the G. I. Bill. Many went to college, obtained basic and advanced degrees, and began to think of themselves and their practices in new, expanding ways.

In hospitals, nurses began grouping patients recovering from anesthesia, or suffering from specific maladies such as heart disease, in clusters that assured them the most concentrated or intensive nursing care.[1] These nurses became expert in managing the care of special populations of hospitalized patients, many of whom were critically ill. Titles like clinical nurse specialist developed to differentiate these expert specialists from their nursing colleagues who functioned in more traditional, general practice roles. Almost simultaneously, visiting and public health nurses increased their expertise in managing the care in clinics, schools, and homes. As the major agents of the nation's widespread public health efforts, these nurses promoted health and prevented disease through patient teaching, immunization services, and widespread public education programs. In the late 1950s and early 1960s, several noteworthy nurse/physician collaborative teams developed in places like Colorado and Rochester, New York, in which physicians mentored experienced nurses to deliver primary care services in clinics. Medical centers like The New York Hospital offered Primex programs to teach nurses the basics of physical assessment and clinical decision making central to delivering primary care services.

The passage of Medicare/Medicaid legislation in 1965 created an expanded demand for health services. The supply and distribution of primary care physicians was unable to meet this demand. In addition, the services demanded were broader in scope than those contained within the domain of medicine prior to the 1960s. Newly empowered consumers organized into advocacy coalitions, such as Grey Panthers, civil rights, and women's movements, sought expanded supportive functions once considered the province of multigenerational families, clergy, and the like. The nursing profession stepped into the breach. Asserting that it possessed the neces-

sary history, organization, and educational facilities, nursing acted to
supply knowledgeable and licensed individuals to meet the growing and
broader demands in primary care practice.

In subsequent years, it became equally evident that clinical nurse specialists contributed, quantitatively and qualitatively, to meeting a large
portion of patient needs in hospitals and acute care. With the explosion
of managed care post-1995, inpatient and acute-care facilities have begun
substituting for physician care, with clinical nurse specialists now unified
with nurse practitioners under the generic term "advanced practice nurses."
The major objection raised about the utilization of nurses in independent
and autonomous roles came from those in medicine, hospital administration, and government who believed that nurses did not have the expert
authority and its derivative, autonomy, on which independent practice
rests.

Application of the principles of authority and autonomy to any human
activity is problematic. In the context of the dynamic interactions of
human experience, authority and autonomy fluctuate as do all processes
that involve people. No one is always and absolutely autonomous, just
as no one is completely devoid of autonomy. What is at issue is a continuum
of authority and autonomy and the contextual boundaries of that continuum. In a subsequent chapter, Marx and Mullinix argue that the debate
about authority and autonomy is really a debate about money; that the
subtext regarding "authority" is that the question how much do you know
really means how much are you worth, i.e., who will be paid, and how
much.

Nursing[2] as an occupational category is also problematic. In the generic
sense, it encompasses multiple levels of philosophy, educational preparation, and practice that have developed over time as society's complexity
increased. Because newer nursing education and practice models did not
totally replace earlier ones, and because nursing has resisted mandatory
university-based preparation that society recognizes as legitimating all
other professions, multiple nursing levels exist. These levels, by definition
and quasi-design, occupy different positions on the continuum of authority
and autonomy, and their differences are not clear to the public. Organized
nursing's inability to enforce stated desired educational entry levels for
basic nursing practice understandably raises questions about its ability to
assure the practice quality of yet another kind of nurse. However, although
variations in the education of nurses seeking to practice in advanced
roles exist, by the 21st century almost all advanced practitioners will be

master's-prepared and ANA advanced practice certification examinations will require master's preparation.[3]

Therefore, the focus of this chapter is the nurse who may have begun nursing education at the diploma or associate degree level, but ultimately received professional nursing preparation at the baccalaureate or higher degree level, and additional specific graduate education to practice in primary care or other advanced practice roles. Because primary care practice by nurses sparked most of the debate about nurses taking independent practice roles, most of the public commentary focuses specifically on primary care. However, over time, the descriptive language that limited primary care practice to outpatient or ambulatory settings has been replaced by general practice and specialty care descriptions of advanced practice, as is evident in various state nurse practice acts.[4] This chapter, therefore, takes the position that all variations of advanced nursing practice rest on the same authoritative base as does primary care practice.

Within the limits so described, this chapter will discuss some philosophical issues raised by nursing's assertion of its claim to occupy independent provider roles in advanced practice and primary care. The discussion will be biased in the direction of endorsing appropriately prepared nurses practicing in independent practice roles.

DEFINITION

In 1994, the Institute of Medicine's Committee on the Future of Primary Care defined primary care as: " . . . the provision of integrated, accessible health care services by clinicians who are accountable for addressing a large majority of personal health care needs, developing a sustained partnership with patients, and practicing in the context of family and community."[5]

Further, the Institute's Committee identified the nature of primary care as including six core attributes:

1. Excellent primary care is grounded in both the biomedical and the social sciences.
2. Clinical decision making in primary care differs from that in specialty care.
3. Primary care has at its core a sustained personal relationship between patient and clinician.

4. Primary care does not consider mental health separately from physical health.

5. Important opportunities to promote health and prevent disease are intrinsic to primary care practice.

6. Primary care is information intensive.[6]

These definitions represent the views of this author and will serve as reference points from which some philosophical issues can be discussed. The definitions suggest three general, fundamental assumptions regarding the primary care role: (1) It is not specific to any one health profession; (2) it is not limited as to population served, health problems encountered, or duration of practitioner-client relationship; and (3) it requires from its practitioners independent and autonomous decision making based on professional knowledge. It is the assumption regarding autonomy[7] that causes the major delays and dilemmas encountered by nursing when it attempts to occupy the primary health care role.

Despite some model legislation,[8] nursing has most commonly been defined legally as a dependent practice that delivers health care services under the supervision of a duly authorized physician or dentist. As the demand for primary care services expanded, many institutions inaugurated solutions in which nurses, under titles such as nurse practitioner, act in primary care roles, but operate under a system of protocols designed in advance in conjunction with physicians. Such compromises cloud the autonomy issue, because protocols are external constraints that suggest the inability of the nurse to choose correctly among "alternative possibilities of action . . . in accordance with [appropriate] inner motives and ideals . . . "[9] Protocols merely extend the distance between the nurse in practice and the physician in supervision. They act essentially as "standing" or "PRN" orders and implicitly reinforce a dependent model of practice for nursing. However true this criticism of protocols might be, expanding managed care programs and the ever-present threat of litigation have spawned protocols in all sorts of clinical arrangements that affect the practice of all clinicians, not only nurses.

The central issues blocking widespread use of appropriately prepared and truly autonomous nurses to meet people's health care needs in a variety of independent, advanced practice roles are political and are hidden behind protests that nursing is not a true profession, capable of safely caring for patients in an independent manner. This chapter will address both the stated and the hidden issues.

AUTONOMY, AUTHORITY, AND NURSING KNOWLEDGE

Independent, autonomous practice rests on the assumption that the agent of such a practice has the expertise from which that agent derives the authority to act.[10] In the case of autonomous practice, this reliance on authority is essential to the protection of citizens in situations where knowledge is utilized about which the lay consumer has little understanding.

There is a substantial body of literature that discusses the notion of authority.[11] Issues of power, morality, the consent of the subject, the limits to authority, and the interactions among the concepts of authority, reason, and freedom form the core of centuries of philosophical debate that cannot be addressed adequately in this chapter. The piece of the debate that seems most applicable here is that which addresses the legitimacy of authority; that is, how an individual or group justifies its claim to an authoritative position on certain bodies of knowledge and the behaviors or actions that derive from that legitimating base. Sociologist Max Weber's conceptual base will be utilized in this chapter to clarify nursing's authority.

Weber described three basic legitimating models for the construct of authority. Legal authority: "the legitimacy of the powerholder to give commands rests upon rules that are rationally established by enactment, by agreement, or by imposition."[12] Charismatic authority: the legitimacy of the powerholder rests on "an *extraordinary* quality of a person, regardless of whether this quality is actual, alleged, or presumed."[13] This personal model has been exemplified by "the prophet with the mark of grace" and has its basis in theological experience.[14] Traditional authority: the legitimacy of the powerholder rests on "the psychic attitude-set for the habitual workday and . . . the belief in the everyday routine as an inviolable norm of conduct."[15] This basis of authority rests on the principle that certain authority has always existed or is alleged or presumed to have always existed. The most important example of this model is patriarchy.

Medicine possesses an authority aura that encompasses all three types described while nursing's authority base is less broad. Nursing is recognized as having legal and traditional authority to a point. It has charismatic figures such as Nightingale, Dock, Wald, and Sanger, but its overall aura is not charismatic in the same life-saving dramatic sense that characterizes the aura of medical practice.[16]

When nursing asserts its claim to practice independently, it invites comparisons to medicine in the extent of its authority to act in that manner.

In that comparison, in the context of the previously described types, nursing is seen as having less authority. But that is a false issue. In comparison to medicine, every profession is seen as having less authority. The important question is does nursing have appropriate, or enough, authority to act independently? Returning to the definition of primary care as the exemplar, the foci of the primary care role are: (1) Providing integrated, accessible health care services by clinicians who are accountable for addressing a large majority of health care needs; (2) developing a sustained partnership with patients; and (3) practicing in the context of family and community. Further, the core attributes emphasize the social as well as the biomedical sciences; the personal relationship between clinician and patient; the opportunity for health promotion and disease-prevention activities; and the integration of mental and physical health care concerns.

These health care goals have been part of modern nursing since its Nightingalean origins. At the 1893 World's Fair, Nightingale's paper described "Sick Nursing and Health Nursing . . . nursing proper is . . . to help the patient suffering from disease to live—just as health nursing is to keep or put the constitution of the healthy child or human being in such a state as to have no disease."[17] At the same meeting, Isabel Hampton (later Robb) spoke of the nurse's " . . . three-fold interest in her work—an intellectual interest in the case, a (much higher) hearty interest in the patient, a technical (practical) interest in the patient's care and cure."[18] Nightingale's focus on environmental conditions, and their manipulation to ensure health, was responsible for her legendary work as a reformer of England's sanitation laws. Nurses were defined as the "ministers of health" who were " . . . not only caring for the sick, but teaching the principles of cleanliness, ventilation and economy" to their patients and the families of patients.[19] The district nurse of nineteenth-century England and the visiting nurse of early twentieth-century America clearly provided primary care services to underserved populations.

The same objectives characterize certain current standards of university nursing education and state Nurse Practice Acts.[20] Therefore, the stated foci of the primary care role have historical, educational, and legal bases in nursing practice, and are substantiated as within the context of nursing's legal and traditional authority. The question therefore must lie not with the existence of nursing authority, but with people's recognition of that authority.

A distinction is drawn between de facto and de jure authority: " . . . de jure presumes a set of rules, according to which certain persons are

competent (authorized) to do certain things, but not to do other things . . . "
De facto exists when one person "*recognizes* [sic] another as *entitled* [sic]
to command him."[21]

Medicine and nursing each possess elements of both de jure and de
facto authority. What matters to the practice of each is the extent to which
each is accepted by the public, and the point at which the practice of
each profession is seen as reaching the limits of its authority. Yet within
each profession there are recognized differences in preparation and responsibility. In medicine, a general practice physician is not expected to perform
neurosurgery, but would be considered competent to suture a small wound.
Similarly, nurses prepared in advanced practice must perform within the
limits of their specific preparation. However, as nurses have expanded
their expertise into independent practice roles such as primary care, they
are seen as pushing the perimeter between the professions of medicine
and nursing. Sociologist William Goode described this process as "encroachment," whereby "a new occupation claims the right to solve a
problem which formerly was solved by another." The claim of the new
group is interpreted by the old as an "accusation of incompetence, and
the outraged counteraccusation is, of course, 'encroachment'."[22]

Nursing's reasons for its advanced practice role should be effective in
defusing the "accusative" nature of its claim to the role. Historically
certain nurses always practiced in an independent way. Currently, nursing
is identifying independent practice more clearly because:

1. Nurses now know better how to assert their rights and claims, and
that they must make overt those practices that have been covert for
generations of the "doctor-nurse game";

2. Nurses have the expertise to meet the expanding health care needs
of society in the face of the declining numbers, not incompetence, of
primary care physicians;

3. Advanced practice presents nursing's qualified members with practice roles more consistent with their rigorous preparation; and,

4. By providing a competitive delivery system, nurses can help contain
health care costs.[23]

The restrictions on nursing's de facto authority derive largely from the
public's lack of knowledge about what nursing is, what nurses know,
do, and are capable of doing. Nurses' expanded educational preparation,
research-based knowledge, and highly sophisticated practice roles are not
generally recognized by the public, which still thinks of nurses at the

bedside, in the maternal, handmaiden role of a much simpler era. Development of expert authority occurs interactionally between the group needing a service and the group providing that service. Medicine has been the group recognized as interacting with society's need for primary care. Nursing's role has been seen as necessary, but secondary and dependent, not primary and independent. When educated nurses present themselves as a group prepared to fill the gap in many health care services, cognitive dissonance may occur for those who have older views of nursing. A new group without nursing's historical image might have less difficulty occupying the role, but would lack the trust that nurses have earned from the public. The term "Nurse Practitioner" has been successful because it manages to keep the nurse-trust component, yet simultaneously presents a new image for nurses in new roles.

Accountability Operationalizes Authority

One way to demonstrate authority is through accountability.[24] One cannot, in justice, be held answerable for behaviors, actions, and events over which one has no authority or control or for which one is not responsible.[25] Therefore, nursing is documenting its perceived areas of accountability through conceptual model development, nursing diagnosis taxonomies, quality assurance programs, nursing audits, outcome-criteria measurement, and legal and legislative action.

These measures demonstrate some areas for which nurses accept accountability. They do not answer other questions regarding accountability, such as to whom is one accountable? When reference groups or issues conflict, to which is one accountable under which circumstances? Must one act counter to one's own beliefs in order to be accountable to the goals of a particular group for whom one is the service provider? Nurses often find themselves in conflicts of accountability. Philosopher Newton described a model[26] which helps to clarify conflictive accountability, based on one's definition of health care:

1. If health care is a commodity for sale in a hospital, the patient is a customer, the physician is an outside contractor, and the nurse is a straight employee with responsibility only to the institution and the immediate supervisor.

2. If health care is a series of medical cases, then the physician is the scientist in charge of the project, the hospital is a laboratory, and the

nurse is a subproject participant or assistant who is accountable only to the physician.

3. If health care is seen as the patient's right to relief from pain or illness, and the hospital is the locus of that relief, then the nurse is accountable to the patient.

4. If health care is defined as promoting the general well-being of persons, " . . . the patient, nurse and physician form a triad around the single enterprise of furthering that patient's well-being. The patient is the focus, but is expected to . . . aid in his own recovery; the physician is primarily a scientist, oriented towards the body's disease; and the nurse is a completely different professional, holistically oriented toward the patient's entire growth as a person. . . . In this conception, the nurse cannot be accountable for her performance as a nurse to any but her own professional standards."[27]

Professional standards begin with the personal ethical system of the nurse as an individual. These standards develop in individuals in the context of their membership in many groups within the larger society. People are socialized culturally in various ways and carry those customs with them into other parts of their lives. Most nurses are women. Their gender carries cultural demands for behavior that affects later, professional behavior. Many nurses are members of groups that have varying experiences of child rearing, socioeconomics, national origin, education, and other factors that influence nurses before they begin the professional socialization process. In addition, each nurse is a member of a social system that legally defines accepted behavior of the nurse as a citizen, resident, and nurse.

The nature of accountability, therefore, is multileveled and complex, and nursing's heterogeneity increases that complexity. The professional level on which nurses hold themselves accountable is most often the last area of accountability to develop. It may carry a weaker personal commitment when in competition with earlier developed senses of accountability; for example, women's accountability as mothers versus women's accountability as nurses. In addition, the nature of accountability changes over time in relationship to changes in the person, the society, and the profession. Conflicts among and between various aspects of accountability have been part of nursing since its earliest years, as this 1893 statement demonstrates: "The superintendent of a training school is under a three-fold obligation: first to the hospital in which she works; secondly, to the patients who are entrusted to her care; and thirdly, to the women for whose education as nurses she is responsible."[28]

Although Hampton encouraged all persons connected with the hospital to "resolve that they will work harmoniously together . . . [that] justice may be done to all"[29] the historical evidence is abundant that accountability to the hospital dominated the others. As times and gender customs changed, nurses became more aware of these conflicts, and more skillful in asserting their professional rights, but the conflicts still exist. A major source of such conflict is the difficulty in quantifying what nursing is, what nurses do, in a system that relies heavily on unquantifiable data. The essence of nursing, caring, defies measurement, and quality of life does not take precedence when survival is at stake, which is often the case in acute-care settings. In primary care delivery circumstances, immediate survival threats are not as likely, which allows "care" and "quality of life" foci to take precedence. Additionally, as the population ages, and increased numbers of people need supportive care for chronic illnesses and acquired immune deficiency syndrome (AIDS), nurses' broader range of practice is in greater demand.

Nursing as a Discipline

The major argument put forth by those who oppose independent nursing practice is that because nursing uses knowledge from the physical, behavioral, social, and biomedical sciences, it cannot be regarded as having its own unique, independent, and professional knowledge base. There is no question that nursing integrates knowledge from other disciplines. But nursing adds its own special knowledge to the gestalt and applies it in practice in a manner uniquely its own. Nurses do for people what people would do for themselves if they had the will, the strength, and the knowledge that the nurse has.[30] Therefore, as a discipline, nursing's recurrent themes and concerns focus on the wholeness of people, the interaction between people and their environments, and nursing's management of people and environment to enhance comfort, quality of life, and general well-being during, and beyond, illness.[31] In fact, and with irony, it must be noted that this very breadth of background is what makes nursing so clearly suited to the primary health care provider role. It is breadth not possessed by any other health care delivery group because, though medicine also integrates knowledge from other fields, the fields are more limited to the biochemical and physical sciences. While the advances created in medicine by the merger of these sciences cannot be denied, concurrent losses of the supportive, caring functions of healing have been significant.[32] Though increased technology has also affected nursing, the supportive, caring functions of healing have continued to be central to nursing. Since doctoral preparation has become more common for nurses, and a corps of nurses have been prepared as researchers, rigorous scientific inquiry into the knowledge that validates nursing action has reduced the relevance and legitimacy of arguments raised against independent nursing practice. Such arguments must rest then, not on concerns for science or authoritative knowledge, but on power considerations.

POWER, PROFESSIONALISM, AND PROTEST

A social process, professionalization, evolved at the end of the 19th century to organize knowledge growing out of the scientific and industrial revolutions. Developed as a means to protect uninformed citizens required to place their trust in expert authorities, professions also controlled valued information and access to that information, which gave them power. Able to choose and socialize new members, the professions became regulating bodies for their practices and reference groups to which society addressed questions regarding certain areas of knowledge. New professions continue to emerge as technological advances create expert knowledge for those activities formerly conducted according to intuition or trial and error experience. Sociologists describe a continuum of professionalism on which occupations fall by virtue of the extent of their unique knowledge base and orientation to service, the two primary characteristics of professions.[33]

As the "new" professions emerge, the balance of power is disrupted, particularly between groups that share clients, content, and workplaces. The territorial protectiveness stimulated in the older group against the "encroachment" of the newer has already been discussed. A new profession that provides a service to a client once "belonging to" another will derive income from and gain influence over that service and client. This economic and political threat is, not surprisingly, fought by the older group. The incongruity of this reaction by medicine to nursing as nurses enter advanced practice roles is that firstly, most of what is changing is the overtness of nurses' activities, and secondly, the physician practitioners being "threatened" are not those actually delivering the disputed service.

Physicians are not providing primary care services in needy areas or in adequate numbers, but they do not want nurses to provide them either— probably because nursing is an increasingly independent profession, with a growing militancy in its refusal to be dominated by medicine. As a consequence, medicine created, and is supporting with its vast resources, physician-extender or assistant groups through which it seeks to maintain control over services and clients without having to use its legitimate professional resources to do so. This creates another irony. Groups clearly labelled "assistant" are given legitimacy to act independently, even to write orders that nurses are pressured to follow.

Such obvious maneuvering led this author toward class and gender interpretations of these power plays. The majority of medical practitioners are more affluent than their nursing counterparts, and constitute an elite, dominant group in American society. Medicine uses its greater economic and influential resources to lobby among legislators and consumers to protect its position. Because medicine has been predominantly male (even with recent increases in women members), while nursing is 94% female, sexism, as a societal and historical feature, contributes its piece to what is, in essence, a political struggle. Related to sexism, but derivative of a technologically worshipful society as well, are the different values attached to the two major functions of health care—care and cure. The nurturant, supportive behaviors fundamental to caring and nursing do not engage the American interest or value to the degree that the more instrumental technology of curing and medicine do. Nursing has only begun to address these concerns in the last two decades, as patient outcomes research documents nursing's significant positive impact on patient care. The complex social history of nursing suggests why nurses avoided political issues and activities in prior eras.

Modern nursing emerged as an acceptable occupational alternative for women during the Victorian era. As single women, living away from their homes, earning salaries, and ministering to the bodily needs and functions of both sexes, usually strangers, 19th-century nurses were social revolutionaries who dared not breach too many more conventions for fear of losing their basic footholds. The notions of self-effacement, deference, long hours of toil for small wages, and political reticence, that began as sociopolitical necessities to establish the work in one generation, became habits and customs associated with, ascribed to, and even required of nursing in subsequent generations. With the rise of science and the professionalization of knowledge at the turn of the twentieth century, certain individuals and groups of nurses became more politically aware and active. But the majority of nurses avoided issues like sexism, power, and politics.

Nursing, as a group, did not support the Nineteenth Amendment (for women's suffrage) in the early 1900s, equivocated on civil rights in the 1960s, and only belatedly and halfheartedly backed the Equal Rights Amendment of the 1980s. With large numbers that could have exerted noticeable pressure, nurses' reticent behavior cost them the reciprocal support of other disadvantaged groups—women, African Americans, even health care consumers—who might have added strength to nursing's political muscle. Isolated in a "Little world of our own,"[34] and often divided amongst themselves as to the best action for nursing to take, nurses have not been effective advocates for their own positions.

Some women's groups, attempting to confront sexism in the professions, recommend increasing the number of the underrepresented sex, such as increasing the number of men in nursing and women in medicine. But that is a false solution and has not worked in nursing. The underlying societal attitudes must change, such as increasing the acceptance of assertiveness in nurses and nurturance in physicians. Otherwise, the stereotypes of relative dominance, achievement, independence, and power remain intact, and the traditionally male, White, elite choices continue to be the more desirable ones.

The negative effect of stereotype-driven choices is confounding in multiple ways. Some women who enter the more prestigious field of medicine experience conflict and disillusionment when they discover that physicians do not spend as much time with patients as they had expected. These young physicians' desire to be supportive and nuturant with their clients may be discouraged and even denigrated. Simultaneously, nursing suffers the loss to its ranks of well-qualified and highly motivated women. Similarly, men who enter the more nurturing field of nursing may experience social and economic discrimination. Society is the ultimate loser in this chain of events.

CONCLUSIONS AND SUGGESTED ACTIONS

The question central to this chapter has been: Do nurses have the appropriate authority to act as independent health care providers in advanced practice roles? The evidence presented supports the conclusion that they do—within the context of specific educational preparation for identified nurses, legal sanction by legislative bodies, and public recognition by consumers of health services. Through these three mechanisms, advanced practice roles for nurses will be accepted and legitimated.

Organized nursing must establish specific educational programs and certification criteria on a national basis. A baccalaureate degree to enter general professional nursing practice and master's degree preparation for advanced practice are essential. Nursing must discriminate among its own levels of preparation and practice in ways that are standard in all other disciplines.

The extension of legislative activity that would permit such practice by properly prepared nurses is necessary in all states. This may require legal encounters that challenge existing restrictions, and it will require some nurses to allow other nurses to earn a different status. Having asserted that some of its members possess specific, independent expertise, nurses cannot then insist that all nurses gain the benefit of that expertise or hide behind physicians when the outcomes of their actions are challenged. In fact, if nurses seek the status of professionals, they must insist on being held accountable for the appropriateness of their actions on all levels.

Public education that alerts consumers to health issues is a well-used and demonstrably successful strategy in the United States. Similar strategies can be employed to familiarize the public with the importance of nursing in health care, and the specific nursing services available from advanced practice nurses. Probably the most important of all actions, nurses must demonstrate the positive health care outcomes and economic value of their practice, and then publicize those results for legislators and consumers through sophisticated use of the media.

Nurses' contributions must be acknowledged, even promoted. How many people know that Margaret Sanger was a nurse; that two previous presidents of Planned Parenthood were nurses (Fay Wattleton and Pam Maraldo); that the Henry Street Settlement was started by a nurse (Lillian Wald); that the first president of the National Organization for Women was a nurse (Wilma S. Heide); that nurses run major government agencies and control 100-million-dollar budgets in medical centers? We have allowed the nurse who moves out of the dependent model to cease being identified as a nurse, thereby tacitly reinforcing the public image we now deplore.

A major concern expressed by some nurses who oppose advanced practice by nurses is fear of loss of the nursing role and identity. This is a worthy consideration. Some nurses who enter advanced practice roles become seduced by the power of the stethoscope to provide instant status. This misuse of the model must not be permitted. A stethoscope is only a tool, as is a pencil or a thermometer, with which competent data can be collected, and the nursing process activated. The best reason for nurses to provide primary care is because they are nurses. Nursing's focus on people; its blend of medical, behavioral, and social science expertise; and its commitment to caring, teaching, counseling, and supporting patients are the characteristics of nursing that make nurses so uniquely qualified to provide advanced practice and primary health care services to the public.

NOTES

1. Julie Fairman and Joan Lynaugh, *Controlling Crises: A History of the American Critical Care Movement, 1940–1990.* (Philadelphia: University of Pennsylvania Press, In Press). See also, Julie Fairman, "Watchful Vigilance: Nursing Care Technology and the Development of ICUs, 1950–1965," *Nursing Research* (1992) 1:52–60. See also Joan Lynaugh and Julie Fairman, "New Nurse, New Spaces: A Preview of the AACN History Study," *American Journal of Critical Care* (1 July 1992), 19–24.

2. Florence Nightingale defined nursing as putting the patient in the best position for nature to act upon him. Virginia Henderson defined nursing as doing for patients those things they would do for themselves if they had the knowledge, the will, and the strength to do them. Dorothea Orem defined nursing as substituting the nurses' actions for the patients' own actions to different degrees, partially, wholly, or supportive/educative. The ANA defines nursing as the diagnosis and treatment of human responses to actual or potential health problems.

3. American Nurses Credentialing Center, *Advanced Practice Certification Catalog* (Washington, DC: Author, 1997). See also, Data Sheets prepared for the American Nurses Association by Winifred Carson, Practice Counsel, entitled: States which recognize clinical nurse specialists in advanced practice; Joint regulation of advanced nursing practice; States recognizing advanced practice under independent acts, separate titles of advanced practice acts, or regulations; and, Continuing education requirements for prescriptive authority.

As of this writing (May 1997), various state nurse practice acts reflect public confusion about nursing's roles. Some states (Alaska and Oregon) give full plenary and prescriptive powers to advanced practice nurses. Other states (New York) limit advanced practice nurses' autonomy, by requiring "nurse practitioner(s)" to practice "in collaboration with a licensed physician . . . " (NYS, Article 139, Section 6902 (3a), 1995). Other states do not differentiate between basic and advanced practice nurses. Regarding American Nurses' Association (ANA) certification for advanced practice, as of the end of 1997, applicants for advanced practice certification examinations will be required to have a minimum of master's level preparation. However, because some nurse practitioners were "grandfathered" into the designation prior to that requirement, all advanced practice nurses may not necessarily be master's prepared until well into the 21st century.

4.   As an example, in New York State, nurse practitioners are authorized with the following language: "The practice of registered professional nursing by a nurse practitioner, certified under section six thousand nine hundred ten of this article, may include the diagnosis of illness and physical conditions and the performance of therapeutic and corrective measures within a specialty area of practice, in collaboration with a licensed physician qualified to collaborate in the specialty involved, provided such services are performed in accordance with a written practice agreement and written practice protocols" (NYS Education Act, Article 139, Section 6902, Paragraph 3a, 1995). Paragraph 3b authorizes nurse practitioners' prescriptive powers with similar restraints.

5.   Institute of Medicine, *Primary Care: America's Health in a New Era.* Molla S. Donaldson, Karl D. Yordy, Kathleen N. Lohr, and Neal A. Vanselow, eds. (Washington, D.C.: National Academy Press, 1996), p. 1.

6.   Institute of Medicine, op. cit., p. 3.

7.   Dagobert D. Runes, *The Dictionary of Philosophy.* (New York: Philosophical Library, 1942), p. 29, defines autonomy as, "Freedom consisting in self-determination and independence of all external constraint."

8.   cf., 3.

9.   Runes, op. cit., p. 112.

10.   Stanley I. Benn, "Authority" in *The Encyclopedia of Philosophy*, Paul Edwards (ed.), vol. 1 (New York: Macmillan and the Free Press, 1967), p. 215 defines authority as meaning: "to possess expert knowledge and therefore the right to be listened to." Further, "The authority of the expert . . . involves the notion of someone qualified to speak. It presumes

standards by which expertise is expressed and recognized, for example, degrees of professional reputation."

11.   Ibid., pp. 215–217 briefly reports on this literature.

12.   *From Max Weber: Essays in Sociology*, translated, edited, and with an introduction by H. H. Gerth and C. Wright Mill (New York: Oxford University Press, 1946, 1958), p. 294.

13.   Ibid., p. 295.

14.   Benn, op. cit., p. 216.

15.   *From Max Weber*, op. cit., p. 296.

16.   Magali Sarfatti Larson, *The Rise of Professionalism: A Sociological Analysis* (Berkley: University of California Press, 1977). On p. 31, the author asserts that occupational tasks that are more familiar in ordinary life have less magical allure, and therefore seem to require less expertise.

17.   Florence Nightingale, "Sick Nursing and Health Nursing." In *Hospitals, Dispensaries, and Nursing*, Papers and Discussions of the International Congress of Charities, Correction, and Philanthropy, Section III, June 12th to 17th, 1893, Under the Auspices of the World's Congress Auxiliary of the World's Columbian Exposition, John S. Billings, M.D. and Henry M. Hurd, M.D. (eds.) (Baltimore: The Johns Hopkins Press, 1894), p. 446.

18.   Isabel A. Hampton, "Educational Standards for Nurses." In Isabel Hampton and Others, *Nursing of the Sick 1893*, Nursing Papers and Discussions taken from the Billings and Hurd book and published under the sponsorship of the National League for Nursing Education (New York: McGraw-Hill, 1949), p. 3.

19.   Irene Sutcliffe, "The History of American Training Schools." In Billings and Hurd, op. cit., p. 511.

20.   For an example of educational standards, see the University of Pennsylvania School of Nursing Statement of Philosophy and Conceptual Framework: "The faculty believes that nursing is an autonomous profession whose focus is caring for persons throughout the life cycle during periods of wellness and illness" and specifies nursing actions in health maintenance, promotion, and teaching as well as therapeutic interventions. For an example of Nurse Practice Arts, see New York's Education Law, Article 139, Section 6902, 1995: "The practice of the profession of nursing as a registered professional nurse is defined as diagnosing and treating human responses to actual or potential health problems through such services as casefinding, health teaching, health counseling, and provision

of case supportive to or restorative of life and well-being, and executing medical regimens prescribed by a licensed physician, dentist or other licensed health care provider legally authorized under this title and in accordance with the commissioner's regulations. A nursing regimen shall be consistent with and shall not vary any existing medical regimen."

21. Benn, op. cit., p. 215.

22. William J. Goode, "Encroachment, Charlatanism, and Emerging Professions: Psychology, Sociology and Medicine," *American Sociological Review 25* (1960), p. 902.

23. Claire M. Fagin, "Nursing's Value Proves Itself," *The American Journal of Nursing* 90 (October 1990), pp. 17–30. See also, Claire M. Fagin, "Nursing as an Alternative to High-Cost Health Care," *The American Journal of Nursing*, 82 (January 1982), pp. 56–60. See also, Monical Wolcott Choi, "Nurses as Co-Providers of Primary Health Care," *Nursing Outlook*, 29 (September, 1981), p. 521.

24. Leon M. Lessinger in *Accountability in Education.* Leon M. Lessinger and Ralph W. Tyler (eds.) (Worthington, Ohio: Chas A. Jones, 1971, p. 29, defined accountability as meaning, "that an agent . . . [agrees] to perform a service [and] will be held answerable for performing according to agreed-upon terms, within an established time period, and with a stipulated use of resources and performance standards."

25. Richard D. Adkins, "Responsibility and Authority Must Match in Nursing Management," *Hospitals*, 53:3 (February 1, 1979), pp. 69–71.

26. Lisa H. Newton, "To Whom is the Nurse Accountable? A Philosophical Perspective," *Connecticut Medicine Supplement*, 43 (October 1979), pp. 7–9. Presented with permission of the author and the journal.

27. Ibid., p. 9.

28. Isabel Adams Hampton (later Robb), *Nursing: Its Principles and Practice for Hospital and Private Use* (Philadelphia, Sanders, 1893), p. 17.

29. Ibid.

30. Virginia Henderson's definition of nursing appears in many sources. In this case, I have paraphrased from her quote in: Ellen D. Baer, *Editor's Notes, Nursing in America: A History of Social Reform* (New York: The National League for Nursing, 1990), p. 1.

31. Sue K. Donaldson and Dorothy M. Crowley, "The Discipline of Nursing," *Nursing Outlook*, 26 (February 1978), p. 113: "A discipline . . . is characterized by a unique perspective, a distinct way of viewing all phenomenon, which ultimately defines the limits and nature of its inquiry."

32.   Edmund D. Pellegrino, "The Sociocultural Impact of Twentieth Century Therapeutics." In *The Therapeutic Revolution: Essays in the Social History of American Medicine*, Morris J. Vogel and Charles E. Rosenberg (eds.) (Philadelphia: University of Pennsylvania Press, 1979), p. 262 identifies the "discontent with medicine today" as related to conflict between ideals of technology and "the Aesculapian Physician."

33.   Everett C. Hughes, "Professions," *Daedalus*, 92 (1963): William J. Goode, "Community within a Community: The Professions," *American Sociological Review*, 22 (April, 1957), pp. 194–200. William J. Goode, "Encroachment, Charlatanism and the Emerging Professions: Psychology, Sociology and Medicine," op. cit.

34.   Nancy Tomes, "Little World of Our Own:" The Pennsylvania Hospital Training School for Nurses, 1895–1907, *Journal of the History of Medicine and Allied Sciences*, 33 (1978), pp. 507–530.

PART II

THE PRACTICE ARENA

Chapter 4

PRIMARY CARE AS AN ACADEMIC DISCIPLINE*

Claire M. Fagin

THE chapter "Primary Care as an Academic Discipline" was originally written at the invitation of the Robert Wood Johnson Foundation for presentation at their first annual symposium highlighting the work of the Nurse Fellows in Primary Care. The title was theirs; the content was mine. I doubt that I would have articulated the view of early ownership of the primary care arena by nursing had I not had the opportunity to reflect on the meaning of the term, "academic discipline," offered me by the Foundation.

It was clear then, and it is even clearer now, that nurses are educated to be superb primary care practitioners; and that the skills and knowledge required to practice are imparted in most of our undergraduate programs and continued in many of our graduate programs. Research over the past two decades has proven that nurses can deliver cost-effective primary care that can substitute for physician care in many situations. Further,

---

*"Primary Care as an Academic Discipline" has been slightly adapted by Claire Fagin from her chapter in *Primary Care: A Contemporary Nursing Perspective*, edited by Ingebourg Mauksch (1981). Originally published by Grune & Stratton, Inc. Reprinted and adapted by permission of the publisher, W. B. Saunders Company.

nurses can provide new and important services in long-term care and nursing homes.

Other chapters in this book bring the numerical record about nurse practitioners up to date. This is not my aim in this chapter. Rather, I would like to put several other issues into a contemporary perspective. First, the issue of direct reimbursement of nurse practitioners: Over the last eight years two nursing groups have been extremely successful, on a national level, in achieving direct reimbursement for their work. They are Certified Nurse-Midwives (CNMs) and Certified Registered Nurse Anesthetists (CRNAs). More recently, advanced practice nurses have gained Medicare reimbursement subject to state nurse nurse practice acts (Capitol Update, 1998). Moreover, there are some examples where nurses have successfully developed independent practices targeted at middle- and upper-middle-class patients (Brenna, 1997). During the 1980s two large-scale reviews of the literature provided evidence that nurses' styles of delivering care are extremely suited to people's needs in terms of health teaching and counseling, follow-up care, use of fewer diagnostic tests, and per-episode costs (Office of Technology Assessment, 1986). Yet, in recent national deliberations, the issue of recommending reimbursement did not benefit much from these exhaustive data. Now new questions are raised as obstacles to reimbursement. They have to do with "sameness" of work and "human capital" theory. However, human capital theory as it applies to nurses seems, at this time, to be referring exclusively to opportunity costs of training. Opportunity costs are not seen as appropriate for differences in physicians' backgrounds.

It is interesting to note that studies have found that there are diminishing returns to education as it increases: the return on elementary school educa- tion is highest and the return on graduate studies (excluding professional degrees) lowest (PPRC, unpublished manuscript). The issues of sameness linked with the human capital theory have not been used in establishing relative costs for different specialties among physicians, clinical psycholo- gists, or limited-license practitioners.

It is hard to believe that these are the true issues which stand in the way of recommending direct reimbursement for nurse practitioners. Nurses are the only group which has produced a large volume of convincing evidence about care and outcomes of care. Yet others have achieved the goal of direct reimbursement without such evidence. Clearly, this issue is still a problem.

Over the past decade we *have* brought primary care into the mainstream of nursing education. Preparation begins at the undergraduate level, and most nurses and others accept the view that graduate education is needed to prepare the nurse practitioner for generalist and specialized roles. A critical mass of faculty *have* been prepared for teaching primary care content. Thanks to the Robert Wood Johnson Foundation, the Kellogg Foundation, the Commonwealth Foundation, and the Joshua Macy Foundation (and others), cadres of nurses have been prepared for both practice and teaching.

While organized medicine's stance in relation to collaboration has not changed significantly (Mangan, 1997), there are thousands of examples of collaborative relationships between nurses and physicians which attest to major change at the patient care level.

There are numerous clinical settings appropriate for learning, and educational resources to provide diverse knowledge and skills in teaching, administration, and research have increased exponentially.

Medical school output has increased markedly and, health systems cost, as predicted, have increased dramatically. Both service-based and provider-based reimbursement are being examined and new payment structures (such as the Resource Based Relative Value Scale) are in place for implementation.

Much work has been done on the relative merits of community care versus institutionalization. Home care alternatives and hospice are part of many third-party reimbursement programs, and home care is found to be cost-effective as compared with hospital care. Early discharge programs for low birth-weight infants have led to replications with other populations, and nursing has led the way in these studies.

Nurses are increasingly involved with the "power brokers" of the health care and political systems. They do sit on boards, and in various national, state, regional, and local policy making bodies.

A new issue that emerged in the 1990s with regard to primary care and the nurse practitioner is the extent to which the international community has come to recognize nursing's importance in meeting health care needs. Work on the international scene in primary care is increasing in importance. United States' nursing's maturity is permitting it to help meet needs of nurses and health care systems in other countries through collaborative efforts. The World Health Organization is cognizant of nursing's role in primary care, and has named several United States universities and programs in other countries as the WHO Collaborating Center. We can expect, therefore, the international activities of nurse practitioners, and CNMs in particular, to increase.

There is more to be done. Given the extraordinary changes that have occurred in the past decade, by the year 2000 it was projected that nursing should be at the point of achievement in primary care where nurses are making the maximum contribution to our nation's health and the international community. This goal has only been partially achieved.

I said in 1978 that primary care is the generic discipline of nursing. Nothing has happened to alter that view. What has occurred is that nursing has proven that statement, in its practice, education, and research, and no longer needs to make a claim as rhetoric that is readily seen in reality.

Primary care as an academic discipline is a vital issue for nursing and medicine to address for reasons that have to do with intellectual considerations as well as political, social, and financial factors. More striking, however, is its importance as an issue that permits the conceptual-ization of a distinction between the medical and nursing models. It should be said at the start that the author does not believe that primary care is a separate academic discipline within nursing nor, based on nursing's history and meaning, should it be. Primary care is an integral part of nursing in all its aspects and is the academic discipline of nursing. How the author arrived at this conclusion will be discussed by defining the term, explaining why the issue is of interest to nursing and medicine, taking a brief look at the major relevant historical events of this century, and examining nursing's past and present focus (Fagin, 1992; Fagin & Goodwin, 1972). It is the author's belief that nursing and medicine have followed, and must follow, separate routes to the goal of primary care.

DISCIPLINES, DEPARTMENTS, AND DISTINCTIONS

To begin from a common understanding of this subject, it is necessary to define what is meant by "academic discipline." There are some cases where semantics *do* make a difference, and this is one of them, since reactions to the concept of primary care as an academic discipline will be based in no small part on the terminology involved. The *Oxford Dictionary* (1990) defines the word *discipline* as "a branch of instruction or education; a department or learning of knowledge"; note that there are two parts of that definition.

Donaldson and Crowley (1978) state:

Disciplines have evolved as a consequence of a distinct perspective and syntax, which determine what phenomena or abstractions are of interest, in what context such phenomena are to be viewed, what questions are to be raised, what methods of study are to be used, and what canons of evidence and proof are to be required. (p. 114)

Looking at primary care within the strict context of such a definition as well as that part of the *Oxford Dictionary*'s definition that describes "a branch of instruction or education," the idea of primary care as an academic discipline seems reasonable. While its body of knowledge has not been fully developed through theoretical exposition and research, the parameters of this area, which lend themselves to investigation and theory development, have been identified by many writers. Thus, the potential for establishing a theoretical body of knowledge that relates to primary care exists, even if all of it is not available to us at the present time.

It is the second part of the definition that is a subject for debate, that is, a discipline as a "department of learning or knowledge." In centers of learning, such as universities, there appears to be a natural transition between the identification of a particular area as a discipline and the belief that this discipline should be administratively or organizationally set up as a department. It is in this area that questions must be raised as to the appropriateness of such an organizational structure for nursing. What are the factors that create, defeat, or blur the formation of content area as an academic discipline, or, in this case, as an academic department? Are these factors dominated by the intellectual force of argument that pertains to the body of knowledge of the area, or are there other considerations?

An examination of the ways in which the basic sciences are organized in medical schools may clarify the point. In examining the organization in medical education of basic science disciplines—"a branch of instruction or education"—one can note from school-to-school the blurring discipline lines and the lack of commonality of discipline groupings; that is, the lack of "a department of learning or knowledge." In one school, for instance, the department of anatomy was closed, and two new divisions were created in cell biology and cytology. In other schools, biochemistry may be linked with biophysics, while still other institutions maintain all of the above as separate departments (Kohler, 1982).

Why this lack of consistency? Various factors, such as competition for support, prestige, historical circumstances, perception of problems, and social interactions, contribute to this situation. So does the power of external forces, such as financial support from governmental and private agencies, that influence the growth and specific labeling of academic disciplines. Medical schools across the country have responded to these pressures by increasing their emphasis on education for primary care. It is interesting to note that a 1977 survey by the American Association of Medical Colleges of trends in primary care education that indicated no well-defined locus for coordinating efforts for institution-wide, primary care training through specific departmental structures (Giacoloni & Hudson, 1977) still applies. While no corresponding survey for nursing has been published, the author is confident that a similar conclusion can be made.

Thus, while both medicine and nursing have shown increasing interest in the primary care area, in most cases the educational component has been discretely organized without a corresponding organization within the school's administrative structure.

HISTORICAL PERSPECTIVE

Two distinct lines of development can be identified as we examine the professional health care scene of this century: These are the public health movement and the growth of medical school–hospital establishments, each of these developments with its own priorities. By the late 19th century, the public health movement had achieved major success in controlling the spread of infection and in microbiology; early in the twentieth century, it began to focus on the health needs of the poor and on maternal-child health care. During this same period, there were a large number of poor-quality programs that prepared physicians. Flexner's report of 1910 had a profound influence on the nature and the content of medical schools and medial education. It set the stage for the stress on research, which later became the *sine qua non* of the quality medical school. The rising professionalism of the medical group coincided with the growing power of the hospital group and the decline in the power of the physicians involved in the public health movement.

In medicine, the forerunner of today's primary care practitioner was, of course, the general practitioner. Although declining somewhat in numbers in the first 30 years of the post-Flexner period, the almost total extinction of the general practitioner on the American scene occurred after World War II. At that time, a variety of developments pushed the health care system into an emphasis on, and power in, the secondary and tertiary care areas. The extraordinary research and technological progress during the decade of the 1940s had stunning implications for the civilian population. There was a growing assumption that the development of technology would be tantamount to the control of illness. With the increase in technology and research, there was a subsequent need for physicians and others to become more specialized as they advanced their knowledge base. It became impossible to know all things about all medical problems.

The financing of hospital growth through the Hill-Burton Act, as well as governmental funding for medical education, grew geometrically during this period. Furthermore, the availability of governmental and private funds for research reinforced the already growing development of an academic role model for the physician-scientist. These faculty members, as the status members of the medical school group, had an enormous influence on medical students who were choosing their future paths. Although attempts were made to revise, or at least maintain, a general practice group within the American Medical Association, these attempts met with little success for reasons such as "the absence of an academic base, the undefined role of the general practitioner in relation to the specialist, and the difference in working conditions and status between the general practitioner and the specialist" (Lewy, 1977, p. 875).

In addition, the decades from the 1940s through the 1960s were dominated by the health care providers, with few consumer efforts to stop the extraordinary growth of the medical and hospital establishment. In later years, however, some countertrends had begun to develop—among them, the notion of the Great Society, with health care seen as a right rather than a privilege. The funding of health centers connected with the Office of Economic Opportunity exposed gaps in health care; in particular, the gap that we now label the "primary care needs of the people."

These developments reawakened medicine's interest in general practice, and during the 1960s several study commissions set out to explore its future. One such commission indicated that the graduate education of physicians for what had now acquired the label of "family practice" required training equivalent to that of other specialties, as well as the development of a specialty board to give certifying examinations (Millis, 1966). The evolution of a new specialty, it was stated,

requires a definition of content, the development of graduate training programs, the development of specialty departments in medical school, the establishment of standards, the development of mechanisms to insure adherence to the standards, the development of continuing education programs to insure maintenance of these standards, and the generation of research programs to further the unique body of knowledge. (Lewy, 1977, p. 875)

It was not easy to establish such programs, especially in universities, since there was no uniform process whereby the content of fields such as community medicine and behavioral science could be taught; besides, there was a severe shortage of qualified teachers in family medicine.

NURSING'S DEVELOPMENT

Nursing's role in the two lines of development in the health scene was in sharp contrast to that of medicine's. Whereas medicine developed its power base in the medical school-hospital establishment, nursing became dominated by the same establishment.

Although the early hospital schools of the late nineteenth century were based on Nightingale's model and were educational apprenticeships, by the twentieth century many became what Joanne Ashley calls "successful instruments for women's oppression" (Ashley, 1977, p. 23). As early as 1915, some leaders in nursing were recommending that nursing education be placed on a professional basis within colleges and universities. Yet well into the 1930s and 1940s, hospitals simply increased the number of students in their schools to meet the demands for immediate nursing service.

There were great leaders in nursing during the first half of the century, but most of these leaders developed outside of the hospital group and were closely aligned with the public health movement, a movement that in nursing is the historical antecedent of the primary care movement. (Lillian Wald, the founder of the Henry Street Settlement and the Visiting Nurse Service, coined the terms *public health nurse* and *public health nursing*).

The first national nursing organization to have a headquarters and a paid staff was the National Organization for Public Health Nursing (NOPHN), which was established in 1912. For quite some time the public health movement in nursing continued to grow in power, to set standards for practice, and to influence education by requiring certain content, including degrees, as a condition of employment. In the 1940s, the National League of Nursing Education established its own accrediting committee, which was a very significant development in the history of nursing. It ended the proliferation of hospital schools and the student labor method of instruction. The influence of NOPHN was very strong on the League, and many leaders in nursing education prior to 1950 came out of the public health movement.

Now, however, it is sometimes difficult to distinguish public health nurses from other university-educated nurses, since more and more nurses work outside hospital walls and nursing education increasingly focuses on a holistic view of patient, family, and community. This can be said despite the fact that nursing followed the medical path in becoming specialized from the late 1940s through the 1960s. The knowledge explosion identified areas of need, such as psychiatric nursing, and federal dollars accelerated specialization in graduate education. But as their knowledge increased, nurses frequently rejected the kind of technical tasks that the new technology created, resulting in an expressed need for different kinds of manpower; that is, technical aides who were task- and physician-oriented. One unfortunate result of this movement was the increase in fragmentation in hospital care; another was the separation of most nursing leaders from the hospital establishment. The absence of bridges from university to nursing service militated against nursing leaders having an influence on improving hospital nursing care. Fortunately, there are new moves in this direction at the present time.

By the late 1960s in fact, nursing programs had become both generalized and comprehensive, stressing public health and mental health. Had it not been for political factors and nursing's resistance to recognizing its own natural progression, nursing could have conceivably moved very rapidly to prepare for primary health care. The few imaginative nurses who carved out roles in primary care were frequently scorned by their nursing colleagues, and other groups jumped in to fill the primary care gap.

Despite this backing and filling within the profession, or perhaps because of it, pressures from governmental and other groups for a rapid method of preparing nurses to meet primary care needs resulted in the establishment of 100 or more "nurse practitioner" programs of varied duration, content, and type. In this situation, as in others before, nursing's adaptation to meet immediate needs solved some problems but created or perpetuated others. Over the past 40 years, close to 100,000 nurse practitioners have been prepared. Considerable funding has also gone into the preparation of other health care practitioners and into increasing the number and capability of medical schools. By now, nursing has changed its stance and sees itself as playing a major role in the delivery of primary health care.

AN ACADEMIC DISCIPLINE

We are now at a point where there is interest in primary care on the part of both medicine and nursing. But are the two fields comparable in this area? The author has tried to build a case that indicates they are not comparable, and the analysis will now be completed.

It has become increasingly apparent that for real change to occur, primary care must be seen as a respected part of the academic scene. The mass of data attesting to influence of high-status medical faculty members on the socialization of medical students supports the importance of establishing the academic centrality of primary care. In both nursing and medical education, in other words, primary care must be part of the mainstream, with its content and faculty constituting an integral part of the academic power structure.

In medical education, however, two problems have been cited as greatly inhibiting the growth and development of comprehensive care. These are the assumptions that comprehensive care (particularly primary care) is solely a function of an attitudinal set and a kind of noblesse oblige that does not require specific training, and "the lack of professionalization of the role required to provide comprehensive care in the role of primary physician" (Magraw, 1971, p. 475).

The Nature of Nursing

Despite the admission by medical educators of the need to educate for primary care, the attitude in most medical centers toward this field, as Alpert pointed out, continues to be condescending (Alpert & Charnay, 1974; Mullan, Rivo, & Politzer, 1993). The subspecialist researchers-clinicians are the tail that wags the dog in every academic clinical department, be it medicine, pediatrics, or obstetrics-gynecology. A conceptual move to equalize the status between the primary care physician and the specialist in internal medicine or pediatrics would have been hard enough. However, since specialists are now considered generalists in their respective fields and subspecialists are the predominant powers, the gaps between the subspecialist group and the primary care group is a wide one indeed. It is therefore understandable that pressures exist resisting the establishment of primary care as an academic discipline within the medical profession. If indeed the establishment of an academic discipline, and subsequently a specific department, to coordinate and develop the primary care component of the curriculum would help to solve some of the political and status issues faced by those devoting themselves to primary care, then this may well be a legitimate goal—for medicine, that is.

For nursing, however—given its natural evolution from a concept of public health and a concern for the individual, family, and community to a concept of primary care—the situation is different, and the solution to the problem is almost the antithesis of the medical solution. In nursing, primary care is *not* low man on the totem pole. Rather, it is increasingly recognized as the integral core of nursing rather than one of its specialties.

The nature of nursing as described by Nightingale and others following her has been too close to the nature of primary care as described by almost everyone else for primary care to be conceptualized as a discrete academic discipline within nursing. Primary care is so multifaceted that it cannot be considered the domain of any one group to cover all its aspects. If we were forced to define it as a separate entity, we would be robbing its strength from all other groups in nursing. What is the body of knowledge for primary care, for instance, that can be differentiated from the body of knowledge needed in nursing in general?

As the author sees it then, primary care as an academic discipline within nursing is *the* generic discipline. The care of people with actual or potential health problems and the manipulation of the environment to contribute to optimal health have long been seen as the generic base of nursing practice. Nursing is defined as including the promotion and maintenance of health, prevention of illness, care of persons during these acute phases of illness, and rehabilitation or restoration of health. Are these not also the functions of primary care described by most writers, and do they not also suggest the knowledge required? As Donaldson and Crowley (1978) stated,

> Nursing has traditionally valued humanitarian service. But in addition, the self-respect and self-determination of clients are to be preserved. The goal of nursing service is to foster self-caring behavior that leads to individual health and well-being. These values and goals, which are intrinsic to professional practice, have shaped the value orientation of the discipline. (p. 114)

Primary care has now moved into the mainstream of nursing education. The stopgap measures to prepare nurses as primary practitioners have accomplished short-term goals. There is a need to continue to incorporate teachers and leaders in educational and service programs who have a strong commitment to primary care. To do this, six ingredients must be present in the educational organization: (1) an understanding of the nature and scope of primary care nursing; (2) faculty prepared for teaching in primary care; (3) philosophical commitment to primary care at the core of nursing; (4) appropriate clinical settings with arrangements for faculty practice; (5) collaborative relationships with physicians that provide for consultation and referral; and (6) educational resources that provide diverse knowledge and skills in teaching, administration, and research. Where nursing faculty in primary care seek and do not find these ingredients, they must help to create them.

Although primary care as the appropriate focus of nursing is a comfortable concept, the issue becomes more complex, more difficult, when one considers the complementary and interdependent roles required to flesh out these concepts. The question of the collaborative or collegial relationships of the two major disciplines involved in primary care—medicine and nursing—is important to study. The lack of coordinated planning in primary care has exacerbated this issue and the situation can be expected to worsen unless it is directly addressed. In the guidelines for federal support of primary care residency programs, the definition of primary care content is virtually identical to every nursing description of this area since 1968. Clearly we must come together in education and practice to utilize the best each discipline has to offer, to build on our individual strengths, and subsequently to collaborate in meeting health needs in a rational manner.

Nurses and physicians involved in primary care have not been sufficiently involved in health-policy making bodies or in health planning. Health planning is an area studied by many. However, in one sentence we can say that, as in 1978 (Falkson, 1978), we have neither a national health policy nor a national health plan or planning process. Proof of this can be found in the way primary, secondary, and tertiary care have developed in the past three decades. If a collaborative and rational plan had been drawn up at the start, it is not inconceivable that a different system of health care could have been organized that would have had a major impact on the nature of primary care services as well as total-systems costs.

If the readings from the professional and public marketplaces are correct, there are three periods of change that relate to identifying and meeting primary care needs. The first one occurred in the 1960s with the recognition of the need, and there were a variety of solutions planned and implemented. All were without any connection to one another or any consideration of their long-term effects in areas such as the nurse practitioner movement, the development of the physician's assistant, and the infusion of money into medical schools to expand enrollment with a heavy focus on preparation for primary care. The view commonly held during this period was that a nurse practitioner was to be prepared as a physician-extender, therefore, a physician substitute.

The findings from the next period of change in the mid-1980s have been very clear in indicating that the nurse practitioner in primary care can indeed fill the vast majority of needs commonly identified. Phase two is replete with studies of the effectiveness of nonphysician providers. Toward the end of this period, we begin to see data that indicate that long-term systems costs can be affected by extended community care versus hospitalization; that is, by assisting people to remain in their own homes through supportive services. On the other hand, the question of how long-term systems costs are affected by the relative expense of educating various practitioners has not been explored.

We are now into phase three, which is the realization that physician-students already in the pipeline have caused an oversupply of specialist physicians in this country. What effect this will have on primary care, on the development of the nursing profession, or on health systems costs is unknown. Several hypotheses can be posed. One is that since physicians control the marketplace, we can expect health systems cost to increase with the abundance of physicians. Economists are examining this issue closely, and various alternatives are being posed, such as service-based (Enthoven, 1993) rather than provider-based reimbursement. Further, the extraordinary expansions of the for-profit sector with a concomitant growth in the percentage of salaried physicians may create other employment possibilities for nurse practitioners. At any rate, in phase three it would be well to examine the issues posed by the already known variables and to pressure for participation in policy development.

It is the author's belief that the expansion of the primary care effort in medicine was in error. This, incidentally, is not because of my lack of good memories about the general practitioners of the late 1930s, but, rather, because the author's consumer bias is to get her money's worth for dollars spent. If indeed, at a maximum of six years, a nurse practitioner can deliver at least as good, or in some cases better, primary care than a physician—whose educational costs are much higher, length of education close to double, and income expectations correspondingly greater—then serious questions must be raised about this kind of luxurious approach (Fagin, 1990). Further, many of the reasons for medical specialization *were cogent*. The explosion of knowledge did indeed make it impossible to know all things about all medical problems. Given the nature of medical education and training, it is entirely appropriate to expect this kind of expertise from the physician. However, this kind of thinking is clearly ex post facto and will have little affect on the present situation. This is all the more reason for a clear identification of where we stand in nursing and medicine in relation to primary care and for a more open and complete discussion of these issues in interdisciplinary and consumer groups.

CONCLUSIONS

Primary care within nursing is the academic discipline of nursing. It cannot be separated from the other components of nursing into a new part but *is* the dominating force of the discipline itself. An examination of the contents and concepts of primary care clarifies the difference between the professions of nursing and medicine in relation to primary care. Primary care is not a focus of nursing; it is nursing's major focus.

REFERENCES AND BIBLIOGRAPHY

Alpert, J., & Charney, E. (1974). *The education of physicians for primary care.* Rockville, MD: U.S. Public Health Service.

Ashley, J. (1977). *Hospitals, paternalism, and the role of the nurse.* New York: Teachers College Press.

Brenna, A. (1997, Oct. 6). Is there a nurse in the House? *New York Magazine.*

Capitol Update. (1998, Jan. 30). Medicare reimbursement: An update. 16 (01), 2. Washington: ANA Publication.

Donaldson, S. K., & Crowley, D. (1978). The discipline of nursing. *Nursing Outlook, 26,* 113–120.

Enthoven, A. C. (1993). A history and principles of managed competition. *Health Affairs, 12,* 24–48.

Fagin, C. M. (1977) Nature and scope of nursing practice in meeting primary health care needs. In American Nurses Association (Ed.), *Primary care by nursing: Sphere of responsibility and accountability* (pp. 35–51). Kansas City: American Nurses Association.

Fagin, C. M. (1990). Nursing's value proves itself. *American Journal of Nursing, 90*, 10, 17–30.

Fagin, C. M. (1992). Collaboration between nurses and physicians: No longer a choice. *Nursing and Health Care, 6*, 25–31.

Fagin, C. M., & Goodwin, B. (1972). Baccalaureate preparation for primary care. *Nursing Outlook, 20*, 240–244.

Falkson, J. L. (1978). We need a national health policy. *Journal of Health, Politics, Policy, and Law, 4*, 311.

Flexner, A. (1910). *Medical Education in the United States and Canada. A report to the Carnegie Foundation for the Advancement of Teaching.* New York: Carnegie Foundation.

Giacolini, J. J., & Hudson, J. I. (1977). Primary care education trends in U. S. medical schools And teaching hospitals. *Journal of Medical Education, 52*, 971–981.

Kohler, R. (1982). *From medical chemistry to biochemistry: The makings of biomedical discipline.* Cambridge, England and New York: Cambridge University Press.

Lewy, R. M. (1977). The emergence of the family practitioner: An historical analysis of a new specialty. *Journal of Medical Education, 52*, 875–881.

Magraw, R. M. (1971). Implications for medical education. *American Journal of Diseases of Children, 122*, 475–486.

Mangan, K. S. (1997). Some medical and nursing schools declare a truce and start to work together. *The Chronicle of Higher Education 44*(17), A10–12.

Millis, J. S. (1966). *The graduate education of physicians.* Report of the Citizens Commission on Graduate Medical Education. Chicago: American Medical Association.

Mullan, F., Rivo, M. C., & Politzer, R. M. (1993). Doctors' dollars and determination: Making physician work-force policy. *Health Affairs, 12*, 138–151.

Office of Technology Assessment. (1986). *Physicians' assistants and certified nurse midwives: A policy analysis.* Washington, DC: U.S. Government Printing Office.

Oxford English Dictionary, Eighth Edition. (1990). R. E. Allen (Ed.). New York: Oxford University Press.

Physician Payment Review Commission (PPRC). Report on nonphysician practitioners. Washington, DC (unpublished).

Schweitzer, S. O., & Record, J. C. (1977). Third-party payments for new health professionals: An alternative to fractional reimbursement in outpatient care. *Public Health Report, 92*, 236–242.

Chapter 5

THE INTERACTION BETWEEN NURSE PRACTITIONER AND PATIENT: A PARADIGM FOR CARE

Joan E. Lynaugh

"PRACTITIONER . . . one qualified by practice . . . a person who practices a profession, art, etc.," so says Webster's New World Dictionary (1994). Not much help to be found there when trying to understand species 'practitioner' of genus 'nurse,' that is, nurse practitioner. Perhaps that is because a practitioner is best defined by being and doing.

This chapter examines the idea of the nurse practitioner, using a three-part analysis. First, and most important, is the encounter between nurse and patient. What counts in clinical nursing is what happens there. Second, using the care encounter as a framework, the emergence and relevance of nurse practitioners will be discussed. Finally, there will be a look at the nurse practitioner in his or her practice environment with its various conflicts and opportunities.

THE ENCOUNTER

Nursing cannot be practiced at a distance; access to patients and time alone with patients are both essential. Thus, the simplest and most fundamental aspect of the nurse practitioner movement of the late 1960s and the 1970s was the establishment of nursing access to some of the time people devote to the care of their health. Time alone with patients in an office with the door closed was a novelty for nurses in ambulatory care even though their colleagues, community health nurses, always enjoyed the intimate care opportunity inherent in their visits in their patients' homes. For patients visiting medical offices or clinics, nursing care was bound to remain peripheral until the care-giving system was reorganized to allow ambulatory patients and their nurses planned time together. What goes on in these encounters?

An ideal encounter between nurse and patient includes at least six elements:

1. The nurse discovers and addresses the need or problem that the patient hoped to solve by seeking health care.
2. The patient tells or shows the nurse what the nurse needs to know in order to understand the patient's situation.
3. The nurse tells or shows the patient what the patient needs to know in order to understand the situation as the nurse understands it.
4. A course of action is agreed upon by both parties.
5. The course of action is implemented and evaluated.
6. An effective transfer of trust and recognition occurs between both parties.

Let me illustrate with an example. Mrs. H refers herself to see a nurse practicing in an ambulatory setting. Mrs. H chose the nurse because her husband was already receiving care from that particular nurse and she found the setting and practitioner familiar and relatively convenient. Mrs. H wants a general checkup because she is feeling fatigued and because "there is a lot of heart disease in my family." She is 50 years old and feels that now is the time she should be getting some advice about her health.

The nurse practitioner and Mrs. H sit down together to review Mrs. H's current health, her past health, her family's health, her social situation, and her reasons for seeking professional care at this time. Then the nurse examines Mrs. H following the traditional head-to-toe format of the physical examination. Next, if appropriate, Mrs. H and the nurse agree to some routine laboratory studies, such as urinalysis, blood work, or an electrocardiogram.

What is happening here is part of an implicit, occasionally explicit, negotiation between two persons; one person seeks help and the other offers it. These people are strangers to one another, yet they will try to establish a trusting relationship. As in all negotiations, each party comes to the meeting with an agenda. In a care encounter such as this, the agendas of the nurse and patient will probably be only partially revealed to each other. Of the two, perhaps the nurse's agenda is the more predictable.

Since the nurse is interested in the life processes, well-being, and optimal functioning of human beings, he or she will try to compare Mrs. H's situation with some concept of health that seems clinically useful. Does Mrs. H present any overt or covert indications of dysfunction or disease? Is she in any other kind of trouble? Does she need to know something about herself or her situation that she does not know that will help her stay well or improve her health? As the nurse analyzes Mrs. H's situation, he or she will make a number of diagnoses (one could substitute the word hypotheses), any one of which could fall not only under the rubric of nursing but also of medicine, social work, education, or psychology.

Mrs. H, on the other hand, may well have a more subtle agenda. Since she sought this encounter with a health care professional, she might safely be assumed to be concerned about some aspect of her health. But whether her objectives for this encounter match those of the nurse is something they both must discover. Personal and social problems beyond the nurse's scope of practice may well be presented by patients. It is crucial that Mrs. H reveal her real reason for seeking care early in the encounter.

An ideal encounter demands excellent verbal and nonverbal communication, a shared goal of decision making, and some degree of trust on both sides. Since the nurse is the professional in the situation, he or she has the burden of creating this ideal encounter.

From the nurse's viewpoint, the most critical first step is to find out, in detail, the story of the problem that concerns the patient. Two obstacles invariably crop up here. One is the requirement of listening and withholding judgment. The second is the problem of taking time. Listening carefully will help both participants identify the real reason that prompted the patient's visit. Problems that interest the nurse can be dealt with, of course, but unless they are urgent they should not take precedence over those that brought the patient to the nurse. Once the story is fully shared, an appropriate examination should be done. The physical examination provides useful clinical information often vital to a correct hypothesis; importantly, in the context of this discussion, the examination reduces the distance between two persons, allows the nurse to touch the patient, and validates for the patient the nurse's competence, concern, and interest.

Only when the patient's story is fully heard and the examination is finished should the nurse explain his or her findings and beliefs about the patient's problem. The discussion should include the nurse's perspective on what is and what is not occurring.

For the patient to understand the situation as the nurse understands it, the patient needs to know what significant hypotheses the nurse has rejected. It is entirely likely that the patient has already thought of the most frightening possibilities and will need clarification before proceeding to the next step, which is the negotiation of a plan of care. The plan may be simple or complex; it may involve more data collection, treatment, referral, or education. Whatever it is, it must be consistent with the objectives of both parties in the encounter.

Numerous constraints limit achievement of the ideal nurse-patient encounter. One major limitation is the knowledge gap between the two parties. The nurse has a conceptual grasp of biophysical and psychological knowledge shared by few lay persons. Some people who seek care lack the ability to absorb new information and apply it to themselves. On the other hand, the patient's social and cultural knowledge may be entirely beyond the experience of the nurse, but crucial to problem identification and the plan of care. Finally, no transfer of knowledge between two persons is absolutely complete, forcing both participants to operate on incomplete data.

There are social and attitudinal constraints as well. Some people, perhaps those of lower income, different language group, or minority status, may feel intimidated by the nurse, the care setting, or the whole situation. If patients feel powerless, it is substantially harder for them to participate effectively in any negotiation. Sometimes patients and professionals assume that the professional knows best what the problem is, what the patient fears, and so on. This yearning for caretaking omnipotence is likely to be ungratified. Unrealistic and unmet expectations will lead to unhappiness on both sides. Shared responsibility in decision making requires shared power. Often the nurse must deliberately insist that the patient accept decision-making power to create more parity in the relationship.

In most primary health care situations, both nurse and patient deal with uncertainty and ambiguity, since clear-cut, correct answers are rare. Mutual participation in care planning is crucial to long-term treatment success.

Still, people seeking care have a right to expect an informed and clear opinion. It is an abrogation of responsibility to abandon a patient to his or her own uninformed judgment. The nurse is required to share knowledge, to teach, to persuade, and to "assist [others] in the performance of those activities . . . that [they] would perform unaided if [they] had the necessary strength, will or knowledge" (Henderson, 1969, p. 4).

What is at stake in a care-giving encounter is the right of the person to his or her personal liberty—a natural and inalienable right in Western culture. The task of the nurse practitioner is to recognize this right while at the same time fulfilling the professional obligation to offer service and do no harm.

To place this task in perspective, both in its simplicity and its vast social obligation, we can review the two functions of what is now called primary health care. First, the primary health care practitioner constitutes the initial contact with the health care system. Second, the primary care practitioner helps patients retain a continuum of care, including maintenance of health, evaluation, and management of common health problems as well as referral to other health care professionals and agencies.

This is responsibility on a broad front indeed. Why should nurses fill this role? Are they competent to do so? This is a good place to turn to a discussion of the relevance of nurse practitioners in primary health care.

RELEVANCE AND CONTEXT

The kind of accessible, continuous, and generalized health care under discussion here was found to be lacking in the late 1960s and the early 1970s. The American public complained that health care was too specialized, too centralized, too impersonal, and too difficult to obtain. In those decades the concept that all Americans had a right to equal access to health care was widely shared and politically popular in the United States.

One of the earliest descriptions of an ideal national system came from David Rogers (1977), then president of the Robert Wood Johnson Foundation. Such a system (paraphrasing Rogers) must be (1) accessible to persons with ordinary medical problems; (2) capable of distinguishing potentially serious problems from innocent or self-limiting problems; (3) able to convey humanistic, scientifically informed support to its clients; (4) capable of continuity; (5) reasonably equitable; (6) able to reward its practitioners and attractive to new practitioners; (7) compatible with the heterogenous lives of Americans across the country; and (8) competitive for the nation's resources against other social demands. It was in the context of these ideas that nurse practitioners emerged.

In retrospect, Rogers' analysis was a very fair statement of the ideal system envisioned by health planners and professionals. It is less clear whether a national consensus on the need for such a system with all its component parts and social and financial ramifications will ever develop in the United States.

Over time our nation has come to agreement on certain social minimums. We now agree on the idea of minimum income for certain specified contingencies. We assume that some minimum level of education is needed for all children. More recently, we have agreed to the exercise of a number of controls to protect our environment. Furthermore, we will support public works, including roads, parks, fire protection, police, and specified public health services. But, as British social historian Brian Abel-Smith (1981) pointed out, it is far less clear that we, as a nation, will ever commit to some minimum level of personal health care for all. Questions of equity, reasonable and acceptable costs, and limitations on freedom of choice delay such a national consensus. Certain groups, such as the aged and the very poor, are eligible for financial assistance for personal health services, but we still seem quite far away from national support for the kind of primary care system so well described by Rogers more than twenty years ago.

Given the vagaries of American social consciousness as related to primary health care, what happened to the new variety of nurse—the practitioner? Oddly enough, though born in the primary health care movement of the 1970s—an only modestly successful social experiment—the nurse practitioner is doing well. Nurse practitioners practice much as the dreamers of 35 years ago hoped they would.

After their appearance on the scene in the late 1960s, nurse practitioners became strongly involved in ambulatory care (Sultz, Zielezny, Gentry, & Kinyon, 1980). A substantial majority practiced in inner-city and rural locations. Nurse practitioners do care for the poor; many of their patients are in the lowest income category. And, most master's level graduates of nurse practitioner programs work full-time, and their employers report that they improve the quality of care while extending primary care services to more patients. Nurse practitioners also help expand the primary care that is available to the aging, especially in home health care and in nursing homes (Aiken & Salmon, 1994; Mezey & Lynaugh, 1991; Naylor & Brooten, 1994).

I submit that the reason the nurse practitioner continues to do well is that there is an excellent fit between the basic interests of the discipline of nursing and the health requirements and desires of a majority of the American people. Elements central in nursing ideology include: (1) concern with life processes; (2) the well-being and optimal functioning, whether sick or well, of human beings; (3) understanding patterns of human behavior in critical life situations; and (4) understanding the processes by which positive changes in health are effected (Donaldson & Crowley, 1978). When the central ideas of nursing are examined together with the requirements generally believed crucial to a care system, it becomes obvious that the group in closest correspondence with the general health care needs of our people is the discipline of nursing (Lynaugh & Brush, 1996).

As British physician Thomas McKeown noted in his influential analysis of modern health care, modifications in care requirements brought about by improved living standards, an aging population, and contemporary therapeutics require reorganization of responsibilities among society's "health servants" (McKeown, 1976). McKeown reminded us that the determinants of health rest largely outside the health care system. Except for exacerbations of acute illness or injuries where physicians' skills are required, the majority of needed health services involve personal care of the sick, a phrase he used in its broadest sense. McKeown detailed his concept of personal care of the sick much as Virginia Henderson defined nursing (1966, p.15), i.e., to substitute for those things the person cannot do for himself. He concluded, as do many nurses now, that nurses should assume major responsibility for primary care services. Accumulated data reported by the Office of Technology Assessment (1986) verified nursing's success in meeting that obligation and achieving positive patient care outcomes.

The talented clinicians whose patient care skills stood up under scrutiny not usually visited upon health professionals gained their abilities through rigorous educational programs and extensive clinical experience. To become a competent, sensitive primary caregiver requires a combination of commitment, effort, and opportunity.

Though virtually all nurse practitioners come to preparatory programs with substantial nursing skills derived from basic programs and practice experience, the sheer scope of work in primary care requires assessment and analytical abilities that require truly committed effort from the candidate. Patients appear at the door of the primary care nurse practitioner uncategorized and unscreened. Earlier in this essay, the two-way nature of the care encounter was emphasized; the nurse tries to pit knowledge and art against the problems confronted by the patient and to engage the patient in their solution. Acquiring that knowledge and art takes time and practice. Preparation for practice is now standardized at the master's level. This evolutionary process was driven by the imperative to assure competence. Schools of nursing found they must educate an expert clinician with a capacity for sophisticated clinical decision making and a repertoire of excellent assessment skills. Primary care education requires opportunities to participate in patient-nurse encounters. Nurse practitioner students need extensive clinical practice experience with quality preceptors. They need to see many different patients, to discuss care problems with teachers, and to learn the art of clinical decision making in the ambiguous world of primary care. As a basis for this practice opportunity, students need excellent courses in science, counseling, assessment, and clinical management. Perhaps most important, primary care practitioners need general knowledge of the world and its culture, history, and wonderfully varied inhabitants. As Donna Diers (1982) so aptly phrased it, "Nurses are invited into the inner spaces of other peoples' existence without even asking . . . " Nurses who practice as nurse practitioners in primary care receive such invitations fifteen or more times a day. To do it well is a career.

ENVIRONMENT FOR PRACTICE

Nurse practitioners work in outpatient clinics, health maintenance organizations, neighborhood health clinics, long-term care facilities, hospitals, occupational health, schools, home care, private practice, and public health agencies. A significant number practice in foreign countries, thereby participating in the worldwide goal of primary health care for all people.

Four major influences affect the practice environments of these practitioners: the needs of patients, time and money; physician relationships; and appreciation of their scope of practice. With the exception of private duty, nurses in the past rarely dealt directly with these issues because most were employees of relatively large bureaucratic organizations. In contrast, the current practice environment is influenced by serial one-on-

one relationships, direct trade of units of time for money, and broad and open-ended accountability to consumers. Now that the nurse practitioner is recognized as a significant provider of care, these environmental issues loom larger.

Trading time for money implies that professional time used to diagnose, advise, teach, or treat can be assigned a price. Nurses quickly learned that time is the unit by which they must measure productivity; they also discovered that to measure out exemplary nursing within a 20-minute visit is difficult, if not impossible. The key to reducing the dilemma is to apportion realistically the number and length of visits, taking into consideration the predictable care needs of one's patient population. Most importantly, a realistic price must be attached to care-giving time. It has often been said, for instance, that no one makes any money doing primary care. This holds true because primary care uses little technology; unfortunately, Americans have long been more willing to pay for x-rays than for advice. Nevertheless, nurses must be reimbursed adequately to maintain themselves and their share of the practice overhead or they will not survive professionally. Any care system must be able to reward its practitioners and attract new ones. This simple premise underlay the drive to obtain direct Medicare, Medicaid, and commercial insurance reimbursement for nurse practitioners. To the extent that this goal continues to be achieved, nurses will be able to fulfill their commitment to the public.

Important linkages between nurses and physicians span the century since nursing came on the American scene in the 1880s; they are characterized by a mix of interdisciplinary struggle and mutual support. This ambivalence persists among nurses and physicians practicing today. The evolution of the nurse practitioner concept in primary care was a direct result of innovation and cooperation between nurses and physicians—Ford and Silver, Lewis and Resnick, and Andrews and Yankauer are but a few examples of those pioneer teams. An interdisciplinary effort to integrate medical and nursing practice developed, inspired by a common goal of improving health care for Americans. The complementary functions of medicine and nursing were stressed in recognition of the fact that many patient needs in primary care settings fell well within the realm of nursing. When personal care, counseling, support, and educative interests of nurses were meshed with the diagnostic and therapeutic interests of physicians, it became clear that the majority of patients in primary care could be fully cared for by nurses most of the time. Within a relatively short time (between 1965 and 1975) worries about the competence of nurses and patient acceptance disappeared from the literature.

Other problems remain, however. There is clear competition between nurses and physicians in those instances where they cannot agree and organize to share patients. Physicians who aspire to support themselves by seeing the 80 percent of primary care patients that could by cared for by nurses will try to prevent nurses from practicing. An equitable adjustment in reimbursement practices to give nurses access to the third-party dollar puts this competition on a fair footing. It is crucial to resolve these conflicts because a truly effective primary care system rests on the availability of both excellent nursing care and excellent medical care to all the people. Nurses and physicians cannot neglect their social obligation to give care because of distractions stemming from territorial infighting. The blurred line between medical practice and nursing practice is always shifting, always being renegotiated. To really understand the phenomenon—nurse practitioner—it may be necessary to remind ourselves that all professionals exist at the bidding of the society that supports them. Nurse practitioners exist because they are needed to provide services to children, to the chronically ill, to the aged, and to the sick poor.

This chapter began with a definition of practitioner and developed around that species of nurse. The transitional form we have come to call nurse practitioner is not only assimilated but now dominant in advanced nursing practice. And the accountable, patient-centered, clinically focused attitude of the nurse practitioner influences curriculum and faculty values while conceptual stimulation and research opportunities strengthen and improve nursing practice.

In many senses, although the analogy is by no means perfect, the nurse practitioner movement is like the trained nurse movement of the 1880s or the visiting nurse movement at the turn of the century. When an opportunity appears, for example, in the form of public desire for hospital care, a social need to help the poor in their homes, or a demand for accessible health care, nurses respond. In the process, nursing and nurses change and so does the society they serve.

REFERENCES

Aiken, L., & Salmon, M. (1994). Health care workforce priorities: What nursing should do now. *Inquiry, 31,* 318–329.

Abel-Smith, B. (1981). Minimum adequate levels of personal health care: History and justification. In J. B. McKinley (Ed.), *Economics and healthcare* (pp. 509–523). Cambridge, MA: MIT Press.

Diers, D., & Molde, S. (1979). Some conceptual and methodological issues in nurse practitioner research. *Research Nursing Health, 2,* 73–84.

Diers, D. (1982). Between science and humanity—Nursing reclaims its role. *Yale Alumnae Magazine, 65,* 8.

Donaldson, S., & Crowley, D. (1978). The discipline of nursing. *Nursing Outlook, 26,* 112–118.

Henderson, V. (1966). *The nature of nursing.* New York: Macmillan.

Henderson, V. (1969). *Basic principles of nursing care.* Basil (Switzerland): S. Karger.

Lynaugh, J., & Brush, B. (1996). *American nursing: From hospitals to health systems.* Cambridge, MA and Oxford: Blackwell Publishers.

McKeown, T. (1976). *The role of medicine—Dream, mirage or nemesis?* London: Nuffield Provincial Hospital Trust.

Mezey, M., & Lynaugh, J. (1991). The Teaching nursing home program: A lesson in quality. *Geriatric Nursing, 10,* 76–77.

Naylor, M., & Brooten, D. (1994). Comprehensive discharge planning for hospitalized elderly: A randomized clinical trail. *Annals of Internal Medicine, 120,* 999–1006.

Office of Technology Assessment, (1986). *Nurse practitioners, physician's assistants and certified nurse-midwives: A policy analysis.* Washington, DC: U.S. Government Printing Office.

Rogers, D. (1977). The challenge of primary care. Doing better and feeling worse: Health in the United States. *Daedalus, 106,* 81–103.

Sultz, H., Zielezny, M., Gentry, J., & Kinyon, L. (1980). *Longitudinal study of nurse practitioners, phase III.* Washington, DC: U.S. Government Printing Office, pp. 26–35.

Webster's new world dictionary. (1994). New York: Simon and Schuster, p. 118.

Chapter **6**

THE ROLE OF A FAMILY NURSE PRACTITIONER IN AN URBAN FAMILY PRACTICE

Rachel Wilson

FROM the coal fields of Appalachia, to inner cities across the country, individuals and neighborhoods pressed for health care, employment, services, and equal rights. My decision to become a nurse and, later, a family nurse practitioner (FNP), was made in this environment three decades ago.

I lived in Southern Ohio among coal miners and their families who were organizing to win benefits for miners who had become disabled with Black Lung disease (pneumonoconiosis). I visited nurses who were both midwives and FNPs at the Frontier Nursing Service in Hyden, Kentucky. The midwives/FNPs traveled by jeep down mountain hollers in order to reach people and provide desperately needed health care. Their example of competent practice was inspiring.

Through loans and scholarships, I went to nursing school in Cleveland, Ohio. While in school, I volunteered at the Cleveland Free Clinic and worked with people from the community, nurses, and doctors to provide primary care largely to adolescents in inner-city Cleveland. I graduated from a BSN program in 1974, and for the next two decades worked as a nurse, close to home in Jersey City, Newark, and New York City. I worked in emergency care, intensive care, general medicine, public health, and high-risk labor and delivery. These health care environments provided an invaluable matrix of experience in preparation for family practice. In the emergency room, I often triaged patients, ordered diagnostic studies, supported the patient and family, and then discussed the diagnosis with a medical resident or attending physician who signed the chart. I longed to expand my nursing practice as a clinician. It was time to return to school.

Like so many nurse practitioner students, I struggled with site placements. My best experience was providing primary care in a high-school-based clinic in Jersey City. There, with the participation of young African-American women and an ob-gyn nurse practitioner, we created a culturally based pamphlet using desk-top publishing and researched its effect. It was the first time I had been involved in a nursing research project. Culturally based care was to become fundamental in defining my practice. My focus as an FNP enabled me to assess the adolescent developmentally and to provide consistent, comprehensive care, which included supporting a young person to work through feelings of anger, loss, or loneliness; providing services such as women's health exams, Pap smears, contraception, prevention and treatment of sexually transmitted diseases; episodic care for minor acute health problems; management of chronic illness such as asthma and sickle cell anemia; and work/school/sports physicals. The broad scope of family practice was an asset in this setting, since the high school student could see the FNP for a range of primary care services.

I was awarded a Master's in Family Primary Care in 1992 and worked in a women's health facility in an inner-city neighborhood in Jersey City. The multicultural environment of Jersey City provided the opportunity to offer primary care to women who grew up in this city, and to women from many different countries. For example, when immigration increased during the war in Somalia, my practice grew to include Somalian women who demonstrated symptoms of war trauma that were similar to those I saw among young women who grew up in the neighborhood of this clinic, who had survived child abuse or other violent domestic trauma. This work increased my interest in the health care needs of adult survivors of trauma and allowed me to experience different cultural meanings for health practices among women of Arabic, Latino, African, African-American, Native, and Eastern European cultures. I also taught in nurse practitioner programs and drew up case studies from my practice.

AN ILLUSTRATION OF FAMILY PRACTICE

My current practice is in New York City at the Sidney Hillman Family Practice (SHFP). SHFP was once the main provider of primary care for garment workers in the Amalgamated Clothing and Textile Workers Union (now UNITE). Today, the practice includes large numbers of garment workers and their families, as well as other unionized workers, and the unemployed. Most patients are insured by one of a number of different managed-care insurance plans, Medicaid, Medicare, or the Ryan White program. Some uninsured patients pay for services on a sliding scale depending on income. I see patients from different cultural backgrounds, including immigrants from Mexico, South America, and the Spanish- and English-speaking Caribbean who work in the local garment industry.

This practice provides care for approximately 26,000 patients annually. SHFP is part of the Institute for Urban Family Health (IUFH). IUFH was founded by a family practice physician and family nurse practitioner. The philosophy of IUFH is to provide interdisciplinary, family primary care to those who need it, and to provide multidisciplinary educational opportunities for students in health professions including nursing, medicine, public health, and social work. There are several IUFH clinics in New York City neighborhoods, housing projects, and homeless shelters and an inner-city birthing center is in development.

The practice of an FNP in family primary care involves care of babies and children, reproductive-age women, young men, and older persons. My scope of practice includes health promotion, care of the person with acute, episodic health needs, and care of the more stable, chronically ill person. On a typical day, I will see people with presenting needs that include arthritis, chronic stable diabetes, hypertension, asthma, anxiety, stress, headaches, and a range of women's health needs such as evaluation of a breast lump, hypermenorrhea, amenorrhea, PAP screening, and follow-up treatment for cervical dysplasia. I treat women and their partners who have sexually transmitted diseases. I see women for contraception, prenatal care, postpartal care, perimenopausal changes, and well-woman care during menopause. I see HIV-infected people, and people with AIDS. I see people with work-related musculoskeletal injuries as well as sports-related injuries. I provide care of the newborn, well-child care, and screen for early developmental delays such as delays in growth or speech. I treat common children's complaints such as otitis media, sore throats, and colds. From the perspective of family practice, I often am able to assess the child's growth in the context of family patterns. I have seen whole families as a unit and individually. On a typical day I see individuals, couples and families, lesbian, gay, and straight.

A significant clinical responsibility is identifying a patient's behavior as a manifestation of risk taking, including sexual risk, drug and/or alcohol use, and cigarette smoking, and discussing a plan of approach with the patient. My particular areas of interest are assessment and change of sexual risk patterns among sexually active people and risk patterns among adult survivors of trauma.

I work at SHFP with several family practice physicians. The practice is not limited to traditional western approaches to health care. Herbs, homeopathy, acupuncture, and other complementary modalities, such as therapeutic touch are available. Patients are able to purchase herbs at SHFP to treat common complaints, and may be referred to a nutritionist. These options attract a subset of patients who are interested solely in complementary care. Many patients have already used herbs to treat common complaints in their home cities of Lima, Mexico City, or Basel, for example.

DISTINGUISHING FNP PRACTICE FROM FAMILY MEDICINE

I view my practice as an expansion of nursing. Sometimes the practice distinctions between a family practice physician and an FNP are blurred, though often they are not. The family practice physicians in this practice are oriented toward health promotion and risk reduction, and are generally focused on the person, not the disease. The focus of nursing is person, environment, health, nursing (Fawcett, 1995). My practice perspective is influenced by the view that the person/environment is integral (Rogers, 1994). The person cannot be explained by looking separately at psycho-social-physical systems. The person is more than a sum of parts and is unitary with the environment, constantly changing, growing, and emerging. Mutual understanding of the patterns in the person's life is necessary for change (Barrett, 1988; Rogers, 1994). As an FNP, I rely on data from medicine, am influenced by psychoanalytic theories, and have a growing interest in the body of literature on posttraumatic stress. However, I make sense of the health needs of patients who see me, and of earlier experiences with patients, through the nursing framework outlined above. I believe that practicing within a nursing framework offers the patient an option to see a nurse practitioner, not a "physician extender" for primary care.

The distinction between MD and FNP may begin with the patient's first phone call to the practice. The appointments are made by patient service representatives (PSRs) who answer the calls. For example, patients will call and ask the PSR to recommend someone to help them with their presenting concern. After the PSR makes the appointment to see the FNP, the person may ask "what is an FNP?" The PSRs describe our role effectively and this has been very helpful in promoting FNP practice. About a year ago, the PSRs asked to learn more about the FNP role so that they could better explain it to patients. At one of the weekly staff meetings FNPs described the FNP educational preparation, philosophy of care, and scope of practice. There were many questions and a lively discussion. The IUFH employee newsletter also featured an interview with FNPs. This has helped to bring clarity.

I always introduce myself to new patients and state I am an FNP. However, I am still occasionally called doctor by patients (and even staff!). I think this happens because people think I would receive this as an expression of appreciation. Whenever I clarify that I am not a doctor, I try to see it as an opportunity to say "You have just been seen by an FNP." In all the time I have practiced as an FNP, I have had only two occasions when a new patient requested to see the physician instead of an FNP. On both occasions, I offered the patient the opportunity to see me and then if the person still wanted to, I would set up an appointment for the person to see a physician. On both occasions the patient declined the physician visit and continued to see me. The nursing staff have demonstrated support for the FNP role as an expansion of nursing, and some have set personal goals to become an FNP or midwife.

PRACTICE METHODOLOGY

My practice is characterized by establishing a therapeutic relationship during the first meeting. Through active listening, and usually over several visits, I look for themes and patterns. Mutual pattern manifestation appraisal and deliberative mutual patterning are methodologies (Barrett, 1988) I use in my practice. Pattern appraisal occurs in the context of the initial structured history. The presenting problem, past medical history, the woman's health history, sexual history, family history, allergies, habits and addictions, workplace, home and community environments, and review of systems, illuminate these patterns over time. The physical exam and diagnostics are usually confirmatory.

I usually see patients for follow-up visits for approximately 20 minutes. Some patients require more time and some less. I am allotted 30 minutes for new patients and for a woman's health exam, for example. The patient's current presenting concerns are rarely routine to me because of the diversity of health needs in family practice. Therefore, organization of history taking is extremely important. New FNPs may find solace in understanding that these skills develop with time. Experience is a requisite for expertise (Benner, 1984).

DIVERSITY OF ROLES

In addition to my practice, I conduct in service sessions with nurses using a case study model. The focus of the case studies is telephone triage of patient's presenting health concerns and triage of patients who walk in without an appointment. The outcome of these discussions is the ongoing development of critical thinking skills in this important area of nursing care. As an FNP I also precept nurse practitioner students. While there are contradictions inherent in providing health care and precepting under the tyranny of time, clinical teaching is a way to share these experiences and grow mutually. Interested in clinical research, I have returned to school to pursue a Ph.D. in nursing.

COLLABORATION

Identifying one's scope of practice is central to FNP practice and is constantly changing. The decisions concerning which patient health needs I will manage with the patient; which patient concerns require collaboration with a physician; which concerns I will regularly comanage with a physician; or which patient concerns are beyond my scope of practice and will be referred by me to a physician in the practice, or to a specialist are based on knowledgeable practice, on the practice agreement signed by myself and the collaborating physician, on the state laws regulating NP practice, and on the federal statutes that regulate health care. Nurse practitioner protocols in obstetrics, pediatrics, and adult care are kept on-site for consultation, and have been approved by the New York State Board of Nursing. There are also ongoing chart reviews with NPs and physicians. Scope of practice is also economically influenced by the reimbursement policies of the patient's insurance coverage or plan. NPs and midwives spend a great deal of time offering primary care services, such as exercise and stress reduction counseling, although these are still not covered by most insurance plans and are generally not reimbursed to the practice. The practice does not bill an NP visit, as these visits (to date) are not generally reimbursed by the commercial plans.

During a day of morning and afternoon sessions, if I see 16 to 20 patients I might collaborate with a physician on one or two of these patients' health concerns. This collaboration may take place informally by consulting one of the physicians during the clinical session, or formally by waiting for the weekly one-hour-long precepting session with a designated physician preceptor. With a more medically complex patient, a physician and I may decide to alternate visits. By alternating visits, I have the opportunity to review the patient's management, continue the plan of care, and explore new issues. I may alternate visits with a physician for patients who have multiple, unstable diagnoses, such as a patient with previous myocardial infarction with unstable angina and poorly controlled hypertension, a patient with poorly controlled diabetes with signs of renal compromise, and a patient with opportunistic infections with AIDS.

On the other hand, there are physicians who refer patients to me. Physician providers may refer patients with patterns that have persisted over time, such as women with a history of trauma and current risk factors, or patients with complex responses to managing their obesity, diabetes, or hypertension. This pattern of collaboration has worked well. It is based on mutual respect. Mutual respect is a prerequisite for collaborati' and is strengthened when it is both interpersonal and structur' the practice.

I do not have admitting privileges in the affiliated hosr' patient requires admission, he or she is admitted to far' affiliated hospital. The attending family practic' teaches in the family practice residency prog' patient, and the family practice team provides t

REFERRALS, CONSULTATIONS, AND INSURANCE COVERAGE

If a patient needs to be referred to a service such as physical therapy or to a specialist, I write out the referral and then it is processed in the practice, usually under the medical director's name. To reduce out-of-pocket expenses, unless the patient prefers otherwise, the referrals are made to specialists who are covered by the patient's managed care plan. When a patient needs diagnostics, such as an x-ray or ultrasound, these are also processed by the referral office under the medical director's name. I order blood tests and these are drawn at a laboratory on-site and sent out for analysis to a laboratory that is covered by the patient's insurance plan.

Since most insurance companies, to date, do not reimburse nurse practitioners' practice, patients will often ask me why another person's name has appeared on the x-ray request. They also ask why their insurance membership card carries a different provider's name. My challenge is to briefly describe the economic restrictions placed upon current NP practice, and to reassure the patients that they can continue to see me for health care, even though my name is not on their insurance cards.

THE CONTEXT OF CARE: PATIENT/COMMUNITY/ ENVIRONMENT

Much of our practice as primary care providers involves participating in changing harmful life style patterns such as smoking, a high-fat diet, lack of exercise, stress, sexual risk, drug and alcohol use. Changing these patterns are fundamental aspects of the care of patients with a personal or family history of diabetes, heart disease, stroke, cancer, addiction, and posttraumatic stress, for examples. These patterns, manifested by millions of people in this country, have social roots; yet the individual is usually the center of analysis in health care research, including nursing clinical research (Chopoorian, 1986). One's social role and economic situation have a far more profound influence on health behaviors than do interactions with the nurse or any health care provider (Butterfield, 1994; Chopoorian, 1986). By viewing the social context as integral with the person, patterns more readily emerge from what otherwise might appear as a maze of 'sconnected complaints.

The following examples are described to emphasize the environmental ʾxt of health and change. Garment workers who do needlepoint piece-work may present with injuries of overuse such as De Quervain's tenosynovitis. Those who spend long hours typing on a computer are prone to Carpal Tunnel Syndrome. Workers who lift heavy objects are prone to rotator cuff injuries to the shoulder joint. Chondromalacia Patellae occurs among runners. I often refer patients with overuse syndromes to physical therapy for pain management and to learn exercises, and the clinicians and the patient mutually assess progress in healing. Natural remedies such as rest, warmth, or cold are often very helpful. I prescribe medications when indicated. Patients learn how to care for and strengthen their susceptible joints against injury, but ever increasing demands for increased production are manifested in recurrent injuries to muscles and joints.

Osteoporosis risk increases among women who are postmenopausal who do not exercise. Following through with regular exercise is often very difficult for women who live in the inner city. Many of the women who see me work from dawn to dusk and then have child care responsibilities. Asking them to get up early to jog in the street sounds unreasonable to us both, so I no longer approach the discussion of exercise in this way. Often what is more feasible is for us to look at the woman's schedule, locating opportunities for exercise and conceptualizing this time as belonging to the woman, who might be able to get off a train or bus one or two stops earlier and briskly walk the additional distance. Many older women have been socialized not to exercise vigorously. Understanding woman's role in society and culture is a crucial departure point for discussing change from sedentary practices to a regular pattern of exercise. These would be examples of pattern appraisal and working toward deliberative mutual health patterning in the context of the person's environment.

Patients respond differently to suggestions of changing their health care practices. Regular exercise, nutrition, and medication (if needed) to facilitate glycemic control are important aspects of care for people with diabetes mellitus. One 65-year-old African-American garment worker who has always managed her own affairs manages diabetes with insulin, nutrition, and exercise and sees me as someone she consults when she feels it is needed.

An overweight, stressed male worker tries to defy his diabetes by eating high fat, simple sugars, rarely exercising, and smoking cigarettes. He comes to see me to confess to eating pizzas as a way to handle stress. Each visit has marked his renewed effort to change these practices. The person's visit is a component of change for him. For myself, the visit involves assessing where this patient is in relationship to change, and mutually searching for ways to perceive and manage stress differently. Another patient with poorly controlled diabetes held on to persistent patterns of missing appointments, eating fast foods, and missing medications. When he was ready to do so, he disclosed an underlying alcohol dependence and began participating in Alcoholics Anonymous. As his alcohol dependence changed, he experienced some of the feelings formerly dulled by the alcohol. His growing understanding of these feelings is changing his relationship with diabetes.

I have been working with a Mexicano patient with poorly controlled diabetes. After a few visits, I began to understand that I needed to cease being prescriptive concerning nutrition, exercise, and medication, and sit back for a relaxed visit with him, even when the time was abbreviated. Relaxing and discussing family, foods, and customs during subsequent visits laid the basis for a healing atmosphere. His glycemic control began to improve and I grew with new understanding. His view of my role was to approach health as a relaxed, informal process, and his view of his own role was to change within this environment.

Stress related to housing conditions, homelessness, unemployment, or overwork and exhaustion are common issues. When the patient adopts a self-blame approach, experience of stress may snowball. Appraising the event from the perspective of its social causes helps shift the person's perspective, free up feelings, and seek potential ways to change the underlying situation. This approach has helped with people who experience insomnia, muscle tension headaches, and gastritis, for example.

There are a subset of patients who repeatedly visit in crisis. One patient visits when he has potentially been sexually exposed to HIV and/or another sexually transmitted disease. I have treated him for urinary tract infection, prostatitis, and scabies, and have spent visits discussing the anxiety he experiences over possible HIV seroconversion. His relationships with men are short-lived, and he is usually the victim of abuse in his relationships. During one crisis, when he indicated he was ready, we looked at his earlier patterns and he drew a connection between the severe abuse he had experienced as a child by both parents, and the current risks. He saw these risks as representing enactments of earlier abuse. He has started psychotherapy and has continued to see me to discuss the events that trigger anxious feelings and to identify old patterns of responding by taking sexual risks. He has become interested in safer sexual expression, attends gay men's discussion groups, and is in a stable relationship.

CONSTRAINTS ON PRACTICE

Having a broad scope of practice is balanced by feeling as a "jack of all trades, and master of none." FNPs may work in a specialized practice, or focus on a broad area such as pediatrics, orthopedics, or women's health. Family practice, however, involves the breadth of primary care, and by the nature of the health needs presented by the people who see you, is a general practice. This concept is appreciated differently among FNPs; some enjoy the generality, others feel frustrated by it.

Referrals must be made judiciously and diagnostic tests kept to a minimum in order for the patient to be reimbursed. These pressures increase the importance of thorough assessment through history and physical exam. However, the combination of time and the need to see numbers of patients are ongoing pressures. I have come to understand that I best manage these pressures by focusing on the moment, giving each patient complete attention, blocking out the other thoughts, concerns, and demands outside my door. When patients present with a long list of health concerns, I encourage them to pick one or two of the most pressing concerns and reassure them that we will address the others in time. I do note these concerns in the chart for upcoming visits. The abbreviation of time accelerates the need for pattern recognition with each patient.

There is also the growing problem that patients' health insurance coverage is changing more often due to lay-offs or due to the company changing its insurance plan. This can be very unsettling for patients who, after establishing a relationship with a provider, have to seek a new provider who is covered under the new insurance plan.

NP control over decisions that will affect the FNP's own practice is structurally limited in an environment where economic demands pressure all of us; there are few NPs in the practice, and the practice bills the service under the physician's title. While nurse practitioners have made significant practice gains, not being reimbursed by insurance policies results in a nearly invisible, seemingly seen-and-not-heard, tucked-away practice. Explaining these restrictions to patients is a difficult, necessary responsibility. However, some insurance plans are beginning to reimburse under the NP's name, and there is growing organized resistance among national and state NP organizations to the traditional forces that oppose NP reimbursement. Linking these efforts to community efforts to organize against cutbacks in overall health care services would increase the strength of this movement. There are important opportunities for growth and activism.

I think future directions for NP practice will be in Centers of Nursing Care in the community; residences which house older people, day care centers, housing projects, schools and free-standing clinics in neighborhoods. These could be affiliated with nursing schools, and with local hospitals. Relationships with local providers of care would be strengthened from mutual referrals. The essential issue will be support for affordable health care as a priority.

REFERENCES

Barrett, E. A. M. (1988). Using Rogers' science of unitary human beings in nursing practice. *Nursing Science Quarterly, 1*(2), 50–51.

Benner, P. (1984). *From novice to expert: Excellence and power in clinical nursing practice.* Menlo Park: Addison-Wesley Publishing Company.

Butterfield, P. G. (1994). Thinking upstream: Nurturing a conceptual understanding of the societal context of health behavior. In P. L. Chinn (Ed.), *Exemplars in criticism: Challenge and controversy* (pp. 152–160). Gaithersburg, MD: Aspen.

Chopoorian, T. J. (1986). Reconceptualizing the environment. In P. Moccia (Ed.), *New approaches to theory development* (pp. 39–54). New York: National League for Nursing.

Fawcett, J. (1995). *Analysis and evaluation of conceptual models of nursing* (3rd ed.). Philadelphia: F. A. Davis Co.

Rogers, M. E. (1994). Nursing: A science of unitary man. In V. M. Malinski & E. A. M. Barrett (Eds.), *Martha E. Rogers: Her life and her work* (pp. 225–232). Philadelphia: F. A. Davis Co.

PEDIATRIC NURSE PRACTITIONER AND PEDIATRICIAN: COLLABORATIVE PRACTICE

Carol Boland and Susan Leib

W E write from the vantage point of a nurse practitioner and pediatrician who have worked together for 7 years in private practice in a community of 20,000 in Connecticut. The practice consists of three pediatricians, and one pediatric nurse practitioner (PNP); a second PNP joined the practice in late 1997. The practice is supported by 10 nurses and 15 administrative and secretarial staff. Patients in our practice are primarily White and middle class. Almost all patients have health insurance, approximately 40% from private pay and 60% through some form of managed care. While pediatric practice is primarily ambulatory, we see newborns and hospitalize children at a 350-bed community hospital.

Our joint reflections: Our definition of collaboration is a relationship of interdependence that requires recognition and respect for complementary roles. There are four components that are integral to successful collaboration.

1.   Mutual respect. What we mean by mutual respect is that the physician and nurse practitioner have respect for each other's individual skills
and for the unique contribution that each makes to the practice.

2.   Trust. Trust is important in terms of the nurse practitioner because
she needs to be able to trust that the physician will give thoughtful input
during consultation, listen to what the problem is, and treat it as if it were
his or her own. The physician needs to trust that the nurse practitioner
knows his or her own limits primarily in relationship to consulting or
referring to the physician as necessary.

3.   Shared accountability. Because this is a joint practice we are both
responsible for all the patients in the practice and are equally accountable
for them.

4.   Joint decision making. The key word here is joint in that if collaboration or consultation is needed, important decisions must be made
together.

Our practice originally consisted of two solo physician practitioners.
Carol joined the practice as the nurse practitioner prior to Susan coming
into the practice. So Carol's role was well established in the practice
before we started to practice together. From the beginning, the PNP was
introduced to the patients and families as a member of the practice, as
someone who could see patients independently and who was seen as an
asset to the practice rather than a secondary provider. We have found that
it is very important that the nurse practitioner be introduced into the
practice in this light.

Another important factor that sets this same tone is that the fee schedule
is the same for both nurse practitioners and physicians. When patients
comment about the fact that they are paying the same price to see a nurse
practitioner as a physician, they are told that the NP is providing essentially
the same services as a doctor and, therefore, the fee schedule is the same.
In addition, overhead is the same in the practice for the nurse practitioner
and the physician. The NP has a nurse who works with her. She has lab
technicians and she has secretaries who provide the same services to her
that they do for the physicians, and, therefore, the fee should be the same
for both the nurse practitioner and the physicians.

Presently in our practice, Carol, the NP, takes after-hour calls once a
week, as do the physicians. Due to her own personal choice Carol does
not take calls on weekends. There is physician back-up provided for the
NP, but this is also true for one of the older physicians who does not

want to admit patients to the hospital. So that is not different in our practice for a NP than for a physician.

Since 1991, Carol has seen newborns in the hospital. Carol was one of the first NPs to be given privileges at the hospital where we admit patients. We explain to parents that they may be seeing her on newborn visits in the hospital. We feel it is very helpful to present our model of the NP as on an equal footing with the physician during the early encounters the patient has with the practice.

We have discussed including the NP in administrative and partner issues. When Susan came into the practice, she assumed that she would be a partner at some point; Carol, on the other hand, did not have similar expectations. If a NP is looking at a practice with the idea of becoming a partner, we feel that issue needs to be discussed prior to accepting a position in a private practice. We would offer the same advice to a physician looking into a new practice as well.

We have found several barriers to the idea of Carol becoming a partner. One is psychological in that, as physicians, we find it hard to conceive of a partner who is not a physician. A second barrier is that, on Carol's part, she is not willing to accept the extra responsibility of becoming a partner in a practice in terms of sharing calls more equally and assuming a more active role in the administrative details of the practice. The other barrier is legal. It is unclear under existing Connecticut laws whether the legal structure of a professional corporation allows physicians and NPs to enter into legal partnerships. If a NP is considering becoming a partner in a practice, she needs to investigate the legal issues in her state.

INDIVIDUAL PERSPECTIVES ON COLLABORATIVE PRACTICE

Carol

The first position I had after finishing my NP program was as a NP in an out-patient, adult medical clinic where there were five physicians and five NPs on staff. The NPs were basically treated in the same fashion as residents. The physicians were available for consultations and for teaching but were not interested in collaborating. Their role in relationship to the NPs was strictly advisory. My second position was at a Planned Parenthood clinic where I was the sole provider at any given time. There was a physician available by phone for consultation. He also scheduled appointments one afternoon a month to see patients that I felt needed further evaluation. He was always available in terms of being willing to answer questions, but would take over the cases rather than the two of us collaborating and making joint decisions.

The third practice I joined was a private family practice with a NP already established in the practice, and involved seeing patients by appointment as well as walk-in patients. When I joined the practice I was not introduced as a colleague; my main role was doing some counseling and educational programs for the staff as well as seeing walk-in patients. This practice advertised for walk-in patients. However, when people walked in without an appointment, they were discouraged from seeing a physician and were told that the NP was the person who was available to see them. It became somewhat of a penalty to see the NP and it became very difficult to develop a caseload of patients.

Then I interviewed for a position with this current practice. I explained to the physician who hired me why I felt my role was not as successful as it could have been in the other practice. I felt that if I were going to be an independent provider and contribute to the economic viability of the practice I needed to be introduced to the staff and patients as a colleague. We accomplished this by developing a pamphlet for the practice which described who I was and what I did. We had a staff meeting with the nurses and receptionists and I explained my role to them. Most importantly, the physician who hired me spent a lot of time introducing me personally to the patients in the practice. He would introduce me as a colleague, bringing me into the room to meet the patient and telling patients I would be doing the same things he did and that they should feel comfortable seeing me for their health care. Also he began to consult with me for patient issues such as breast feeding, rashes, and asthma, thereby helping patients to see that I had specific new skills to offer to the practice.

Consultation between the physician and me is really an important issue. Basically, I choose to consult for two reasons. One is to confirm my suspicions about a diagnosis or a treatment plan. The second reason is the case of a complicated situation that requires physician input. Whom I choose to consult with depends on a lot of different factors. I may decide to consult with the physician who is generally most familiar with that patient or family. I will consult with the physician that the patient usually sees if he or she is in the office. I may consult with a physician depending on his level of expertise in a specific area; some physicians are better at specific problems. Third, and probably the most important reason, is that I tend to consult with the physician who shares my point of view. All providers practice differently. Some physicians tend to do more testing than I like to do or they want to prescribe medication when I am more willing to monitor a child's condition. I will choose to consult with the physician who shares my approach to patient care.

Consultation with specialists has not been a problem. Most have been willing to discuss cases over the phone and see my patients when indicated. Because I have not been accepted on many HMO provider panels, referrals are made under a physician's name. Most often, the correspondences from the specialist will be addressed to that physician, interfering with my follow-up of the patient. This frustrating communication gap has yet to be remedied. The most important aspect of consultation in a truly collaborative relationship is knowing how to consult with a physician without losing your own credibility or having the physician usurp your authority. There is an art to this. Basically when I need to consult I ask the patient "Do you mind if I consult with one of my colleagues on this problem?" I will ask the physician to come in and take a look at the patient. After the physician examines the patient, he or she will always stop outside the patient's room before rendering an opinion. When we have come to a joint decision I go back in to the patient and implement the plan of care. In the past, I have been in situations where, if I ask to consult, the physician says "Why don't you go on and see your next patient and I will take care of this." This type of situation will destroy your credibility with the patient. They will think the physician has more authority in the relationship.

Conflict in terms of consultation rarely happens in this practice. Because I am a seasoned practitioner, I do not consult often. If I do seek consultation it usually means I do not know how to proceed with the problem and I am usually going to follow the physician's advice. If I really disagree with that advice I may seek a second opinion with someone else in the practice. We talk about it and work it out.

Susan

I want to address physician and patient acceptance of pediatric NPs. Physicians' acceptance of NPs is dependent, to a great extent, on what past experience the physician has had with a nurse practitioner. In general, in both my residency training and medical school, I had limited exposure to nurse practitioners. As a resident I had a limited supervisory role of nurse practitioner students both in the Emergency Department and in the clinic setting and some experience with nurse clinicians and nurse practitioners on the wards in their capacity of dealing with patients. Older physicians have even more limited exposure to nurse practitioners. Lack of exposure definitely affects a physician's acceptance of a nurse practitioner, in the sense of not knowing what they do and what they are capable of.

It probably has been easier for me to accept a NP as compared to other physicians because I practice very similarly to a NP in that I have an interest in teaching about developmental and behavioral issues and in empowering parents through patient education. These are areas that nurse practitioners have traditionally focused on. Physicians have usually been more treatment oriented. Carol and I tend to practice very similar medicine. An older physician or a physician without this kind of focus might have a bit more difficulty integrating a NP into a practice. Initially in our practice Carol's role included more patient education. However, as she has become busier and as the practice has become busier we really can't afford for her to do only that. We need her to provide direct patient care and to incorporate the education into her everyday practice.

In terms of patient acceptance of NPs, a lot is set by how the physician and staff approach the NP. If a secretary says to a patient on the phone "the doctors are all busy but you can see the NP" that is a very different message then saying "Mrs. Boland has a spot available." The tone is set first of all with the secretaries and how they approach it. Our secretaries are very supportive of Carol so that they do a very good job of directing patients and making them see the positive aspects of seeing a NP. Being able to see newborns in the hospital is helpful. Carol also participates in the practice's prospective parent conferences. So parents meet Carol at their initiation into the office. Therefore, they know it is expected that she will be participating in their care just the way the physicians will. We do make an effort when we see new patients, both expecting parents and new patients with older children, to describe Carol's role to the patients, explaining what she does in the office, her training, and that she functions the way the physicians do in the office.

We have had a couple of complaints or issues in the past. We have had some patients who have insisted they will see Carol but that an MD must also see them. In these situations we have explained that Carol will discuss with us any issues that she feels she cannot handle, but that otherwise she is perfectly capable of handling the situation. We have had a few patients who have called and asked that the physician review Carol's prescriptions. We have agreed to do this but we reemphasize quite strongly that Carol has written out the prescription appropriately. The biggest issue we generally hear about is fees.

Some patients feel that because they are seeing a NP, not a doctor, they should not have to pay the same price. We explain that Carol provides the same service, the overhead is the same, and, therefore, the fees are the same. I have occasionally heard from a patient "Why do I need a doctor?" and I have explained that often they don't need a doctor. While my training is more extensive than Carol's in pediatrics I do not need such advanced training to manage sore throats and ear infections. If Carol comes across a problem she is not able to handle, we are there as back-up. In most cases Carol's training is more than adequate to deal with the general pediatric illnesses and well-child care that we see.

I think what is most important is that we continue to assure our patients that we have the utmost confidence in Carol's capabilities and decision making. We trust that she knows her limits, just as we as physicians know our limits in handling more complicated cases. We trust that she will recognize when she needs to consult with a physician to provide the appropriate care for the patient.

THOUGHTS ON CURRENT AND FUTURE PRACTICE

As we mentioned before, Carol is probably the only NP at our hospital right now to hold privileges in the Pediatric Department. Her applying for these hospital privileges actually stimulated the Pediatrics Department to look at their policies for credentialing what they call "non-physician" providers. It then sparked a whole reevaluation of the department's use of providers other than physicians. Carol has also recently been working with the insurance companies and HMOs, and we have been working with the individual practice associations that have sprung up, in an attempt to get her admitted to the panel of providers so that she can see patients and bill for them under her name rather than under the physician's name. Unfortunately, as providers, we have not gotten very far, although the state nursing associations are working on these issues, and Carol continues to work closely with these associations.

We have dealt with the insurance companies by being very up front with them. Carol is here, she is in our practice, she is seeing patients. She is not going to stop. She practices under a physician's supervision, consistent with state law requirements, but she is seeing patients independently. In some cases insurance companies have just said to go ahead and bill for her under a physician's name. A few have allowed her to bill under her own name. In the future it is possible that insurance companies will allow Carol to bill in her own name but for reduced fees. As stated before, this goes against our present office policy of charging the same fees for MD and NP services.

Billing the pediatric NP visits under the physician's name has some implications in terms of managed care because labs and referrals that Carol makes are recorded under the physician's name. This makes it hard to sort out individual utilization patterns, who sent to the lab and why it was done, and creates some issues for our staff, but in general it has worked fairly well. Sometimes we have had patients question why a lab bill came back to them in the physician's name when they saw Carol. We have had to explain that these are insurance issues that can be a little tricky.

We have some strong feelings about billing and insurance. The problem has do to with credibility of the individual provider. If you are seeing patients and you are supposed to be capable of taking care of them, it is very difficult to put someone else's name on the insurance bill. While this may seem like a technicality, little things like this are important to patients; it makes them question whether they really should be seeing a NP versus a physician. At any rate, we do not have a lot of control over the insurance issues right now. In terms of administration within the practice, the NP is usually included in all decision making regarding how the office is run, who does what, and particularly in any decisions that need to be made that affect practice patterns. We feel it is important to involve her in business decisions as well as in the day-to-day administration of the office.

Nursing staff issues have not been a problem in our practice. Again, this is because of the way that the PNP was introduced right from the start. It was made clear to the nurses as well as receptionists who the nurse practitioner was, what she could do, and what kind of expectations the patients and this staff should have concerning Carol's practice. In other practices, however, we have seen the NP run into a wall with nursing staff in terms of their not wanting to assist the NP in various procedures, such as giving immunizations and that type of thing. Again, we feel that you can head this off by talking with people and allaying their fears and letting them know what their and your expectations should be.

CONCLUSION

In summary, a NP and physician who are going to begin a collaborative practice need to discuss and agree upon these specific practice issues ahead of time. They need to do a lot of planning in order to make the collaboration successful and importantly they need to be sure the nurse practitioner is introduced to patients and staff as a professional colleague. The nurse practitioner and physician need to understand each other's role. It is important that the physician understands the nurse practitioner's capabilities and limitations. It is especially important that the practitioners work out their method for consulting with the physicians on day-to-day patient issues. How such consultations are carried out is, in many ways, symbolic of the face that the practitioners seek to portray to patients.

Chapter 8

ADOLESCENT FAMILY PRACTICE

Ann L. O'Sullivan

M y professional career has been spent almost exclusively in positions that combine opportunities for practice, teaching, and research in pediatric primary care nursing. Following diploma and baccalaureate education, I worked as a staff nurse at a large metropolitan children's hospital until completion of a master's program as a pediatric clinical nurse specialist. On completion of this program, I accepted a position that combined responsibility as a nurse clinician with that of instructor in the graduate division of a family nurse clinician program. At the same time, I continued a 4-hour-per-week collaborative practice with a pediatrician in order to maintain skills as a nurse practitioner. In 1978 I was accepted as a Robert Wood Johnson Foundation nurse faculty fellow, spending the subsequent year in the Primary Care Department at the University of Maryland.

It has been gratifying to continue to maintain clinical and faculty activities since completion of the fellowship program. In 1983, I was able to add research with adolescent mothers and their infants to my faculty role. My practice experiences have included those of a pediatric nurse practitioner and director of a Teen-Tot Program, while faculty activities have centered around participation in a Primary Care Family Nurse Clinician Program. My dissertation capitalized on my clinical interests and consisted of case studies using qualitative methods of interviewing to describe how six adolescent mothers decided to return to school after the birth of their first infant. Each of the six families, including the adolescent mother, the baby's grandparents, friends, school nurse, counselor, and gym teacher were interviewed several times until I was able to describe how the adolescent mother made decisions regarding herself and her infant.

Even after 14 years, adolescent mothers' behavior regarding returning to school, delaying second pregnancies, and providing appropriately timed immunizations for their infant continues to provide me with incredible challenges as teacher, clinician, researcher, and community advocate.

PRACTICE WITH ADOLESCENT FAMILIES

Characteristics and Components

The practice with which I am currently involved services the special needs of adolescent families. Located within the ambulatory clinic of a large teaching hospital at their satellite office just five blocks from the main hospital, the practice addresses comprehensive health needs of both the babies and mothers. Presently, most young mothers choose to use the family planning clinic, also located at the satellite building, for their own care, or the hospital's adolescent clinic. Formerly funded by the Robert Wood Johnson Foundation, Mary D. Rockefeller, and The PEW Memorial Trust, and presently by the National Institute of Nursing Research, the project consists of a randomized control study of mothers and infants who attend either a special care program (the Teen Mother Program) or a routine community clinic and are followed for 18 months after the birth of their infants. Infants over 18 months from former programs are followed on a separate day at the same setting. Level of immunization and development of the infant, and whether the mother is immunized, has used condoms and hormonal contraception, and has delayed a subsequent pregnancy are the outcome measures assessed at the end of each study.

Our current caseload includes 258 mothers, 15 to 19 years of age, and their babies. The practice consists of myself, a safety counselor/community outreach worker, a social worker, and a pediatrician working together in a collaborative practice arrangement for infant care. Another team made up of a pediatrician, a family nurse practitioner/midwife, and community health nurse/case manager gives care to the mothers.

The practice is structured so that the safety counselor and either the nurse practitioner or the pediatrician see the adolescent family on every first visit to the clinic setting. Patients see either the pediatrician or the nurse practitioner on the first visit to the clinic, which takes place 2 weeks after discharge of the baby from the hospital. This visit is scheduled in order to make an early assessment of the mother and baby and to provide an orientation to the health care setting. The scope of the clinic services and the practice model are described, including an explanation of the home visit to the teen mother and baby's grandmother or the women in the adolescent mother's life who help her make decisions. A 30-minute time slot is customarily set aside to allow for adequate interaction and questions. This introductory visit eases the family into the system and helps to prevent abuse of the emergency room for common problems, such as low-grade fever, spitting up, and other primary care problems of the newborn period. An additional 30-minute visit is scheduled for the mother if she would like to be seen on the same night as her infant for her postpartum follow-up visit.

Whom the patient sees after that depends on which one of us is free. The nurse aide, after weighing and measuring the infant, places the charts in a rack in the order of arrival at the clinic. Those families with problems with their medical assistance card coverage are seen by the social worker prior to the visit by a clinician. We try to arrange alternate visits, so that if I see the chart of a client whom I have just seen the last two or three times, I switch it to the pediatrician's door. Occasionally, if a client asks to see one or the other of us, we accommodate that request. Then we explain to them why we might not have scheduled them with me or with the pediatrician, and that if they want to participate in this program, it is to their advantage as well as ours that they see both nurse and physician providers. But there are just some days when somebody wants to see one or the other of us for some personal reason, and the practice group feels it necessary to meet that need.

The nature of the practice is such that truthfully 95% of the problems could be managed by the skill and knowledge of a nurse practitioner. Nevertheless, while the practice is wellness oriented, what we are trying to accomplish with adolescent mothers is more than providing wellness care. Within this context, and given the aura that still exists around physicians, there is a real need to have a pediatrician integrally involved in the practice. In actuality, there is very little that differentiates the pediatrician's practice from my own, either in areas of management or referrals. This degree of overlap between the role of nurse practitioner and that of physician is not restricted to our practice, but seems to be true with pediatricians in general. Pediatricians tend to be easier to work with than other medical providers, perhaps because of the nature of the patients served and the ambulatory work environment, as well as the personal preferences of persons choosing a pediatric specialization.

Consultation and Referrals Among Providers

Because of the interaction of the client with several health providers, the mechanism for introducing new management strategies and for referrals must be explicit and adhered to by all of the practice professionals.

In the practice both the nurse and physician treat illnesses as they arise, and therefore there is no differentiation in who does the initial screening. Based on our practice model, the pediatrician and the nurse practitioner are expected, whenever possible, to deal with the problems at hand. One level of consultation involves the confirmation of findings that must take place during the patient encounter. For example, if I think that a burn ought to be treated with antibiotics, I seek consultation with the physician at the moment. In such a situation, the burn is a medical problem beyond my skill and knowledge and I want to make sure it is managed appropriately. Other kinds of problems for which I might seek immediate consultation include orthopedic problems of the hip or feet, and suspected pneumonia in infants under 3 months of age.

A second level of consultation is that of referral to another provider during a return or subsequent visit. If a problem is not urgent and needs more than a two-minute consultation, then the client is asked to make a return visit. This situation typically arises concerning problems of toilet training, spanking, and other disciplinary issues for which the physician might schedule the next or an interim visit with the nurse practitioner. Another example in which we use purposeful alternating visits is in determining the possibility of child abuse. In such a situation the pediatrician will finish up the visit and say something like, "Now the next time I think you ought to come in and see Ann. The routine visit is scheduled for 2 months, but we are going to have you come back in 2 weeks because we have some concerns about the things we talked about today."

There are two major reasons for the way that referral patterns have evolved in the practice. In the first place, the pediatrician and I know and feel comfortable with each other and we recognize and capitalize on each other's strengths. Unfortunately, every time a team member changes, this trust, which forms the basis for collaborative practice, must be reestablished. Because of physician mobility and the development of a family planning practice for mothers, we have had changes in pediatricians over the years that I have been in the practice. Our present pediatrician is a 40-year-old male who has no children of his own and has been with us for one year. Previously two of our pediatricians were female, each staying only six months during residency; and one was male, 55 years old, who had grown children of his own and stayed for three years. Role negotiation and establishing trust, therefore, is a process that absorbs a large amount of both individual and group consultation time.

The second reason underlying our current referral pattern relates to the environment in which we practice. Specialty clinics are accessed only through the primary care referral, based on federally funded managed care in our city. Because these specialty clinics are located at the main hospital, both the pediatrician and I refer out problems that in other settings the pediatrician might be more prone to handle on his or her own. This has helped to establish a practice model in which the practice boundaries for the pediatrician and the nurse are virtually identical. I am not seen as less of a provider than the pediatrician because of an inability, for instance, to ligate extra digits with a suture. We both take full advantage of the available specialty support staff.

The Teaching Program

Much of what we both do in the management of adolescent families includes informal teaching concerning such issues as feeding problems and formal teaching sessions. While we have always recognized the need for a strategy for formal teaching, our initial notion as to how to present content has changed markedly since the inception of the program. Originally, we attempted to conduct a class at each clinic visit. We literally shut down the clinic and had the providers and the clients come into the teaching setting. People came at 12:30 p.m., were seen by the social worker and pediatrician, and then attended a class that lasted from 2:00 p.m. to 3:00 p.m. Other people came at 2:00 p.m. and had appointments scheduled following the class. Constant disruptions further added to the chaotic atmosphere. The providers were rattled, the infants exhausted, and the mothers worried about keeping their appointments. No one could pay attention to what was going on and it just did not work!

We then tried a series of eight classes. The content was primarily a mother-infant stimulation program whereby mothers were encouraged to be the primary teachers for their newborns. This series of classes covered the growth and development phase of the infant, beginning at 5 weeks to 3 months of age and continuing until the child was 14- to 16-months old.

The content was based on a series of 20 classes developed by Dr. E. Badger, at the University of Cincinnati. The series has been used successfully for about 20 years in Cincinnati and has been replicated around the country. We incorporated components of those 20 classes into our series, along with additional content intended to build up the adolescent mother's self-esteem and to provide additional information about contraception. The series provided for repetition of content. Infant stimulation, strategies for handling and managing a baby, and the importance of the mother as teacher were incorporated into each of the eight sessions.

Older parents "goo" and "coo," stick out their tongues, play peek-a-boo, and in general carry on a show-and-tell scene with their infants. Adolescents are too inhibited to behave this way with their newborns. It takes a lot of work to teach adolescent fathers and mothers the importance of these behaviors to their babies' development. Reinforcement of the class content, therefore, was done during each clinic visit. Regretfully, the attendance at the classes was so poor, whether in the summer, fall, spring, or winter, early or late in the afternoon, that we have returned to our earliest model of informal teaching. This is done by the nurse in the waiting room based on the age of the infants present, or by a special discussion after a short video on such topics as safety, birth control, or sexually transmitted diseases. In addition, graduates of the research program (18 months and older) are invited to a 1 hour weekly play session on the floor of the waiting room with the safety counselor and nurse. This weekly session models the appropriate play to develop fine motor and language skills for these infants and toddlers. Our site has also become part of the Read-Aloud program—so that at each visit from 6 months to 5 years a book is given to the infant or child, with a prescription for several minutes of reading aloud each day based on the age of the child. Understanding comes in small doses and requires ongoing attention on the part of all the practice participants.

Collaborative Practice Issues

It is the nature of practice with adolescent families that they need a sense of regularity, continuity, and a similar expression of concern irrespective of who is providing their care. These attributes, therefore, become the basis for the group practice.

One of the things that people bring up frequently about interdisciplinary provider groups is that it is difficult for the client to integrate into the group and adjust to the different approaches of group members. Our clientele could, potentially, have such a difficulty but for the fact that we as a team are particularly aware of the problems inherent in interdisciplinary practice. My practice and that of the pediatrician are similar. We ask the same questions and stress the same issues. Therefore, the client has a very similar experience on each visit and the practitioner's approach does not overwhelm the visit. It is our experience that adolescents can get used to more than one provider as long as the approach remains relatively consistent.

The practice is therefore a concentrated effort on the part of four individual providers with special interest in adolescent families. If one of the providers is not interested in adolescents, the practice does not hold together. This becomes especially apparent when an alternate provider substitutes for one of us when we attend meetings or are on vacation.

The importance of uniformity of philosophy, communication style, and ability to come to some general consensus as to management of adolescents is especially visible during the group conferences. At the end of each clinic session, the four of us sit down and go over *all* of the charts of the families who have been seen that evening to identify problems that have come up since the past visit and to identify special resources that might be needed. We also meet to share information obtained by the social worker and other providers, since by sharing we are able to pull together information not necessarily available to each individual provider.

The decision-making process in the group conferences is very fluid. The primary care providers take turns presenting what they have found on history and physical examination of the infant and the psychosocial information they have gotten from the mother. The social worker and safety counselor add to that profile. Subsequent discussion is aimed at resolving differences in management styles. Sometimes the nurse practitioner or physician is more alarmed by a lack of weight gain or an actual loss of weight than another provider. Sometimes I may want to bring someone back in 2 weeks and the pediatrician would not bring them back for 4 weeks. Provider differences in dealing with clinical problems usually are resolved in some compromise agreement. Sometimes it is the nurse who is pushing toward acceptance of his or her position on an issue and sometimes it is the pediatrician, depending on the issue. The important determinants of the process rest on the ego strengths of the participants. Disagreement is healthy. When my decisions are questioned, it does not mean that the other person is challenging my overall ability or me as a person. Rather, the challenge is to my knowledge or skill in handling a specific incident, and if I am unable to substantiate my position, then the challenge is warranted. The same is obviously true when the nurse questions the pediatrician's actions. But you cannot challenge people nor can you yourself be challenged unless everyone in the situation feels competent in their practice and comfortable with themselves.

The issue of competency and comfort within true, interdisciplinary practice is one that must be addressed from the time of the provider's initial contact with the practice. Practice positions must be filled by people who hold similar practice philosophies. During the hiring process it is important to identify the desired practice group and behavioral style of the providers, including the expectations for the nurse practitioner, pediatrician, social worker, and safety counselor/community outreach worker. Professional competency, personal self-confidence, trust, and communication are equally important attributes for successful interdisciplinary practice.

Perception of Primary Care Practice

Although I am enjoying pediatric practice, I do not think that you can do primary care nursing 9 to 5, five days a week. There is a tendency to get bored with full-time practice. When you have seen 98 mothers or young children and number 99 comes through the door on Friday afternoon at 3 o'clock, it is extremely difficult to listen attentively to the problems at hand. I do not mean to imply that primary care is less energizing for nurses than for other providers. Rather, any full-time practice can become routine or unsatisfying unless, of course, you view it as just a day's work and do not aspire to anything more. When you do the same job day in and day out, there is a tendency to become stagnant, and for your inquisitive tendencies to be blunted.

If physicians are more likely than nurses to find satisfaction in full-time practice, their motivation often stems from financial incentives, incentives not operative for most nurses in primary care practice. Furthermore, physicians are more socialized than nurses to engage in entrepreneurial activities. They recognize that in order to develop an ongoing practice, it is necessary to establish rapport with patients. While some physicians establish rapport because they genuinely care for people, others become somewhat artificial and theatrical in their approach, feeling that this is necessary in order to keep patients.

Lacking the financial incentives, nurses need to seek other ways of making practice exciting and varied. Special projects often serve this purpose. A project, whether administrative, clinical, or teaching, such as precepting students, helps to maintain enthusiasm about practice. Similarly, it is important to develop a special clinical interest, for example, new mothers, single parents, divorced couples, or children of divorced couples. In my own situation, my interest in adolescent families enriches my practice and involves me in new areas of knowledge and with new groups of practice. As consultant to a national study examining nursing in hospitals, I had the opportunity to speak with staff nurses throughout the country. I was impressed with the differences in the attitudes of those nurses who did only their job and those who took on additional activities, such as committee work. When you give more, you feel better.

While stagnation and job "burnout" may occur irrespective of setting, the problem is more evident in primary care because of the character of the practice of most nurse practitioners. In contrast to hospitals, where the routine is less predictable and the patient problems more varied, nurse practitioners work primarily in ambulatory settings. In such practice settings, health providers draw strength and rewards from patients whom they come to know over time. For example, if you are a primary care provider for a patient population with chronic illness, you see people frequently and they make you feel needed. On the other hand, nurse practitioners who work primarily with well populations, for example, with well children and young adults who have episodic and infrequent contacts with a health provider, may not feel as much satisfaction with their practice. For these reasons it is especially important for nurses in primary care to seek out alternative activities that provide a sense of reward, satisfaction, and recognition. For myself this year, working with adolescent mothers attending a 26-week program to obtain their graduate equivalency diploma (GED) and job skills before starting new jobs was very exciting.

It gave me another opportunity to talk about the importance of school, whether for the teen mother or her preschooler, as well as the importance of immunizations for mothers and children alike.

FUTURE OF PRIMARY CARE PRACTICE

The future of primary care practice for nurses is greatly dependent on the positive resolution of reimbursement issues and prescription issues. Without reimbursement and prescriptive authority it will become increasingly difficult to sustain nurse practitioners in traditional ambulatory practices. There are already limited job opportunities in some states, in Health Maintenance Organizations (HMOs), clinics, and the few remaining private physicians' offices. While jobs are still available in rural areas, these too will become scarcer as physicians redistribute from urban to rural settings in search of new practice opportunities. Nevertheless, there are several trends that may increase future employment opportunities for nurse practitioners.

In the first place, the possibilities for transferring the knowledge and skill gained in primary care into settings that have not traditionally provided health care have increased over the last few years. In truth, the potential practice options are as yet unknown for those nurses sufficiently creative to exploit corporate, industry, community, and church interest in providing health promotion, disease prevention screening, and education for their constituencies. Due to an increase in federal funding for the health services for children, I expect a much greater demand in the future for the Pediatric Nurse Practitioner in primary care than we see today.

Secondly, while some nurse practitioners continue to seek work as generalists, there is increasing interest in specialization within primary care. As people familiarize themselves with one area of knowledge, their interests tend to narrow. Typically, nurses have more than one practice interest during the course of their professional careers. In essence, they become specialists in several areas of practice. With each shift in emphasis, they draw on old knowledge, the increasing self-confidence that comes with experience, and the ability to engage in life-long learning gained in their generalist preparation. For example, within my area of practice, I have specialized in the care of the infants and children of adolescent mothers. Yet, even within this focus, there is ample opportunity for further specialization, not only because of increasing physical-biological knowledge, but also because of the need to consider changes in psychological and cultural responses in managing adolescent families.

Regardless of practice setting, the notion of flexibility is crucial to nursing practice. One of the positive results of shifting interests among nurses is the recognition that you can never have, nor do you need, all of the answers. I take the position that when I am in a new practice setting, professionals and clients alike have a responsibility to help me learn those things that will help meet their needs. I have become increasingly confident in admitting the things I do not know and seeking answers from others. A spirit of trust, cooperation, and candidness between client and provider is crucial if nurses are to maintain the level of good will that currently surrounds the delivery of primary care.

Another area of collaboration I want to discuss is the use of nurses with primary care skills in tertiary and geriatric care settings. Nurses can work within institutions on designated units and assume the same authority and responsibility for caseloads of clients that they have had in ambulatory settings, including management of ambulation, nutrition, sleep, and bowel and bladder function—care problems of interest to and best managed by nurses. One current practice in tertiary settings is for nurses with various specialty interests to join together in providing comprehensive care to clients in a manner similar to multispecialty physician group practices. We look to nursing to provide for the whole patient and family. On the other hand, it is unrealistic to expect each individual nurse to be uniformly competent in all areas of practice. Nurses whose skills and interest complement each other should team together.

For example, a primary care nurse and tertiary care nurse can assume joint responsibility for a caseload of patients. They would make rounds together and divide the work based on their specialty interests. The tertiary care nurse would assume the major responsibility during the critical care phase of the hospitalization, while the primary care nurse would be more involved during the recovery phase. The services rendered would be documented, and billing would reflect both nurses' contributions and time expenditures.

The most exciting trend I see in practicing as a primary care provider is the use of the theories of behavioral change and the process of change, coupled with improved communication skills, in an effort to bring about a behavioral change for our clients.

CONCLUSION

There are many practice arenas that would potentially benefit from the introduction of nurses possessing primary care skills. Success in exploiting these opportunities will be dependent on the receptivity of nurses, agencies, and funding bodies.

Chapter 9

PRACTICE IN A CHILD WELFARE AGENCY: AN INTERDISCIPLINARY VIEW

Henry L. Barnett, Ginny Strakosch, Jodee Tolomeo, and Betsy Mayberry

HEALTH supervision of children in foster care encompasses the major principles and practices of primary and secondary care for children with special needs. In this chapter, the provision of primary care for children in out-of-home placement by Pediatric Nurse Practitioners (PNPs) is described and assessed. The foster care medical services of the Children's Aid Society (CAS) are the models presented here.

THE CHILDREN'S AID SOCIETY

CAS is a private, nonsectarian child welfare agency with a 144-year history of providing innovative social, educational, recreational, and health services for underprivileged children in New York City. The agency has a strong commitment to the provision of high-quality health care. There are approximately 50 full-time health professionals on staff. The health staff participate in most of the agency's services, which include foster care and adoption, Head Start and community school-based health programs, summer day camps, a sleep-away camp for disabled children, and a mobile medical/dental van. Although PNPs are involved in all of these programs, this chapter will focus on the comprehensive primary health care clinics for foster children.

Foster Care Medical Clinics

A description of the development of the health services at CAS over the past 20 years reflects the profound changes that have taken place in the health needs of children entering foster care and the environment in which these needs are met. Before that time physicians and nurses attended the medical clinic a few days a week and the social service staff coordinated referrals and follow-up. In the late 1970s the first PNP was recruited to provide well child care for children placed in foster care through the Emergency Foster Boarding Home Program. This program was designed to remove children quickly into a safe home while allegations of abuse and neglect were investigated by the Child Protective Staff.

By 1980 it had become clear that a more comprehensive health care system was required for the increasingly serious and complicated health needs of foster children and their families. From previous experiences of the senior author as a loyal pediatrician and especially as a strong advocate of the special professional skills of PNPs, it was decided that a system staffed primarily by PNPs with on-site pediatric consultants would be the most effective medical model for these disadvantaged children. Two PNP models were developed: the Foster Care Medical Clinic (FCMC) caring for the majority of the children, and the Medical Foster Boarding Home (MFBH) caring for children with more complicated chronic illnesses. The FCMC and MFBH are divisions of the Health Services of CAS.

In FCMC the most common diagnoses in children at time of entry into foster care in 1988 are shown in Table 9.1. A review of the distribution of diagnoses in 1997 revealed several striking changes, including increasing numbers with tinea capitus and asthma (Evans *et al.*, 1997), both of which reflect national trends. The number of children with a history of positive toxicology to cocaine has also increased following the renewal of the policy in New York of considering this finding maternal neglect and placement of the infant in foster care while the mother's drug abuse

TABLE 9.1   Most Common Diagnoses Among Children
Entering FCMC (1988)

Diagnoses	Percent
Lack of health history	66%
Lack of immunization records	60%
URI/pharyngitis	35%
Dermatologic conditions	24%
Positive toxicology to cocaine	16%
Evidence of physical/sexual abuse	11%
Acute ear condition	11%
Developmental/behavioral problem	11%
Dental decay—obvious	11%
Weight less than fifth percentile for age	10%
Heart murmur	9%
Asthma	7%

is investigated. There is an accompanying increase in the incidence of neurologic abnormalities, low birth-weight, and developmental delay in these infants.

In MFBH the most common diagnoses are shown in Table 9.2. The medical complexity of the children taken into care has grown over the last 10 years to include children with tracheostomies and children on home peritoneal dialysis. This increased ability to manage increasingly compromised children at home is a result of a variety of factors, including the institution of a training program providing selected foster parents with the level of medical skills required for the care of individual children; the greater confidence of the MFBH nursing staff in supervising these parents; the greater availability of subspecialist evaluation and treatment and of orthopedic and rehabilitation equipment.

More than 95% of these children in both groups were African-American or Hispanic. The ages ranged from newborn to 21 years; the majority were under the age of 5 years.

The Role of PNPs in the Foster Care Medical Clinics

In the FCMC program, the current census is approximately 500 children. The PNPs manage about 75% of these children with the pediatrician

**TABLE 9.2   Most Common Diagnoses Among Children
Entering MFBH (1997)**

Diagnoses	Percent
Chronic:	
Mental retardation/Developmental delay	83%
Cerebral palsy	43%
Asthma	30%
Seizure disorder	27%
Vision problems (including blindness)	15%
Gastroesophageal reflux	12%
Microcephaly	9%
Hydrocephalus	7%
Scoliosis	
Fetal alcohol syndrome	6%
Hearing loss	
Acute:	
Otitis media	34%
Pneumonia	6%
Tinea corporis/capitis	4%
Bronchitis	3%

providing care to the remaining 25%. On an average day, each PNP sees 10–12 children.

Children are admitted into foster care on an almost daily basis and each child requires a physical examination within 72 hours of admission. The PNPs' schedule must be flexible enough to allow time to examine all newly admitted children, many of whom are sibling groups of three and sometimes four children. These children arrive with no health history and often have acute illnesses requiring treatment. The Agency assumes all of the follow-up responsibilities that a parent would assume in private practice. Thus, as the health provider, the PNP spends a large amount of time in following up and managing these complex cases.

Policies and practices in the clinic are formulated by the PNPs and the full-time staff pediatricians who also serve as general pediatric consultants. The PNPs work closely with staff members of *many* other services at CAS, including social workers, dentists, psychiatrists, developmental psychologists, and educational and vocational specialists.

All children are seen on intake and discharge from foster care. Routine care is provided according to the schedule in Table 9.3. Appointments

**TABLE 9.3   Schedule of Regular Foster Care for Children
in the FCMC of CAS**

The Intake Visit:
— Complete physical exam within 72 hours of placement
— Treatment of any acute conditions

Two-Week Follow-up:
— Developmental assessment
— Bloodwork (CBC, Hgb electrophoresis, STS, lead)
— Urinalysis
— PPD
— Vision and hearing screenings
— Immunization update
— Dental referral
— Update health history records
— Follow-up discussion with foster parent and child

Routine Care:
— 0–6 months: every 2 months
— 6–12 months: every 3 months
— 1–3 years: every 3 months
— 3–21 years: every 6 months

The intake exam is a "no hurt" visit, which begins to establish a trusting relationship with these fragile, often frightened children and their foster parents. Children are seen more frequently than recommended by AAP guidelines to monitor their condition more closely.

---

for episodic illnesses are scheduled as needed. Children needing urgent care during evening or weekend hours usually are seen in the emergency room at Mt. Sinai Hospital. Each E.R. visit is followed by a telephone call to the foster parent to check on the child's condition. Records are obtained from the hospital and revisits are scheduled at the FCMC.

Care of foster children is often complicated by the fact that a child's past history is unknown. Obtaining past medical records is often difficult as care has frequently been fragmented or nonexistent. New York City now has an immunization registry where all providers are required to complete a form on every immunization given to a child. This information is computerized and is immediately accessible on a child's admission to foster care, eliminating the need to re-immunize children whose records cannot be found.

In addition to providing direct services, obtaining medical histories, making referrals, and planning discharges, the PNPs coordinate *all* health-related activities of children coming into care; they serve as case managers, educate parents and social service caseworkers about health issues in special training sessions; they are available for telephone consults and testify in court cases of abuse and neglect.

In the MFBH Program the current census is about 100 cases. The role of the PNP here is primarily administrative and supervisory, rather than clinical. In this program the pediatrician is the primary health care provider with the PNP available for urgent care and other clinical services in the pediatrician's absence. The PNP's primary responsibilities in the MFBH Program include facilitating intake of new children into the program and supervising a staff of six nurses who provide case management of medical services for the children.

Intake responsibilities of the PNP include screening telephone and written referrals of children to determine their appropriateness for the MFBH program; matching referred children with foster families best able to provide them with the level of care needed; making preplacement hospital visits to review medical records and initiate foster parents' medical training by hospital staff; arranging for necessary medical equipment to be available in the foster home. The PNP is also responsible for working with foster families when emergency placement of children is needed during evenings or weekends; this includes telephone contact and home visits as necessary.

The nurses who work as case managers for the medical care of the children in the MFBH Program have the following responsibilities: training foster parents in medical procedures (e.g., tube feedings, catheterization, colostomy care), administering medications, and recognizing signs and symptoms related to the child's illness; scheduling all medical subspecialty appointments; completing written referrals for subspecialty appointments; attending subspecialty appointments with foster families and ensuring that recommended follow-up (e.g., radiologic studies, initiation of physiotherapy, etc.) is completed; ensuring that children are provided with all necessary rehabilitation equipment and assistive devices (e.g., orthotics, wheelchairs, prone standers); attending interdisciplinary school conferences as needed and maintaining communication with school nurses and therapists; completing school/camp physical exam forms to be signed by the PNP or pediatrician; visiting each child in his or her foster home a minimum of four times per year; working with social workers on recertification of foster homes; completing the necessary documentation for the Administration for Children's Services (ACS), the public agency that stands "in loci parentis" for these children; and sharing on-call responsibility for 24 hour, seven-day beeper coverage.

These responsibilities are carried out under the direction and supervision of the PNP. There is a team approach in which the pediatrician, PNP, RN, and social worker work together to address the medical, psychological, educational, and social needs of each child. When discharge of a child to biological parents is planned, the nurse is involved in assessing the parents' ability to care for their medically complex child, as well as in training them to do so.

The PNPs in both programs are board certified and active in local and national professional associations. They are involved currently in establishing a Special Interest Group (SIG) for children in foster care within their professional organization (NAPNAP). They are often invited to give lectures on the special needs of foster children and how these needs are met by the medical services of CAS. The PNPs are salaried members of the staff of CAS. All children are covered by Medicaid. For each child in care the agency receives a per diem Medicaid rate which differs according to the medical condition.

Consultation with Pediatric System Specialists

It has become increasingly difficult for all child welfare agencies to obtain acceptable consultation with pediatric system specialists for foster children. Delays in scheduling appointments, excessive waiting periods, and, especially, poor communication with primary care providers are encountered frequently in hospital specialty clinics accepting Medicaid. These problems are especially troublesome for foster care children and their parents. Previously, CAS had established a roster of practicing pediatric system specialists who were interested in and sensitive to the needs of foster children and their families and who accepted fees below their usual charges. The children were seen by appointment as private patients and the care and especially the communications with the referring PNP were excellent.

Preparations for Medicaid managed care for foster children have required changes in arrangements for consultations. Consultations of CAS are now being obtained at Mt. Sinai Hospital. A system is being developed whereby the children are seen promptly for consultation, a timely report is sent to the referring PNP with findings and recommendations, and there is an opportunity to discuss the plan of care with the consultant.

MANAGED CARE

In anticipation that managed care would eventually include foster children in New York State, CAS began talking with major medical institutions about developing a model of managed health care for foster children and exploring their interest in collaborating in its implementation. In 1994, CAS and Mt. Sinai Medical Center (MSMC) began a relationship that has evolved over the past 3 years from one of sharing information to one of collaborative practice in the provision of medical, mental/behavioral health, dental, and early intervention services.

Recognizing the need to build strong support for policies that were realistic, MSMC and CAS sought a planning grant from the New York State Department of Health to bring together more health providers currently serving foster children. In the fall of 1996, MSMC, CAS, the Administration for Children's Services (ACS), the public agency responsible for foster care, and representatives of other voluntary foster care agencies in New York City began a planning process that will result in the establishment of standards in primary medical and behavioral health care and the development of an institutional infrastructure that will allow these standards to be implemented. The focus will be on the provision of quality health care in an environment that emphasizes the need to be cost-effective.

CASE STUDIES OF CHILDREN IN FCMC AND MFBH

The following FCMC case represents a typical newborn admitted into foster care directly from the hospital. These babies require frequent visits to the medical clinic to teach foster parents how to care for their special needs and to monitor their progress. They are referred to an early intervention program as well as to any other specialty that is deemed necessary.

AC was a premature infant born to a 41-year-old mother who received no prenatal care. His mother smoked cigarettes, drank alcoholic beverages moderately, and abused marijuana and cocaine throughout her pregnancy. At birth, AC required resuscitation and was placed on 100% oxygen. He later became apneic and had to be mechanically ventilated for 24 hours. He was treated with IV antibiotics for group b strep and received phototherapy for hyperbilirubinemia. His urine toxicology was positive for cocaine, but he did not require medication. He had a ligation of an extra digit on his left hand and was medically cleared for discharge at 2 weeks of age. He remained in the hospital as a "social-hold" until foster care placement could be secured.

At examination on admission to CAS, AC was 2 months old. He was developmentally delayed, with head lag present and hypertonicity. He also had a functional heart murmur. He was referred to the early intervention program and the PNP gave the foster mother detailed instructions on how to care for a drug-exposed infant.

AC was seen frequently over the next few weeks for constipation, neonatal acne, a blocked tear duct, upper respiratory infections, and gastro-esophageal reflux. He was started on nebulized albuterol for reactive airway disease. This regimen required extensive teaching of the foster mother regarding the procedure for administering the medications. She was given detailed instructions on signs and symptoms requiring treatment. AC was also seen 3 times in the emergency room for treatment of various forms of his reactive airway disease. Frequent telephone contact was maintained with the foster mother to monitor his condition and to support the foster mother who was becoming more and more anxious about caring for this baby.

At his 4-month well-child exam, AC was noted to have laryngotracheo-malaci. This condition proved to be too overwhelming for the foster mother and within the week, it was decided that a new home would have to be found.

AC was transferred to a new home where the foster mother had experience in caring for a child with asthma. The PNP gave the new foster mother intensive instruction on caring for a drug-exposed infant with reactive airway disease and once again maintained frequent telephone contact.

This case illustrates the complexity of issues involved in caring for a drug-exposed baby with reactive airway disease. The PNP collaborated with the pediatrician, the emergency room physician, the social worker, and the early intervention therapists to provide care for the medical and developmental needs of this infant. In spite of all our efforts, the baby required transfer to a different foster home, but is presently 6 months old and thriving. He has tripled his birth weight and his reactive airway disease is under control. There have been no emergency room visits since his transfer.

MA was a child admitted to MFBH with cerebral palsy, spastic quadriplegia, seizure disorder, mental retardation, and gastroesophageal reflux who was brought to this country by her parents from their native Pakistan in search of better health care. She was admitted into an MFBH foster home at 2 years of age following hospitalization for gastrostomy and a Nissan fundal plication procedure. The foster mother became adept at administering tube feedings, changing the gastrostomy tube, and using a variety of orthopedic equipment. The PNP, through home and office visits, instructed the foster mother as necessary and coordinated MSMC's multiple pediatric subspecialty clinic visits, as well as outpatient diagnostic studies when indicated. MA developed into an obviously happy, medically stable child; her biological parents continued to visit her regularly at CAS. After MA had spent 3 years in foster care, however, her parents were still unable to take her home, so the decision was made to transfer her to a skilled nursing facility (SNF).

While MA was in the SNF, the PNP and social worker from CAS visited her at regular intervals, with the expectation that they would eventually be involved in her discharge to her biological parents. When her parents appeared ready to plan concretely for this event, MA was transferred from the SNF to a CAS Agency-Operated Boarding Home (AOBH). The AOBH is a residence for six children, under the MFBH program, where care is provided by child care workers under the guidance of the PNP. While MA was in the AOBH, the PNP trained her biological parents in her care, including gastrostomy tube feeding, and facilitated their obtaining the equipment they needed to care for her at home. When MA went to live with her parents on a trial discharge basis, the PNP made several visits to their home to assess MA's adaptation. The PNP accompanied MA and her mother to her initial appointment to a local hospital ambulatory pediatric clinic to ensure that all the necessary services were procured for the family and that MA's medical history was effectively communicated.

MA's story is one of a medically complex child with many needs thriving in foster care and then being successfully discharged to the biological family. The availability of a PNP to interface with medical providers from beginning to end of this process and to work with the family in the community as well as with the agency, contributed significantly to MA's eventual reunion with her family.

THE PNPs' VIEWS

Promoting health and preventing disease are what nurses are all about and working as PNPs in a social service agency such as CAS has provided the opportunity to put our clinical skills into practice, while always keeping in mind the psychosocial aspects of care and how it impacts on the total health of a child. Since health care is not the main focus of the agency as it is in a hospital or clinic setting, there is less competition between the different health professionals. Instead, a kind of camaraderie exists among pediatricians, nurse practitioners, health staff, dentists, hygienists, and support staff. This setting eliminates the barriers that have affected other physician/nursing relationships, particularly those barriers created when each person feels they are crossing professional boundaries. Many of the cases at CAS are so medically and socially complex that collaboration between the PNP, pediatrician, and social worker comes naturally as professionals provide their individual expertise, with the result that the child benefits from the insight and experiences of each professional.

The rewards of working as a PNP in a social service agency are many. Serving needy children is of course paramount, but having the opportunity to develop mutually satisfying working relationships not only with pediatricians but also with professionals in other disciplines including social work, mental health, and education is also important. As advanced practice nurses providing primary care to children in foster care, we are cognizant of the fact that managed care has arrived and will affect our future. We anticipate many more changes ahead, but look forward to the opportunity to affect change in a positive way by being involved in making the decisions that will impact upon medical services in a managed care environment.

Work for us must be stimulating to be rewarding and the position of PNP in a child welfare agency has afforded us the opportunity to be challenged in ways we never could have imagined when we graduated from our PNP programs. Our education as PNPs did not cover extensively, in either theory or practice, the primary care of abused children or those with developmental disabilities. However, providing primary care cooperatively, not only with pediatricians, but also with social workers, mental health and educational professionals has been a valuable learning experience for us. Primary care, collaborative practice, and case management were once terms to be studied in school. They are now the foundation for our practice as PNPs in a foster care setting.

THE PEDIATRICIAN'S VIEW

The views expressed here are those of the senior author's (Barnett's) experience of 16 years working with both PNPs and other pediatricians providing primary health care to children in foster care. The high quality of the comprehensive primary care provided by PNPs in this setting has been demonstrated in many identifiable ways. PNPs are excellent clinicians, fully capable of diagnosing and treating the medical problems in ambulatory pediatric practice, and they are well informed about recent advances. They are keenly aware of more complicated conditions that require consultation with a general pediatrician or a pediatric system specialist and which they seek in a way that encourages good communication and cooperation with the consultant. Most impressive is their extensive theoretical knowledge and practical experience in diagnosing and treating psychosocial problems, especially in the area of early childhood development. Here, too, they handle less severe problems effectively and recognize the need for consultation and cooperation with psychiatric and psychological consultants when it arises.

Many children now entering foster care present problems of so-called social pathology, such as physical and emotional abuse and neglect, including sexual abuse, substance abuse, unwanted teenage pregnancy, homicide, and suicide. The PNPs at CAS, working with social workers and relevant specialized consultants, handle these difficult problems as effectively as possible. They also have become "street smart" in coping with the complex systems of child protective agencies and the courts. It is in these areas that the need to work effectively with social workers and related staffs in mental health and education and in administration is so essential.

By virtue of the education and training of PNPs in psychosocial aspects of health care, their role overlaps with that of social workers in several areas, and it could be anticipated that interdisciplinary conflicts with social workers would increase. On the contrary, through better mutual understanding of the professional roles of each of their disciplines, PNPs and social workers at CAS have been able to complement their services effectively. Although medical care has assumed a greater share of the needs of foster children, it is recognized and accepted by the medical staff that primary responsibility for the overall care of foster children and their families must remain with social services. The effectiveness of the care of foster children and their families by PNPs at CAS is enhanced by the location of medical and dental clinics, social services, mental health, and educational services in the same building. This fortunate arrangement is not only a great advantage for the clients ("one-stop-shopping"), but also facilitates contact and communication between services.

During the last 16 years, Dr. Barnett has worked with 16 PNPs and 7 pediatricians at CAS. Generalizing from this small sample, he boldly

offers the following impressions, assumptions, and recommendations.*
The NP/pediatrician model meets not only the medical but also the psychosocial needs of foster children and their families more effectively than
other models. The special professional knowledge of both pediatricians
and PNPs is used in the formulation of professional policies and clinical
practice. In the FCMC the PNPs provide basic, comprehensive primary
care for most of the foster children, while a general pediatrician is available
for pediatric advice and consultation. In the MFBH, in which foster
children with more complicated chronic medical conditions are placed in
homes with specially trained foster parents, the pediatrician is responsible
for primary care which he shares with a PNP and a staff of RNs. Recent
assessment of the experience with this system of having two comprehensive medical clinics for foster care children for illnesses requiring different
levels of care suggested that it should be continued with two modifications:
for some children in MFBH whose chronic illnesses have become stable,
the PNP would assume primary responsibility with advice and consultation
with the pediatrician; other children in MFBH not requiring such intensive
care could be shifted to FCMC; conversely some children in FCMC who
begin to require more intensive care could be shifted to MFBH.

Experience with these two models illustrating different roles PNPs play
at CAS in providing health care for foster children depending on the
children's medical condition may be of general interest. The PNP is the
primary provider of comprehensive health care for well child care, for
children with most illnesses, and for children with more complex medical
conditions that have become stable. In this model, the general pediatrician
and pediatric system specialists are readily available for advice and consultation. For children with chronic illnesses requiring more complex medical
care, the general pediatrician is the primary provider working closely with
a PNP and a staff of RNs.

---

*Not all pediatricians would agree with some of these views. To aid the reader in assessing them,
it seems desirable to describe relevant aspects of Dr. Barnett's earlier professional career. Except
for 3 years of general pediatric practice as the pediatrician at Los Alamos from 1943–1946, he was
in full-time academic pediatrics until he came to CAS in 1981. He was on the faculty of Washington
University School of Medicine, Cornell University Medical College, and Albert Einstein College of
Medicine, where he founded and served as first Chairman of the Department of Pediatrics and later
as Associate Dean for Clinical Affairs. One of his first steps in starting the department at Albert
Einstein was to establish an ambulatory, comprehensive primary care clinic as a major part of the
teaching and training program for medical students and pediatric residents. Experiences in this clinic,
directed by the late Lewis M. Fraad, M.D., and in which PNPs played a major role, attracted many
of the best residents into a career in pediatric primary care.

In these models of care for foster children, both PNPs and pediatricians are practicing in the professional roles for which their education and training have prepared them. The PNPs are able to incorporate their basic nursing skills and insights into their practice of primary care in this setting and they feel that their professional goals are being achieved. These aspects of their work at CAS may account for the success of the agency in recruiting and retaining highly qualified PNPs.

The personal attitudes of some pediatricians working in the FCMC at CAS have been more complex. They enjoy serving as general pediatric consultants to the PNPs and as primary physicians for children with chronic illnesses and serious physical problems. When they themselves are the primary care providers for foster children with less serious physical problems and especially those with complex psychosocial disturbances, they appear to be less comfortable and satisfied.

SUMMARY

The authors' assessment of PNPs in a child welfare agency is that primary health care of foster children and their families is provided more effectively by PNPs working with general pediatricians than by other models, and that providing primary health care for foster children in a child welfare agency is a professionally rewarding and personally fulfilling career for PNPs.

REFERENCE

Evans, D., Mellins, R., Lobach, K., Ramos-Bonoan, C., Pinkett-Heller, M., Wiesemann, S., Klein, I., Donahue, C., Burke, D., Lewison, M., Levin, B., Zimmerman, B., & Clark, N. (1997, February). Improving care of minority children with asthma: Professional education in public health clinics. *Pediatrics, 99*(2), 157–164.

Chapter 10

NURSE PRACTITIONER PRACTICE IN THE SURGICAL INTENSIVE CARE UNIT

Sabrina D. Jarvis

I have been a nurse for over 20 years. I have worked in a wide variety of settings including medical, surgical, emergency, and intensive and critical care nursing. In 1990, I graduated from a family nurse practitioner master's program and began working in hospital-based home health. I quickly realized that while I enjoyed home health nursing, I truly missed the acute-care setting.

At the time there were no inpatient positions for acute-care registered nurse practitioners (RNP) at the medical center where I was working—the only openings were in the clinics and in home health. Fortunately, the master's program I attended had a core program that provided the educational background I needed to also function as a clinical nurse specialist (CNS). Over the next several years I worked as the surgical/surgical intensive care unit (SICU) clinical nurse specialist. I provided clinical support and resource to the staff and surgical nurses and was involved in clinical research, staff development, and patient and staff education. I often helped with patient care in the SICU. As an advanced practice registered nurse (APRN), my role changed over time to include NP functions. In the evenings I was often called to see unstable patients when the primary physician was not available. I used my nurse practitioner skills to assess, diagnose, and treat the patient until the physician could arrive. I also used my NP education to develop and implement complex plans of care for surgical patients.

As the medical center restructured to maintain quality of care within budget constraints and staffing cutbacks, the emphasis shifted to caseload management and realignment of health care resources. Our affiliation with the medical school was also affected. For many years, there was a resident available to provide patient coverage in the SICU, but this position was eliminated when the medical school curriculum changed. In an attempt to provide medical coverage while the surgical teams were operating or away from the unit, I was asked to pilot the role of the SICU NP.

ROLE TRANSITION

My first step was to try and find other NPs working in the acute-care setting. I completed a literature review and networked with several nursing education programs providing acute-care educational tracks. This was unsatisfactory, as the available literature was very general in role development and the educational programs did not provide consistency in training. The NP students' training often appeared to be based on what the physician NP preceptor was willing to teach.

I talked with other NPs who were working in such diverse settings as neonatal intensive care and emergency rooms. I was interested in clinical competencies and documentation of training. Several of the NPs were in the process of developing their own roles and there was diversity in both role description and what clinical skills were required for their particular jobs. I studied the job description for the SICU resident position and met with the SICU nurses and surgeons to determine what role functions they valued.

COLLABORATIVE PRACTICE ISSUES

Initially I met with resistance from both medical and nursing staff. One fundamental problem was the lack of a well-defined, written job description for the SICU nurse practitioner position. Initially I was very cautious and limited the skills I would be willing to learn. The job description was written in generalized terms to allow expansion of the role over time. Some of the physicians had not worked with NPs and identified conflicting areas of responsibility. They were concerned that I was learning and performing such procedures as intubation; placement of central lines, arterial lines, pulmonary artery catheters, and chest tubes; reading x-rays; and prescribing vasoactive and cardiac medications. They saw these activities as crossing into the physician practice domain.

As I have become more comfortable with my role and defined my responsibilities and skills, the physician resistance has decreased. I proactively educate the residents and medical students on the role of the NP. In working collaboratively with them, on a day-to-day basis, I demonstrate my ability to decrease physician workload and to enhance patient care. I am also privileged to work with an SICU intensivist who values my abilities and encourages educational opportunities.

My relationship with the SICU nurses was difficult at times as the new role evolved. Many nursing staff members, including the nurse manager, were very supportive. They were patient and understanding as I worked through the transition period and gained the advanced clinical skills I needed to succeed in the role. It was difficult to develop the NP role in the same unit I had served in as a CNS. There was confusion among the nursing staff as to the difference in the roles. As a NP I could no longer spend as much time teaching at the bedside and helping with routine patient care.

I felt like a neophyte NP despite having worked as an acute-care NP for several years. Initially I was insecure, hesitantly made clinical decisions, and often sought to validate my decisions with others. I lacked the advanced training to do the complex procedures that were required in the SICU. I was, also, initially having to report every intervention to the residents, which added one more step in the communication chain.

Several nurses voiced concerns that I was performing the role of "supernurse" but was unable to write transfer orders or perform the procedures the SICU resident had always done. Some of the nurses did not inform me that there was a patient problem and called the team physician directly rather than involve me.

These problems resolved over time with frank discussion of mutual expectations and as I gained the clinical knowledge, skills, and decision-making ability required for the SICU NP position.

My relationship with the nurses has changed in other ways. As the CNS, I often helped with patient care, and still try to do this as time permits. However, my new responsibilities are such that I have much less time for staff nurse duties and need to focus on other duties. I am asked many questions during the course of the day and need to stay informed about each patient's condition. This means reviewing lab and microbiology results and following through on interventions. I also meet with the surgical ward nurse liaisons and nursing staff to review the medical and nursing plan of care for patients transferring out of the SICU to the surgical wards. I try to make time to visit with the SICU patients who have been transferred out to the surgical wards. Many times, the patients and their families have dependency and care issues and concerns because the nurse ratio is different on the ward. I review the plan of care with the patient, family, and nursing staff to promote continuity of care. The nurses will often consult me regarding patient care issues or concerns.

I bring a unique perspective regarding collaborative practice to the various teams. I have worked for many years with the surgical nurses and I appreciate and recognize their dedication and hard work. I have also developed an appreciation and understanding of physicians, their unique work, and their communication philosophies. The physicians are ultimately responsible for the patient's care, including accountability for morbidity and mortality data that are used by the medical center to compare against national averages. At times, I am able to facilitate resolution of patient issues, discussing them openly and objectively so that both the nurses and the physicians understand each other's perspective. This leads to decreased conflict and improved patient care through mutually supportive decision making.

In the SICU, I am able to spend time visiting with patients and families to establish and maintain a trusting relationship and to determine needs and health care resource allotment. Often families are in emotional and financial distress. I work with the nurses to determine which resources would best benefit the patient and family. This means consulting with other team members in the areas of nutrition, rehabilitation activities, family support, wound management, visual and hearing impairment, and patient and family teaching.

During surgical team rounds, I participate in patient care planning and review any findings and interventions I have implemented. Rounds are also an opportunity to participate in educational discussions as the medical students and residents review the cases and medical interventions and the attending surgeon poses questions. I have found that many of the physicians in other areas, such as radiology, nuclear medicine, rehabilitation, cardiology, and so on, are very willing to teach and provide informal consultation as needed.

CHARACTERISTICS AND COMPONENTS

I currently base my practice in the SICU and formally work 10-hour shifts from 11:00 to 21:30 Tuesday through Friday; however, I actually work 40 to 50 hours a week. My caseload includes up to 10 SICU patients. I often see patients on the surgical wards and provide follow-up care on four to six patients who have transferred out of the SICU. This caseload is manageable but keeps me very busy.

I am the only NP on the unit; therefore, I do not take call and do not serve as the primary caregiver. I work with seven rotating teams who have admitting privileges in the SICU. The vascular and general surgery teams are large ones and manage their own patients. I provide input on care and manage problems when these teams are away from the unit.

The neurosurgical, cardiothoracic, urology, ENT, and orthopedic services are much smaller and are appreciative of the support I provide. I usually round with these teams and participate as a team member. I write orders on these patients and monitor care provided. Several times a day, I visit with the patients and their families. Often families are in crisis and small issues, if not discussed, become very stressful. A trusting relationship usually develops and I provide follow-through for any issues that the physician may need to deal with.

I have a close working relationship with the SICU intensivist and review patients with him at least once a day. Often the intensivist leads team rounds which are used as a learning experience for the residents and myself. If a problem develops, I routinely consult with the intensivist as needed.

If a patient's condition deteriorates, I will manage the patient and notify the responsible physician. Interventions may include intubation, ordering of vasoactive medications, placement of arterial and central lines, ordering appropriate lab and radiographic studies, and so on.

In the evenings there is an in-house resident or intern who covers the surgical service. They are often busy seeing consults or may need to assist in emergency surgeries. I continue to provide coverage in SICU and will respond to pages from the surgical wards. At the end of the shift, I report off to the resident or intern.

I have developed my job description and maintain a clinical log of advanced clinical procedures I perform. I have also developed clinical competencies and reviewed these with the intensivist. I have clinical privileging through the medical center's professional board and each year I update my clinical skills list as I learn new procedures.

Every year, my performance is evaluated based on the federal proficiency system which is divided into clinical performance and professionalism/leadership activities. The proficiency also includes a current list of my advanced clinical competencies. After a self-evaluation, my proficiency is completed by the intensivist, SICU nurse manager, and the associate chief of the surgical care center.

PERCEPTION OF ACUTE-CARE PRACTICE

It has been a very rewarding and educational experience to professionally develop and then actually transition into the role of SICU NP. I enjoy working with the SICU nurses and team physicians and feel that I contribute to quality patient care. I enjoy the challenge of managing seriously ill patients and participating in the plan of care and dealing with emergency situations that occur.

Several issues continue to impact on the NP role. The first issue is prescriptive privileges. Currently, according to state law I can only order Schedule III–V controlled substances. This is a problem because I work in an intensive care setting and perform potentially painful procedures, yet am unable legally to prescribe morphine or Demerol.

Another issue is resident rotations. The medical center is a teaching facility which means the residents rotate every month or two. As soon as I have developed a working relationship with the current residents and medical students, the teams change, leaving me to establish new relationships. This interrupts continuity of care. It is balanced by the availability of the SICU intensivist, attending surgeons, and strong, permanent relationships with other medical center team members, such as social workers, dieticians, occupational and physical therapists, and chaplain services.

Finally, sometimes it is difficult being one of two inpatient NPs. I work closely with the neurosurgical NP and often discuss role concerns with her. I also visit with the other NPs who work in the outpatient setting. They are supportive and encourage role development.

FUTURE OF ACUTE-CARE PRACTICE

I believe that as medical centers reorganize in an attempt to contain costs and streamline patient care services new and exciting roles will develop in the acute-care setting for NPs. It is an exciting time, but also one rife with stress and uncertainty. The entire American health care structure is under scrutiny. Health care providers are faced with many changes beyond their control as they struggle to continue to provide quality patient care.

As these new NP roles evolve, it will be the responsibility of nursing leaders to encourage standardization of education for the NP based on which acute-care setting the NP will be practicing in. This means the development of standardized clinical competency statements that provide consistency in education and training.

I also believe that NPs need to belong to a strong nursing organization that would oversee the political and educational needs of its members. We do ourselves a disservice by having several organizations which currently offer membership and different certification testing for NPs. Strong nursing leadership is needed in the political arena. Our nurse practice acts need to be written to allow growth and expansion in practice and to expand the scope of prescriptive practice privileging. The reimbursement issues need to be clarified and structured for fair compensation.

Acute-care NPs need to develop strong collaborative relationships with physicians to provide optimal patient care and services. Understanding that physicians are going through a time of stress and uncertainty as they are asked to move away from specialty areas to family and general medicine practice is important for NPs. Many physicians are unhappy and frustrated as health care moves into corporate health care organizations dictating physician practice and salaries. This has created increased stress in the relationship between physicians and NPs. It is essential to work through differences and support each other so that the ultimate outcome is improved health care for the patient.

I believe that in the acute-care setting, patients are more ill and require the skills of both the physician and the NP working in collaborative practice. As NPs learn more advanced skills, the training is often done by the collaborating physician.

My personal practice philosophies include the following beliefs:

1. There is a defined difference between physician practice and APRN practice; and that
2. APRNs bring a different philosophy to health care, based on a holistic nursing model rather than a medical model.

CONCLUSION

There are a growing number of NPs moving into the acute-care setting, including the intensive care area. It has been exciting and challenging to develop the SICU NP role in a collaborative practice with the SICU intensivist. Despite challenges and difficulties, it has been a wonderful opportunity for personal and professional growth.

Chapter 11

PRACTICE WITH PATIENTS WITH HIV/AIDS

Jo Anne Staats

I have been an adult nurse practitioner for 15 years and have cared for people with Human Immunodeficiency Virus (HIV) infection for the past 10 years. The first 8 years of my nursing career were spent in public health nursing in New York City. Becoming a nurse practitioner seemed like a natural extension of public health nursing and gave me the opportunity to care for patients more comprehensively. For 5 years after completing the nurse practitioner program, I worked in a variety of primary care settings. I then made a decision to become involved in HIV/AIDS care. Since January of 1987 I have worked in four different HIV/AIDS programs. The first was a residential facility for persons who were homeless and had HIV infection. The next was an infectious disease clinic of a hospital with a large HIV/AIDS population. I then moved on to a HIV-related research project. And currently I am in a clinical setting with a significant number of women with HIV infection.

EPIDEMIOLOGY OF HUMAN IMMUNODEFICIENCY VIRUS INFECTION

In the United States, from 1981 through 1996, 573,800 persons over the age of 13 with AIDS were reported to the Centers for Disease Control.

Forty-four percent of AIDS cases were attributable to men having sex with men (MSM), 26% to injecting drug users (IDU), and 12% to persons infected through heterosexual contact (Centers for Disease Control, 1997). From 1992 to the present there has been an increase in the number of non-Hispanic Blacks, Hispanics, and women reported with AIDS. In 1996, non-Hispanic Blacks exceeded, for the first time, the number of non-Hispanic Whites with AIDS. And women accounted for 20% of adults reported with AIDS. Intravenous drug use is also the major means of transmission of HIV infection to the heterosexual and, as a consequence, to the perinatal population.

In 1993 the Centers for Disease Control expanded their AIDS-defining diseases to include any individual, whether asymptomatic or symptomatic, who has a CD4+ T-lymphocyte count <200 cells/µL or CD4+ T-lymphocyte percentage of total lymphocytes of <14, has had pulmonary tuberculosis, bacterial pneumonia more than two times in one year, or invasive cervical cancer. This change resulted in a large increase in the number of AIDS cases reported for 1993, followed by declines in numbers of AIDS cases reported for 1994 through 1996. However, the number of cases reported in 1996 was 47% higher than the number reported in 1992.

During January to June of 1996 the estimated number of deaths from AIDS was 13% less than the number of deaths during the same time period in 1995. This applied to all racial/ethnic groups except for women, who had a 3% increase in deaths, and to all risk/exposure categories except for a 3% increase in persons infected through heterosexual contact. The decreased death rate is probably attributable to recent improvements in medical care, better prophylaxis against opportunistic infections, and the use of combination therapy with antiretroviral agents.

MEDICAL CARE OF HIV-INFECTED INDIVIDUALS

AIDS is now only used to refer to the end stage of HIV infection. HIV infection includes the spectrum of disease from diagnosis of positivity to death. With the advent of combination therapy and new antiretroviral drugs individuals with HIV infection are living longer, healthier lives. In addition, prophylaxis against certain opportunistic infections (e.g., Pneumocystis carinii pneumonia, Mycobacterium avium complex) has prevented the development of these diseases. The development and increasing availability of viral load testing provide an additional way to monitor disease progression and the effectiveness of antiretroviral therapy. With the rapid development of new drugs and treatment modalities for HIV infection providers must be well informed.

As the number of persons with HIV infection continues to increase, the availability of HIV specialists to care for these patients decreases. Many primary care clinics and providers are caring for persons with HIV infection rather than referring them to specialists. However, one study has shown that patients of physicians with the most experience in caring for persons with HIV infection had a 31% lower risk of death than patients cared for by physicians with the least amount of experience (Kitahata et al., 1996). This argues for patients to seek care with providers who have extensive knowledge in the care of persons with HIV infection. In many inner-city areas, though, there is a dearth of providers with this experience. As a result, there is a need to provide ongoing continuing education to providers to keep them abreast of the newest developments in HIV care.

Nurse practitioners can and have stepped into the role of primary health care provider for those infected with HIV. Many of these nurse practitioners are exclusively HIV providers and have an extensive knowledge of HIV infection. In New York City, nurse practitioners currently care for persons with HIV/AIDS in a variety of settings. Some of the sites are a HIV-oriented community health clinic, HIV/AIDS day treatment programs, residential programs, HIV/AIDS skilled nursing homes, infectious disease clinics, and inpatient HIV/AIDS-designated units.

DEVELOPMENT OF THE ROLE OF HIV NURSE PRACTITIONER

I moved into the challenging world of HIV/AIDS in 1987 when I accepted the position of part-time nurse practitioner at Bailey House. Bailey House is a supportive group residence for homeless persons with AIDS that is located in Greenwich Village, New York City. It was opened in December of 1986. At that time it received funding primarily from New York City with some other monies coming from the state and federal government. The remainder of the budget was supplemented by fund-raising. The facility accommodates 44 residents, each with his or her own room, bathroom, television, and telephone. Three meals a day are served in a common dining room.

The original staffing plans for Bailey House included a part-time nurse practitioner, a master's-prepared social worker, two case managers, a substance abuse counselor, a recreational therapist, a pastoral care counselor, an intake coordinator, personal care assistants, receptionists, residence managers, housekeepers, kitchen staff, office personnel, an administrator, and an assistant administrator. This staffing pattern has changed over the years as a result of a decrease in funding.

When I began at Bailey House it had been open only 1 month, had only seven residents, no policies or procedures, and was not fully staffed. It was my responsibility to monitor and coordinate the health care of the residents, supervise the personal care assistants, and function as a member of a multidisciplinary team. Over a period of 5 months we became fully staffed and gradually filled the 44 rooms. During this period of time the team developed a record-keeping system, developed admission criteria, and determined reasons for residents to be placed on probation or discharged.

My initial steps were to establish liaison with the local hospitals with AIDS clinics and develop patient data forms. Through my contacts it was possible to get appointments and contact providers when residents were ill. I developed a history and physical examination form to be used when each new resident was admitted. This helped me to establish a baseline for future comparison of functioning and for the team to use in developing a plan of care for the residents. During the initial interview, the client's understanding of the disease process, medication, the need for medical care, and knowledge about safe sex and self-care were assessed, and a plan for monitoring and teaching developed.

Within a month after I started it became clear that my position needed to be full-time, and after 4 months funding was found to increase my hours. It was also evident that I required an assistant to track clinic appointments, arrange transportation to clinics, and order supplies. It was not until 2 years later that funding was found for that position.

The Visiting Nurse Service of New York (VNS) provided an on-site nurse at Bailey House. Some residents required intravenous infusions of AIDS-related medications (e.g., ganciclovir, amphotericin B), regular dressing changes, or injections, and were referred to the VNS for those services. In addition, residents who were debilitated, such that they required more assistance with ADL than our staff could provide, were referred to the VNS for a home attendant or home health aide. The VNS on-site nurse was responsible for supervising those aides and monitoring the resident. The visiting nurse and I collaborated to provide coordinated care for the residents. As a result it was possible to keep many residents at Bailey House, despite repeated hospitalizations, until they died.

In 1988 Bailey House was approached by St. Vincent's Hospital and Medical Center's Community Medicine Program about the possibility of providing us with the services of one of their physicians, Dr. Gabriel Torres, who was trained in the care of persons with HIV infection. Dr. Torres would consult at Bailey House 2 half days a week and would arrange to see residents during his clinic sessions at St. Vincent's Hospital. Prior to Dr. Torres's coming to Bailey House, I was somewhat isolated from other AIDS caregivers, and what I had learned about AIDS was by experience and reading. My knowledge of HIV infection and ability to care for persons with AIDS was greatly enhanced by working with Dr. Torres.

Residents referred to the physician had problems that did not require an emergency room visit but could not wait until the next clinic visit. Dr. Torres would see these residents and arrange for appropriate testing or prescriptions or contact the primary care physician. With the early intervention provided by Dr. Torres we believe it was possible to manage many medical problems in the outpatient setting before hospitalization was required (Torres & Staats, 1989).

Dr. Torres and the other HIV clinic physicians at St. Vincent's were readily available by telephone during the times that Dr. Torres was not at Bailey House. Through my increasing knowledge of the management of HIV disease and the use of protocols developed by both the Harvard Community Health Plan (1983) and the New York State Department of Health (New York Statewide Professional Standards Review Council, 1989), it became possible for me to manage many of the residents' medical problems that had previously required an emergency room visit. Not surprisingly, the more knowledgeable I became about HIV, the fewer residents needed to see Dr. Torres during his afternoons at Bailey House. Because we were not a medical facility, I was not able to order tests and alter treatment appreciably, so I still required his assistance in this area. I was not the primary care provider of record.

Over the 4 years that I worked at Bailey House I also developed increasing expertise in the area of chemical dependency. Many of our residents had a history of chemical dependency, whether their risk factor was homosexual/bisexual contact or injecting drug use. A prerequisite for admission to Bailey House was an ability to live drug- and alcohol-free. A potential resident's chemical dependency history was reviewed by the intake worker during the initial interview with the resident. Applicants with questionable motivation were discussed by the entire team and a decision on acceptability was made by the team.

We became more adept at identifying those residents who were using drugs and/or alcohol and at offering them various options to maintain sobriety. Very few residents needed to be discharged because of an inability to stop using drugs. I also became more experienced at distinguishing those symptoms that might be AIDS-related from those that might be related to substance use.

At the end of 1990 I was approached by Dr. Torres about the possibility of participating in the newly developed New York State AIDS Institute HIV Clinical Scholar's Program. The purpose of the program was to train physicians, nurse practitioners, and physician assistants in the delivery of primary care to persons with HIV infection. St. Vincent's Hospital was one of four New York City sites selected to participate in the Scholars Program and had two openings. I and another nurse practitioner were accepted for the 15-month training program. I felt that the program would provide me with the opportunity to learn more about the medical management of persons with HIV/AIDS.

The Scholar's Program at St. Vincent's Hospital focused on following a panel of patients in the infectious disease clinic. The patients ranged from HIV-positive asymptomatic to end-stage AIDS. When our patients were admitted to the hospital we would continue to follow them as inpatients and make recommendations to the house staff regarding their care. The Program had a full-time physician who served as mentor. The physician was available during clinic sessions and made rounds of our inpatients with us. In addition to direct patient care, she arranged placements for us in specialty clinics related to HIV care.

My new role was challenging and daunting. At Bailey House I did not have complete responsibility for the medical care of the residents. And prior to Bailey House I had worked in traditional nurse practitioner settings. I had followed stable, chronically ill patients who had few serious, acute medical problems. Caring for persons with HIV, particularly patients with end-stage disease, required more medical knowledge than I had needed in my previous positions. During the Scholar's Program I learned to care for persons with various opportunistic infections, many of whom were seriously ill and required hospitalization. During those 15 months I became more confident in managing complicated medical problems. I learned to integrate my new skills into my role of nurse practitioner. For example, the other nurse practitioner and I seemed to be more comfortable than the physicians when it came to caring for patients who were dying. We were better able to accept a patient's wish to end treatment and die. Most of the physicians were more committed to aggressive treatment right to the end. I think our nursing experience and ability to listen to the patient were great assets for HIV/AIDS care.

Upon completion of the Scholar's Program both I and the other scholar were offered full-time positions in St. Vincent's Hospital AIDS Program. We each had the same responsibilities for patient care that we had as scholars except that we had more clinic sessions resulting in an increased caseload. We always had access to one of the AIDS Center physicians for consults regarding patients we were following. We also had weekly case conferences with Dr. Torres. In addition, the AIDS Center had a weekly journal club where providers took turns presenting an HIV/AIDS-related journal article.

After 4.5 years at St. Vincent's I realized that I needed a change. I wanted to stay in HIV/AIDS but wanted less patient care. I was feeling the strain of caring for many patients who were seriously ill and dying. I was told of an opening for a nurse practitioner at the Women's Inter-agency HIV Study (WIHS) at their Bronx site. WIHS is a longitudinal cohort study designed to determine the effect of HIV disease on women. There are six WIHS consortia sites with a combined enrollment of 2,080 HIV+ women and, as controls, 575 HIV- women. The position at the Bronx site required the nurse practitioner to do a physical and gynecological exam on the participants every 6 months. I was also offered the option of spending 40% of my time doing clinical care at another site or becoming site coordinator for the Bronx site. After 8 years of direct patient care it was very appealing to be offered a position with an important study that would require no patient management. All the women seen in the study had primary care providers. I also opted for the site coordinator position, again because I wanted less patient involvement. For the first 3 months it was enjoyable to see patients, spend time talking with them but not have responsibility for their health care. I also enjoyed learning more about the study and assuming some administrative responsibilities.

However, it was during this time that studies were being completed on the new protease inhibitors and there was excitement among providers over their use. Without actually managing patients I was finding it difficult to keep abreast of the newest treatments in HIV/AIDS care. I felt that these new developments were passing me by. I was also beginning to miss the management of patients and the relationships that I had with my patients. Despite the importance of the study I felt that I was not using my skills and was becoming further removed from HIV/AIDS care.

It was at this time that I met Dr. Laurie Solomon, the Director of the Ambulatory Ob/Gyn service at Bronx Lebanon Hospital Center. She had been instrumental in developing comprehensive primary care services for women with HIV infection. In conjunction with the Division of Pediatric HIV Services, funding was obtained from the New York State AIDS Institute/Department of Health to form the Division of Women and Children's Services, a family-centered model of care. This became known as the Co-located clinic. Dr. Solomon had been looking for a nurse practitioner or certified nurse midwife to coordinate HIV primary care education and research within the program. The position would also include several clinic sessions following adults infected with HIV in the Co-located clinic.

I was anxious to become involved in patient care again although not to the extent of my involvement at St. Vincent's. The position appeared to be a good combination of patient care, education, and research, giving me some of everything. When the position was offered to me, I accepted with enthusiasm. It has taken almost 1 year to define my role. I have five clinic sessions, one of which is a GYN session for women with HIV infection. Through the HIV Primary Care Training Program at Bronx Lebanon Hospital Center, an AIDS Institute-funded program to provide HIV education to community health care providers, I am giving lectures to various community agencies. Our goal is to keep community primary care providers abreast of the newest developments in HIV care. In addition, the Division of Women and Children's Services has several ongoing HIV-related research studies. The potential studies related to the interruption of perinatal transmission of HIV have been of the most interest to me. Bronx Lebanon had been involved from the beginning in the clinical trial (ACTG 076) that determined the effectiveness of AZT in preventing perinatal transmission of HIV. I work closely with the midwife who manages the pregnant women who are infected with HIV. If they are stable in relation to their HIV infection, she manages them until after delivery. If their HIV infection is not well controlled we manage the patients jointly. After delivery, I become their primary care provider.

Looking back on my experiences in caring for persons infected with HIV, I realize I have followed the epidemic. Both at Bailey House and St. Vincent's most of my patients with HIV were men who had sex with men. Several years into my work I was seeing more people who had contracted the virus through injecting drug use. This was true for both the men and women who were IDUs. However, over the past 2 years with my two positions in the Bronx I now care for many more women than men. And over the past few years of the epidemic we have seen more women become infected, particularly in areas such as the Bronx. And most are becoming infected through heterosexual contact. As a result, the potential risk of perinatal transmission has increased. But the use of antiretrovirals during pregnancy has been extremely significant in preventing perinatal transmission. With newer antiretroviral agents being used in pregnant women, it is anticipated that the risk of perinatal transmission will be reduced even further.

During the years of my involvement with HIV I have met many nurses and nurse practitioners who have been dedicated to the care of persons with HIV. The Association of Nurses in AIDS Care (ANAC) has been instrumental in my connecting with others. ANAC was founded in 1986 by a group of nurses committed to HIV care and a desire to bring together other nurses with the same commitment. I was pleased to serve for two years as treasurer on one of the early Boards of Directors and was a co-founder of the Greater New York Chapter of ANAC. ANAC has developed into a national organization with approximately 2000 members, an increasing number of local chapters, a newsletter, and a journal (Journal of the Association of Nurses in AIDS Care; JANAC). And beginning in November 1996, ANAC offered its first HIV certification exam to nurses who wanted specialty certification in this area.

I remain committed to HIV care. I am excited by the new developments in HIV care: new antiretroviral therapies, better prophylaxis of opportunistic infections, and viral load tests. As a result of these developments I have had significantly fewer patients with serious, life-threatening illnesses, and have had fewer patients die. The challenge for me now is to refocus. For many years I have tried to help patients cope with a terminal illness. I have managed serious medical problems and cared for patients when dying. We are not able to say we have a cure for AIDS. However, I find myself looking at my patients (particularly those with more compromised immune systems) and thinking that this person will probably live longer than I would ever have expected even 2 years ago. And they will be healthier while living. It is a new and exciting challenge.

REFERENCES

Centers for Disease Control. (1997). *Update: Trends in AIDS incidence, deaths, and prevalence—United States, 1996, 46.*

Harvard Community Health Plan. (1983). *Guidelines for clinical practices.* Boston: Harvard Community Health Plan.

Kitahata, M. M., Koepsell, T. D., Deyo, R. A., Maxwell, C. L., Dodge, W. T., & Wagner, E. H. (1996). Physicians' experience with the acquired immunodeficiency syndrome as a factor in patients' survival. *New England Journal of Medicine, 334,* 701–706.

New York Statewide Professional Standards Review Council. (1989). *Criteria manual for the treatment of AIDS.* Albany: New York State Department of Health.

Torres, R., & Staats, J. A. (1989, June). Primary care at a residence for persons with AIDS. Paper presented at the Fifth International Conference on AIDS. Toronto, Canada.

Chapter 12

PHYSICIAN AND NURSE PRACTITIONER RELATIONSHIPS

William Kavesh

INTRODUCTION

THE extraordinary changes that have occurred in the health care system in the past 5 years have affected every sector of the practice environment, including—in my experience at least—the relationships between physicians and nurse practitioners. I first started working with nurse practitioners almost 25 years ago in a neighborhood health center in South Boston. It was a time of great ferment and concern about health care costs. President Nixon had just introduced rigid cost controls which had significantly reduced the rapid inflation of health care expenditures, although the fundamental organization of health care remained intact.

But as much as health planners were concerned about costs, there was an equal concern about extending health services to the underserved, and creative mechanisms to deliver those services were welcomed. In Boston, this included a neighborhood health center system to replace the dwindling inner-city cadre of physicians. The goal of this system was to offer community residents a longitudinal relationship with a health care provider to replace hospital clinic and emergency room visits that entailed a constantly changing set of physicians—usually physicians in training. Neither the planners of this new system nor the community residents had preconceived notions about the type of provider they saw as long as the person was attentive, competent, and caring. Nurse practitioners were an early, integral part of this vision.

It is interesting to look back at this early 1970s model with a late 1990s lens. In the 1970s, we evolved a fairly standard, relatively leisurely approach to seeing patients. I saw all new patients and then referred to the nurse practitioner the ones who had fairly stable medical problems, such as hypertension and diabetes, that were amenable to management by a set of guidelines which her teachers had written. We scheduled six patients for me to see in a 3-hour session and four or five for her. She was able to spend a lot of time doing detailed histories and examinations, but we also had enough time for us to talk and discuss any problem situations. The patients loved it.

I have a certain nostalgia for those days. We had a truly collaborative practice. There was lots of time to see our patients and talk about them together. We had ample opportunity to educate the patients about their medical problems and the medications which they needed to take, although the nurse practitioner usually spent much more time then I did on these tasks. The standard 10-minute managed-care visit had not yet evolved.

However, there were some features of our collaborative practice that foreshadowed changes in health care practice, which are still evolving today. One of the more interesting changes has been the evolution of practice guidelines. Guidelines are structured protocols for the evaluation and treatment of specific health conditions which are agreed upon by the physician and nurse practitioner. In the 1970s, we had an ambivalent approach to guidelines. Both the nurse practitioner and I were aware that our guidelines, or any set of guidelines, could not begin to describe all the nuances of patient care which she encountered. The guidelines served as educational tools and road maps for typical situations. But many situations were not typical. If the nurse practitioner called me in for every problem which didn't precisely fit one of the guidelines, I would have seen most of her patients a lot more frequently than I did. We sometimes viewed the guidelines as important tools to keep us out of trouble with state regulators, although I don't recall anyone ever asking whether we followed them.

Then came the 1990s and the metamorphosis of guidelines from what some regarded as "cookbook medicine" into tools for the improvement of quality and efficiency. Clinical pathways, as they are now often called, are detailed protocols for the care of a patient with a particular diagnosis, usually in the hospital setting. Starting with the emergency room visit, they may describe the day-by-day care practices ranging from the type of assessment to the treatments to be implemented, activity permitted, patient/family education, criteria for discharge, and even expected outcomes. The goal is to standardize care using the best available evidence from the literature. Some might argue that this approach also fits well into the cost-cutting environment fostered by managed care. Whatever the rationale or mix of rationales, acute-care pathways are becoming ubiquitous at major teaching hospitals like the Hospital of University of Pennsylvania which has over 30 guidelines completed or in the course of development (D. Shulkin, personal communication, 1997).

Hospital protocols may end with educational guidance to be given to the patient and family at discharge. However, chronic care—which includes much of geriatric care—does not stop at the doorstep of the hospital. Recognizing the critical importance of transitions planning to the success of hospital treatment, the Lutheran Hospital system in Arizona began work in the early 1990s to develop extended care pathways. Working together with physicians, nurses at two Lutheran hospitals and a home care program developed algorithms for members of the health care team to use in the evaluation and treatment of patients with a large number of DRG diagnoses. These algorithms include specific plans for post-hospital follow-up (National Chronic Care Consortium, 1992). Recent work has validated this concept for at least one common condition, that of congestive heart failure. A study in Philadelphia showed that intervention by a nurse specialist after discharge can prevent complications and early hospital readmissions for congestive heart failure, lowering overall costs in the process (Naylor et al., 1994).

In my experience, nurse practitioners are probably the ideal people to bring coherence to the long-term-care system, providing the continuity and communication that are so necessary to the successful care of the chronically ill as they move from one site to another in the health care system. My experience began 20 years ago when I was working with the Urban Medical Group, a nonprofit group practice specializing in long-term-care and geriatrics. The Urban Medical Group operated an innovative nursing home care program which at that time was serving over 400 residents of about a dozen Boston area nursing homes. In addition, we provided medical services to several coordinated home care programs, which cared for 500 frail elders in their own homes. Two members of the group developed a home-based program for a younger, disabled population with spinal cord injuries and other neurological disorders (Master et al., 1980; Meyers et al., 1989).

The key to success of these programs, and of similar programs which I have encountered in Philadelphia and elsewhere, is the nurse practitioner. Physicians find the time constraints of a typical office and hospital practice inimical to the responsiveness necessary to attend to acute problems in nursing homes and at home. It is virtually impossible to drop everything and run to a nursing home or make a home visit. On the other hand, this is a perfect job for a nurse practitioner whose full-time role includes the flexibility to move from one home to another as necessary or from nursing home to home. Numerous studies have demonstrated the cost- and quality-effectiveness of such programs (Kane et al., 1991; Meyers et al., 1989). The nurse practitioner, through early intervention, often kept patients out of the emergency room and out of the hospital. When the patient did require hospitalization, or movement to another element of the care system, the nurse practitioner's thorough transfer of clinical and social data facilitated better care and avoided "reinventing the wheel" at the new clinical site.

Nowhere is the nurse practitioner's critical role as a care facilitator better demonstrated than in the care of patients with AIDS. In the early 1990s, it was apparent that patients with AIDS were heavy users of the hospital system. This was probably due, in part at least, to the fact that their primary providers were infectious disease specialists who were hospital based and used the hospital as the primary care modality of choice when the patient became sick at home. One of the founders of Urban Medical Group set up an organization to develop an alternative method of providing care for this population. Based heavily on the use of nurse practitioners, the program offered a continuum of services ranging from home to respite care, to foster care and residential hospice. The program demonstrated a high level of patient satisfaction and a striking savings in health care costs. Because of the intensive involvement of the nurse practitioners in the different settings and their focus on communication with each other and other health care providers—including taking night call—the program assured the successful transfer of information vital to continuity of care and the avoidance of hospital care unless absolutely necessary (R. J. Master, personal communication, 1997; Glover, Master, & Meyers, 1996; Master, 1996).

Although there are certain similarities in the physician-nurse practitioner relationship in all health care settings, there are enough unique elements to each arena that it is worthwhile to consider the relationship of the physician and nurse practitioner in several of the major settings.

HOME CARE

Home care is one of the most popular care options for the elderly and disabled. Studies consistently show that 85% or more of the elderly would rather receive care in their own homes than go to a nursing home (Kavesh, 1986). The abortive Health Security Act of 1993 touted a commitment to the expansion of home- and community-based care (although the eligibility requirement that a person have at least three dependencies in activities of daily living insured that the actual expenditures for such a program would be limited) (White House Domestic Policy Council, 1993). In the 1980s home care seemed the ideal alternative to expensive nursing home care. But as Medicare expenditures for home care have grown by over 30% per year since a 1988 court ruling requiring the Health Care Financing Administration to liberalize its rules, efforts are under way to curb home care expenses.

One of the things that has not changed since 1988 is the difficulty most home care nurses have in getting physicians to participate in home care. A typical VNA nurse still spends hours on the phone updating different physicians and getting new orders. This still occurs despite the fact that reimbursement for physician home care visits has significantly improved and probably will continue to improve over the next few years (though it is still more efficient for a physician to see several office or hospital patients than to take the same amount of time to drive to a patient's home) (Bayne, 1997).

Coordinated care programs, which often use nurse practitioners to provide primary care, are one solution to this problem. A team of professionals, including nurse practitioners, physicians, and social workers, are the key providers of care in such a program. Joint meetings serve as a major vehicle for communication about patient issues. If the home care program has a significant amount of shared responsibility for particular patients with an Area Agency on Aging or some other organization that deals with financial or social issues, staff from the agency may be invited to attend the meetings on a regular basis. In between meetings, the nurse practitioner serves as the primary provider and coordinator of care. A sophisticated nurse practitioner will assess changes in a patient's status and make changes in medications and other treatments as necessary. She will review these changes with the physician at the next joint meeting or page the physician if necessary.

A barrier to making full use of the nurse practitioner's role in home care has been the need for physicians to sign off on many of the things they do. A few years ago, I moved from a state where nurse practitioners have prescribing authority in home care settings to one in which they must get a physician's signature for prescriptions. I haven't seen any improvement in the quality of care that has resulted from practicing in a more restrictive environment. What such rules generally do is make this kind of practice unpalatable to physicians because it is so cumbersome (perhaps this is the goal in the minds of some) or it encourages physicians to take the risk of giving the nurse practitioner a signed pad of prescriptions. This practice, which was common in Massachusetts in my experience before the passage of the nurse practitioner prescribing law, pretty much disappeared after the law was passed. I see the same thing happening in Pennsylvania, where the more restrictive rules still apply. I don't see any evidence that the patients are better served by having the nurse practitioner chase after the physician for a prescription instead of using that time to see another patient.

One of the changes that has occurred over the past few years is the acceleration of pressures for early hospital discharge. As a result, the home care programs with which I am familiar are caring for sicker and sicker patients. Not only are the patients coming out of the hospital more unstable, we are now providing care at home for new or recurrent problems which would have resulted in a hospitalization a few years ago. For example, we treat pneumonias and other infections at home with IV antibiotics and respiratory treatments. This is possible because, at least in many urban areas, there are many more diagnostic tools available at home. A big industry has developed which offers X rays, blood tests, oxygen saturations, EKGs, and even ultrasounds at home. Reports are available the same day if necessary. Thus, we no longer automatically have to send patients to the emergency room just to evaluate a fever. On the other hand, because many of these patients have multiple concurrent medical problems—CHF, renal insufficiency, diabetes and dementia are a typical mix—the decision making may be much more complicated and not always readily addressed by a single guideline. Thus, the nurse practitioner and I spend a lot more time on the phone discussing the nuances of a particular acute problem in light of all the data we have available. The most difficult issue we address is often whether the patient needs hospitalization for initial evaluation and treatment. This decision needs to take into account multiple factors in which the expertise of both the nurse practitioner and myself is tested. First, we have to assess the significance of the physical findings which she has noted as well as the laboratory data which has been obtained. That is sometimes the easy part. The key decision often is whether the support system—which could be family, neighbors, professionals, or others—is capable of providing the level of support to monitor and care for the person at home, given the intensity of the illness. Here, the nurse practitioner's judgment is often critical.

Reimbursement changes at the federal level now offer enhanced opportunities for nurse practitioners to practice in home care settings. Although Medicare has always paid for health-related home care visits since its inception, Medicare coverage was, until recently, limited to physician visits or visits performed by nurses employed in a Medicare-certified home care program. If a home care program wanted to use a nurse practitioner to upgrade the quality of home care services, she could only be reimbursed at the level of a registered nurse. Legislation enacted as part of the Balanced Budget Act of 1997 (Public Law 105-33) and effective Jan. 1, 1998, now allows direct Medicare reimbursement for nurse practitioners in all settings, including home care (also see chapter 20 for additional information). The law, which expands a more limited 1989 law for Medicare nurse practitioner reimbursement that I was pleased to have a role in facilitating (Kavesh, W., & Bachrach, S., 1990), permits nurse practitioners to be reimbursed for home visits at 85% of the physician rate. In a period of federal cutbacks for traditional Medicare home health agency services, nurse practitioner reimbursement may allow agencies to continue to provide quality care to patients who might otherwise lose home health coverage.

Despite the gradually changing health care environment, certain basic roles of the physician and nurse practitioner in home care remain much the same, as follows.

1.   Home care is a nursing program. It is usually run by nurses and nursing is a key component of home care in the eyes of regulators and

third-party payers. Despite the physician's role mandated by regulators, the nurse practitioner operates in a nursing setting. She is involved in supervising other staff such as home-health aides, and delegating responsibilities to other professionals, such as therapists.

2. For the patient and family, the nurse practitioner becomes the primary provider and contact. She makes most of the home visits, is the first call for emergencies, and serves as the focal point for the activities of the team.

3. The physician continues to play an important role at various stages of the home care experience. If the physician has been the primary provider prior to the onset of home care, he or she plays a key role in legitimizing the role of the nurse practitioner. The tendency of the patient and family will be to call the physician first for problems. If the nurse practitioner is going to feel invested in the patient's care, the physician must delegate most of these problems directly to the nurse practitioner. If the physician has not been the primary provider, it may be easier to get the patient and family to view the nurse practitioner as the first call.

4. Once the relationship with the patient and family is established, the physician still has overall responsibility, but needs to permit the nurse practitioner to have sufficient independence in making decisions that she remains satisfied with her role. No matter what a set of guidelines may say, personality and experience play a big role here. Some physicians are comfortable delegating a great deal of responsibility, especially as it becomes clear that the nurse practitioner can deal with problems independently but has the self-awareness to know when she is running up against her limits. Other physicians worry more about being sued if a problem arises and therefore want to be much more involved in details. I have personally had a good deal of success in delegating fairly liberally.

5. In any case, the physician must back up the nurse practitioner by being available by beeper for problems and by being supportive if families try to undermine the nurse practitioner's role by calling on the physician to second guess what the nurse practitioner has done. There is nothing more destructive of the nurse practitioner's self-confidence than a physician who countermands an order when it really is a judgment call as to what the preferred option might be.

6. The physician must be available to take over the care of the patient if hospitalization is necessary. The physician should certainly stay in touch with the team to get their input around difficult decisions regarding limitations of care or issues of possible institutionalization rather than a

return home. But regular progress reports at the team meeting are also valuable so that everyone can keep up with what is going on in the hospital.

7.   The physician must be prepared to work with nurse specialists in the development and implementation of extended care guidelines for hospitalized patients. The physician may need to structure time at the end of the hospitalization to interface with the nurse practitioner to be certain that the transition back to the home setting goes smoothly and that all services are in place. In a practice where the physicians rotate inhospital responsibilities, the nurse practitioner. and hospital attending physician may need to talk at the time of admission and at other critical points as well.

8.   The nurse practitioner must be aware of her key role as the hub of the care wheel and the need to keep everyone else informed as to any changes in the patient's condition. The physician's comfort level with the nurse practitioner will be directly related to the degree to which she keeps him or her informed as to potential problem situations—especially at the end of the day when overnight coverage will usually be provided by the physician.

9.   The nurse practitioner must be sensitive to the limitations of her knowledge and skills. This is not a problem unique to nurse practitioners. Physicians also need to know when to call in a subspecialist for a consultation. But since the collaborating physician will be held accountable for any problems that occur with a patient jointly cared for with a nurse practitioner, the nurse practitioner needs to be mindful of the need to consult frequently for problems that approach her limits.

NURSING HOME CARE

I have been caring for nursing home patients for over 20 years and have worked with nurse practitioners in that setting for almost all of that time. In retrospect, the advantage of such a team arrangement would seem to be obvious. With some exceptions, physicians do not make nursing home visits in a timely way. The physician may make routine scheduled visits to the nursing home. However, a physician in the office or at the hospital may find it almost impossible to leave a busy practice and run out to see a patient with a new fever or change in mental status. In that situation, the physician may order tests over the phone and go to the nursing home at the end of the day or send the patient to the emergency room for evaluation. If the physician waits until the end of the day, precious hours may be lost while an infection or cardiac problem worsens. If the patient goes to the emergency room, then he or she is thrust into an unfamiliar environment where the staff may not know the nuances of the patient's needs and a lot of duplicate effort is put forth to assess the patient's problems. Studies in emergency rooms have shown that emergency room staff feel that they often have inadequate information to help them evaluate and manage elderly patients.

A nurse practitioner with a practice based at one or more nursing homes, or a practice combining home and nursing home care, is the ideal person to prevent these types of problems from occurring. Studies of a Health Care Financing Administration-sponsored program which used nurse practitioners and physician assistants in nursing homes throughout eastern Massachusetts demonstrated significant positive results. Not only were administrators and directors of nursing more satisfied with the program, but multiple quality indicators showed that the program resulted in care that was as good or better than care provided by physicians alone (Buchanan et al., 1989).

Based on the positive results found in such studies, Congress authorized reimbursement for nurse practitioners working with physicians in nursing homes. Since 1990, Medicare has reimbursed nurse practitioners at 85% of the physician rate. Since physician reimbursement for nursing home visits has significantly increased over the past 5 years, a practice employing a nurse practitioner should be financially viable.

I started working with nurse practitioners in Massachusetts nursing homes in the 1970s and 1980s. For most of the past decade, I have been in Pennsylvania. In some ways, the experiences have been very similar. But there also have been some significant differences related to the complex interplay of a number of regulatory and financial constraints that I shall describe further below.

The basics of nurse practitioner and physician relationships have not changed much over the past few years. The roles of the nurse practitioner and physician are outlined in Tables 12.1 and 12.2. The physician must establish for the nursing home administration that the nurse practitioner will be readily available to the nurses and therefore will take first call for all problems within regular working hours. The staff also need to know that the physician is readily available to the nurse practitioner if necessary.

The nurse practitioner establishes her credibility in the nursing home by making regular visits to the facility at least once or twice a week and

TABLE 12.1   Role of the Nurse Practitioner in the Nursing Home

1. Primary Onsite Provider

   • Takes first call from nursing home
   • Visits to patient
      a)   Initial within regulatory time limit
      b)   Regular periodic
      c)   Episodic/emergency at request of staff

2. Relationship to Physician

   • Works in collaboration with physician
   • Practices within scope of written guidelines
   • Telephone backup by physician
   • Regularly scheduled rounds
   • Regularly scheduled patient examinations
   • Feedback between physician and nurse practitioner

3. Relationship to Nursing Home Staff

   • Responds to requests of staff
   • Coordinates management of emergencies and critically ill patients
   • Case conferencing
   • Training sessions

4. Relationship to Patient's Family

   • Establishes communication with family
   • Interval contacts

by making emergency visits at the request of the nursing staff. The physician should visit at least once a week to see problem cases and make visits that are required by regulation. The nurse practitioner usually establishes a good working relationship with the staff nurses fairly quickly by being responsive and a source of informal education. Families may initially expect more physician involvement, but the ready availability of the nurse practitioner usually overcomes any concern they have, since it is easier for them to get information about the resident from the nurse practitioner.

Even though I have noticed that these aspects of the relationship between the nurse practitioner and the physician have remained the same over the past few years, certain things have changed. Going from Massachusetts

TABLE 12.2   Role of the Physician in the Nursing Home

1. Backup and Call Accessibility

   - To the NP
   - To the nursing home
   - To the family

2. Collaborative Relationship With NP

   - Reinforce role of NP
   - Initial examination of patient
   - Convey involvement with patient
   - Onsite visits—regularly scheduled, usually weekly
   - Consultation to NP

3. Relationship to Administration of the Nursing Home

   - Responsible for patient
   - Compliance with state and federal regulations
   - Medical Director, committee

4. Connection to the Hospital/Consultants

to Pennsylvania increased my paperwork load enormously. Pennsylvania still requires physicians to sign off weekly on every order and progress note the nurse practitioner puts into the nursing home chart. Furthermore, to meet regulations having to do with Medicaid reimbursement in Pennsylvania, the physician was required to make a personal visit to many patients on a monthly basis, even if the nurse practitioner had already seen the patient. This physician visit rarely added to the nurse practitioner's evaluation, but since we doubted that Medicare would look kindly on reimbursing for two routine visits month after month, we were only able to bill for one of the visits. We have tried various options, including using a joint visit form or having the physician do the monthly visits. But if the physician does the monthly visits and the nurse practitioner makes problem visits, the nurse practitioner may lose touch with residents who are not frequently unstable and not have as satisfying a practice. (Pennsylvania has recently adopted the federal guidelines for visits, so that stable patients can be seen every 60 days; perhaps this will improve matters.)

At the same time, we are laboring in an environment of increasing pressure for early hospital discharge. In my experience, nursing home residents are much more unstable now than they were a decade ago. Patients are increasingly returning to the nursing home partially treated or sent back because all treatments have failed at the hospital. It is not unusual for a nurse practitioner's monthly note to refer to 10 or 15 problems. We now use intravenous antibiotics and fluids to treat infections and dehydration in the nursing home. At the same time, health care employers are much more concerned with insuring that we use our time on reimbursable activities. Taking care of an unstable patient often requires a great deal of time on the telephone discussing the plan of care. The pressures on both the nurse practitioner and physician are much greater.

Despite all these problems, the opportunities for creative collaboration between physicians and nurse practitioners remain bright. In the nursing home arena, capitated systems of care such as the Evercare model which is being replicated around the country, emphasize the importance of communication and provide resources to provide care for the patient at the most appropriate site, which may well be the nursing home. In one of these programs with which I am somewhat familiar, the administrator of the program is a nurse practitioner, as are many of the providers. Home care is increasingly likely to head in the direction of capitation as well, and the opportunities for nurse practitioner and physician collaboration seem equally promising.

A FINAL PERSPECTIVE

I suppose that I cannot conclude a discussion of physician and nurse practitioner relationships without commenting on the exchange of opinions in the *New England Journal of Medicine* regarding the role of nurse practitioners which took place in 1994 (Kassirer, 1994; Mundinger, 1994). The editor of the Journal and an academic nurse practitioner debated who was most appropriate to lead this country forward as health care moves to expand primary care practice. I was surprised at Dr. Kassirer's assertion that nurse practitioners may not always appreciate the seriousness of a clinical problem and may fail to refer the patient to someone more expert. Frankly, in many years of practice at some of the best academic medical centers in the country, I have been astounded at how often very smart physicians let their egos get in the way of referring patients appropriately or even listening to other doctors when they are headed down the wrong path. I have seen this with specialists in teaching hospitals who, as ward attendings, become the primary care physicians for a group of patients, and I have seen this with generalists. Twenty years ago, when I was teaching at Boston City Hospital, I confessed to a renal specialist that I was a bit jealous of his role as a teacher. As a generalist, I could never be sure that I spoke with final authority about any highly technical matter. I suggested that when he rounded with the house staff, and talked about renal problems, he knew the field in depth and could be relied upon to have mastered his field, to which he responded that he didn't feel any better than I did, because once he got out of his field, he didn't have the breadth of knowledge that I did about a lot of other areas. I think the issue of when to refer is as much a matter of the traits of the individual as it is a matter of expertise. Knowing when you don't know requires humility. My renal colleague, who actually knew a lot of general medicine, had that humility. Most nurse practitioners have it as well.

At the same time, I can't fully agree with Mary Mundinger's idea that nurse practitioners can simply do primary care in loose collaborative practice with physicians. The problem is that primary care—at least in the challenging types of home care, nursing home care, and even office practices that I see as a geriatrician—doesn't fit her description of primary care where the nurse practitioner bears the principal responsibility for the diagnosis and management of uncomplicated illness and uses the primary physician as a consultant. The nurse practitioners with whom I work are not seeing uncomplicated illness. They are increasingly seeing people with multisystem disease who are often unstable and don't fit into neat protocols. Yes, they do bear the day-to-day responsibility for the diagnosis and management of these patients and I usually have no doubts about their skills. But, what we really seem to be engaged in is a series of collaborative partnerships—with each other; with the specialists whom we sometimes need to consult; with a whole array of other professionals, nurses, social workers, and therapists; and with patients and their families or other important people in their lives.

Ironically enough, hospitals, the bastion of physician independence, have become increasingly preoccupied with limiting the roles of physicians through credentialling and requiring specialist consultations before certain medications can be used or procedures authorized. Some of this has to do with saving money, but it is also indicative of how complex the interplay between various practitioners has become. The kind of practice which I have requires ongoing close collaboration between the nurse practitioner and myself. At its best, we provide superb care to our patients, using the nurse practitioner's skills to recognize problems early, initiate treatment, and communicate with patients, families, and other professionals; and my skills to try to sort out some of the nuances that my experience has trained me to see. As the health care system for the chronically ill evolves into an interconnected continuum of services, the collaborative model which I have experienced seems to be a good model for the new health care future.

REFERENCES

Bayne, C. G. (1997). New home visit codes and higher payments to begin January first. *American Academy of Home Care Physicians Newsletter, 9*(2), 1–2.

Buchanan, J. L., Kane, R. L., Garrard, J., Bell, R. M., Witsberger, C., Rosenfeld, A., Skay, D., & Gifford, D. (1989). *Results from the evaluation of the Massachusetts Nursing Home Connection Program.* Santa Monica, CA: The RAND Corporation, #JR-01.

Glover, M., Master, R. J., & Meyers, A. (1996, Autumn). Boston's Community Medical Group and Community Medical Alliance Health Plan. *American Rehabilitation,* 1–9.

Kane, R. L., Garrard, J., Buchanan, J., Rosenfeld, A., Skay, D., & McDermott, S. (1991). Improving primary care in nursing homes. *Journal of the American Geriatric Society, 39,* 359–367.

Kassirer, J. P. (1994). What role for nurse practitioners in primary care? *New England Journal of Medicine, 330,* 204–205.

Kavesh, W., & Bachrach, S. (1990). Nursing home innovation in the public arena. *Journal of Aging & Social Policy, 2*(2), 87–106.

Kavesh, W. N. (1986). Home care: Process, outcome, cost. *Annual Review of Gerontology and Geriatrics, 6,* 135–195.

Master, R. J. (1996). Pneumocystis pneumonia in a prepaid care system caring for a Medicaid-covered population with AIDS. *Journal of Ambulatory Care Management, 19,* 38–45.

Master, R. J., Feltin, M., Jainchill, J., Mark, R., Kavesh, W. N., Rabkin, M., Turner, B., Bachrach, S., & Lennox, S. (1980). A continuum of care for the inner city: Assessment of its benefits for Boston's elderly and high-risk populations. *New England Journal of Medicine, 302,* 1434–1440.

Meyers, A., Branch, L. G., Cupples, L. A., Lederman, R. L., Feltin, M., & Master, R. J. (1989). Predictors of medical care utilization by independently living adults with spinal cord injuries. *Archives of Physical Medicine and Rehabilitation, 70,* 471–476.

Mundinger, M. O. (1994). Advanced-practice nursing—good medicine for physicians? *New England Journal of Medicine, 330,* 211–214.

National Chronic Care Consortium. (1992). *Extended care pathway component project* (Draft). Minneapolis: National Chronic Care Consortium.

Naylor, M., Brooten, D., Jones, R., Lavizzo-Mourey, R., Mezey, M., & Pauly, M. (1994). Comprehensive discharge planning for the hospitalized elderly. A randomized clinical trial. *Annals of Internal Medicine, 120,* 999–1006.

White House Domestic Policy Council. (1993). *The president's health security plan.* New York: Times Books.

PART **III**

EVOLVING MODELS OF ADVANCED NURSING PRACTICE

Chapter 13

ADVANCED PRACTICE NURSING IN MANAGED CARE

Patricia M. Barber and Marina Burke

NURSE practitioners (NPs)[*] first delivered primary care in the 1960s when there was a shortage of physicians combined with rapidly expanding services due to the inception of Medicare and Medicaid. Currently, there are more than 100,000 advanced practice nurses nationally, of whom 36,000 are NPs; approximately 3,500 NPs enter the workforce annually (Fitzgerald et al., 1995).

Managed care, with its focus on health care reorganization, cost containment, and the efficient delivery of quality care, has created a renewed interest in advanced practice nursing. Nurse practitioners, clinical nurse specialists (CNSs), and certified nurse-midwives (CNMs) are increasingly viewed as providers who can deliver cost-effective, quality care.

This chapter provides an overview of the current climate in managed care, explores opportunities that exist for NPs, and presents some of the challenges they face as they try to make their mark in a time of dynamic change in health care.

---

[*]Nurse practitioners in this chapter are used to denote advanced practice nurses.

OVERVIEW OF MANAGED CARE

Managed care can be defined as an alternative to the traditional fee-for-service delivery of health care, involving, in most cases, capitated arrangements with networks of physicians, hospitals, and ancillary facilities. The focus is on delivering quality care that is cost-effective to groups of individuals. The growth of managed care has been and will continue to be a painful but challenging process for hospitals and health care professionals alike.

The need for health care reform is undisputed. During the 1980s, health care costs skyrocketed. The percent of the gross national product (GNP) that went to health care in 1994 was 13.7 as compared to 8.9 in 1980. The projection for the proportion of the GNP that will go toward health care by the year 2000 is 18.1% ($1.7 trillion) and, if left unchecked, 32% (16 trillion) by the year 2030 (Weil & Jorgensen, 1995).

Although the so-called managed-care revolution has reduced the rate of increase in health care costs by creating a more competitive price environment, creating a more effective health care market is very much a work in progress that will affect and be affected by both political and market changes occurring over the remainder of the century (Drake, 1997). Nearly one in five Americans is now a member of an HMO. At the end of 1997, the total HMO enrollment was projected to be at least 58.5 million people and may reach 66 million (Solovy, 1996). With the recent growth of Medicare, HMO enrollment could top those projections. These statistics indicate that the traditional fee-for-service indemnity method of delivering health care is a thing of the past and that managed care will continue to evolve and have an impact on and be impacted not only by Managed Care Organizations (MCOs) and employer groups, but by consumers, government, and providers.

Managed-care organizations compete with each other for members, the best network of physicians and hospitals, and competitive prices. At the same time, employer groups strive to obtain low premiums and quality networks of physicians and hospitals for their employees' benefit plans.

Consumers

It is the opinion of some that consumers are driving the health care system. The consumer is more knowledgeable about health care now than in the past, and medical coverage has become an important commodity and an expensive one. There is a certain amount of distrust of health plans due to the cost containment initiatives and the "lack of choice." Consequently, consumers put pressure on employers to contract with health organizations where there are broader networks and out-of-network options. In response to this pressure, payers are becoming creative in the products that they offer. For example, the nongatekeeper approach to health care delivery is gaining popularity and will most likely be a model for the future. Government is responding to consumer fears of managed-care efforts to contain medical costs by passing an explosion of consumer protection legislation.

Government

The managed-care concept is strongly endorsed by public officials and providers as a way to reduce Medicare and Medicaid costs and to improve quality. Managed-care plans have experienced an annual increase in enrollment of 13.5 %, rising from 45.2 million in 1993 to 51.3 million subscribers in 1994 (Weil & Jorgensen, 1995), and state governments and HCFA are increasingly looking for risk arrangements with MCOs in order to contain costs and ensure quality controls.

Government and the managed-care trend have encouraged the creation of integrated delivery systems that provide a comprehensive continuum of health care services to a community within a defined geographic region. Such systems are financially integrated and involve a centrally managed network of health care providers (see Figure 13.1). The goal of these systems is to reduce length of hospital stay and provide a more efficient and better quality of care to patients for an extended period of time—care that seeks to avoid costly hospital admissions (Medical Alliances, 1993).

Providers—Hospitals

Evidence of cost containment as a result of MCO expansion is readily apparent. Hospitals are averaging 68% of bed capacity and it is estimated that by the year 2000, 50% of all hospitals will have closed (O'Neil & Riley, 1996). Surviving hospitals are merging to form integrated delivery systems and are working to streamline their internal operations with a

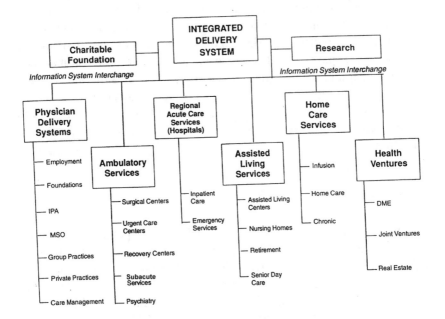

FIGURE 13.1   IDS functional organization chart.

Source: Copyright © 1993, Medical Alliances, Inc., Alexandria, Virginia. Printed with permission.

focus on clinical pathways and outcomes. A shift to the outpatient arena has expanded the use of ambulatory care and home care, and has encouraged the utilization of alternative levels of care in the hospital setting. For example, national statistics show that in 1995, 860.9 million visits were made to physician offices, hospital outpatient departments, and emergency departments (National Center for Health Statistics, 1997). In addition, in 1996, $30 billion was spent on home care (National Home Care Monthly, 1996).

Length of stay is still the most accurate indicator of a hospital's financial stability. As length of stay and occupancy decrease, hospitals are looking for creative ways to utilize beds. As a result, subacute care and observation units are becoming viable alternatives. With this approach, hospitals can provide an alternative level of care that is more appropriate for the patient and obtain income from beds that were previously unused. Along with these changes, hospitals are defining and redefining the roles of health care professionals resulting in a loss of jobs for some, the increase in use of unlicensed personnel as substitutes for professional nursing staff, and a merging of responsibilities across the spectrum of health care professionals.

Providers—Physicians and Other Health Care Professionals

Physicians are beginning to realize that there must be collaboration among all participants involved in the delivery of health care in order to adapt and be successful in this new environment of integrated health systems. Physicians are aligning themselves with the large integrated systems in the form of Physician Hospital Organizations (PHOs), Independent Physician Organizations (IPAs), and Preferred Provider Organizations (PPOs). The increase in monitoring by MCOs and hospitals for quality and good utilization has made such organizations more accountable for their individual physician practice patterns.

Physicians are also entering into risk arrangements with MCOs, where they assume financial responsibility for delivering care to their patients under a global capitated arrangement, with a resultant profit or loss. As these arrangements between physicians and MCOs become more common, and as physicians increasingly assume risk for ambulatory and acute care, they are forced to reexamine their practice patterns and to demonstrate (through outcomes) quality, cost-effective, and efficient care. Oxford Health Plans, an MCO on the East Coast, currently has 20 partnership arrangements where physicians care for patients and share risk and resulting surplus or deficit with Oxford. This model encourages physicians to monitor utilization and to practice quality, cost-effective medicine. In addition, it provides a cohesive bond among the physicians, which is critical in an environment where all entities are vying for control. Oxford has made a commitment to its physicians enabling them to maintain autonomy and control over their practices through this partnership model, emphasizing the need for local medical management and information support.

In addition to changing practice patterns of physicians, integrated health systems change the incentives for the employment of NPs in ambulatory settings and hospitals. While discussed at great length in the remainder of this chapter, an example is illustrative of these changes. In hospitals, shortened lengths of stay and the emphasis on cost containment have resulted in the loss of registered nursing jobs and the increased use of unlicensed personal assistants. These changes have also led to the increased hiring of NPs and physician assistants (PAs) as substitutes for physicians. A recent survey (Riportella-Muller, Libby, & Kindig, 1995) found that 60% of hospital medical directors of 144 teaching hospitals had experience with PA or NP physician-substitution in their hospitals. One third of the hospitals said they were planning to increase the number of PAs and NPs. The trend for NP and PA substitution for physicians is particularly apparent in New York City, where, in response to a HCFA mandate, hospitals will decrease the number of medical residents by 20% to 25% within the next five years.

In summary, as the negative press and controversy surrounding the concept of managed care continues, it is incumbent upon MCOs and providers to balance the quality/cost dilemma. All involved need to work together to ensure that the key components of quality and access are not compromised and remain priorities. For NPS in particular, managed care offers both unique opportunities and unique challenges.

THE NURSE PRACTITIONER MODEL IN MANAGED CARE

It is not difficult to see why NPs are so attractive as providers as managed care grows. The emphasis that managed care places on health promotion, disease prevention, and continuity of care is consistent with the training and expertise of NPs. If NPs are truly "uniquely qualified to meet the complex needs of patients" (Parr, 1996), then they can play a key role in the future of health care. Managed care offers NPs an opportunity to elevate and expand their scope of practice, attain greater autonomy, and assume leadership roles in many settings, thereby increasing their impact on the delivery of health care going forward (see Figure 13.2).

Hospital Setting

The expansion of managed care will lead to an increase in cost-containment strategies, resulting in changes within hospitals that will favor the employ-

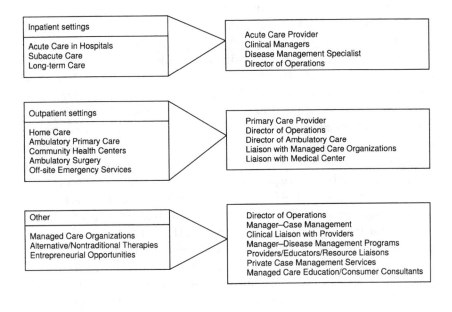

FIGURE 13.2   Opportunities for nurse practitioners.

ment of NPs. As hospitals close and combine patient care units, nurses now must care for a mix of patients with diverse needs and they must master more difficult technologies, often without proper training. The patients are sicker than in the past and the patient/nurse ratio is higher. Even though the length of stay is decreasing, the readmission rate for some of the sickest patients is higher. The increase in the utilization of unlicensed personnel is a cause of anxiety for many nurses as they are ultimately liable for their work. Lastly, the amount of paperwork continues to increase, which takes away time for patient care. Within this climate, NPs have been used successfully by hospitals and by MCOs as case managers to coordinate timely inhospital treatment and discharge.

In their effort to contain costs, hospitals are hiring NPs to substitute for house officers on medical units, where NPs are now delivering 80%

of the care formerly provided by medical residents (Knickman et al., 1992). Many NPs are hired onto attending teams, where they manage patients whose care is less acute and more palliative. It has been shown that NPs reduce length of stay, provide quality care, demonstrate high patient satisfaction, and are less costly than residents, and that they remain on staff (Cintron et al., 1993). Academic medical centers in New York City plan to hire more NPs, CNMs, and PAs as a result of the HCFA agreement to cut residency slots over the next five years. Hospitals predict that NPs will enhance cost-containment efforts because, in contrast to house staff, they focus more on discharge planning and coordination of community resources. Discharge planning by NPs has been shown to decrease the number of hospital readmissions and emergency room visits (Parsons & McMurty, 1997). Because shortening lengths of stay is one of their major goals, MCOs and hospitals are interested in having NPs organize the inhospital care of their patients. How to maximize the coordination between inhospital NPs and MCOs remains a yet unexplored area of practice. Some NPs (and RNs generally) have moved away from direct patient care and are assuming managerial positions in interdisciplinary teams. The interdisciplinary team is an approach that hospitals are increasingly using to coordinate the transition of patient care from inpatient to outpatient.

Subacute care, an area in health care that is rapidly expanding, promises to provide a more appropriate level of care for patients who are stable, but who still have acute-care needs and cannot be treated at home. Subacute care offers NPs an opportunity to utilize their expertise in chronic care, prevention, rehabilitation and palliative care. Health Partners' Transitional Care Center in Minnesota has shown positive patient satisfaction and low hospital readmission rates using a collaborative effort of geriatric nurse practitioners and geriatricians in subacute care (Micheletti & Shlala, 1995).

With fewer house officers and more NPs, departments of nursing will assume a more prominent role in hospital operations. This in turn will enable NPs to function more effectively and have a greater impact on the hospital bottom line. They can take advantage, for example, of opportunities to manage the care of patients in specialty units where they use their advanced training to function as case managers and educators (Parr, 1996). At Mount Sinai Hospital in New York City, NPs have managed the care of patients in their 15-bed respiratory unit since 1995, when the house officer slots were decreased. Four NPs collaborate with an attending pulmonary physician and RNs to manage all aspects of patient care, including patient and family education and discharge planning. The NPs are currently developing clinical pathways and outcomes measures specific to that unit.

Ambulatory Settings

As managed care expands and the shift from inpatient to outpatient care accelerates, NPs are assuming a greater role in ambulatory settings. They practice independently and/or collaboratively with physicians in community centers, hospital and free-standing clinics, schools, MCOs, and private physician offices.

It is expected that NPs will move into salaried primary care positions as preferred providers in HMOs and as PCPs in pilot programs (Scheffler, Waitzman, & Hillman, 1996). Their transition to this type of practice arrangement will be relatively smooth compared to that of physicians because capitation may not be as threatening to them. Nurses have always been salaried, while physicians historically have been self-employed and accustomed to fee-for-service.

Kaiser Permanente North West, a large group-model HMO in Portland, Oregon, employs 360 NPs, primarily for the Family Practice and Internal Medicine Departments. The NPs function collaboratively with PAs and MDs in shared-practice modules. Within these modules, the providers determine how patients are managed, depending on demands for care and provider expertise. For example, an NP who has specialized in diabetes might manage the diabetic patients of that practice. The Health Appraisal Program, a program that is responsible for performing routine physical examinations and providing preventive services, is managed exclusively by NPs (Hooker, 1993).

Nurse practitioners from the Columbia University School of Nursing have contracted with Oxford Health Plans to provide primary care services to its members in the New York City area. The NPs are listed in the Oxford roster as providers, work collaboratively with physicians, and are reimbursed at the same rate as Columbia physicians and have hospital admitting privileges. This is unique in that it is the first time that NPs have independent provider status. Oxford and Columbia have made a commitment to measure productivity and outcomes, as there is very little in the literature about NP independent practice outcomes under managed care (Bitoun Blecher, 1997). As managed care expands and as the roles of NPs increase, measuring outcomes of the NP scope of practice will become increasingly imperative.

Pace University School of Nursing in New York operates a nurse-managed primary care center, consisting of three clinics for students, faculty, and alumni under a contract with Aetna-U.S. Health Care (an HMO). Nurse practitioners have preferred provider status and provide all primary care services; they cannot, however, refer patients to specialists. The NPs in this practice are actively pursuing other managed care contracts to increase their patient care load. At NYU, NPs provide primary care in three school-based health clinics and in one site serving persons referred by the court.

Home Care and Community Health Centers

Nurse practitioners will continue to move into home health care as the shift from inpatient to outpatient care increases. There is substantial evidence that primary care for people with chronic illnesses can be best managed in the home by NPs in collaboration with physicians and other health care professionals, such as RNs, physical therapists, and social workers (Loveridge, 1995).

Medicare members are enrolling in managed-care plans at a rate of 100,000 per month (Etheridge, Jones, & Lewin, 1996). This trend will provide more opportunities for NPs to manage the elderly and chronically ill in the home. Full patient assessment and review of medications are services that can be performed optimally by NPs. Sending an NP into homes to explain medication regimens and encourage compliance has been found to be "the single most effective strategy to reduce hypertension" (Hadley, 1996). California MCOs regularly send NPs into the home as soon as they enroll a new Medicare patient. The chronically ill will benefit most from NP providers who have been shown to be especially attuned to the effects of chronic illness.

Opportunities exist for NPs as primary care providers, either independently or in collaboration with a physician, in underserved areas, such as Federally Designated Shortage Areas, where the ratio of physicians to the general population is 1/3000; less than half the recommended ratio. The government has failed to entice medical students and primary care physicians into rural primary care and is looking to nonphysician providers such as NPs and PAs to provide this care.

The Community Health Centers are the focal point of health care delivery in shortage and rural areas. Most often, funding sources for these practices are some combination of governmental, academic medical center, and, increasingly, MCOs. The Abbotsford Clinic in Philadelphia is a model of a federally funded independent nurse-managed clinic. At Abbotsford, FNPs who provide primary and preventive care to public housing residents have demonstrated higher patient satisfaction, less emergency department usage, and fewer inpatient days than comparable family practice physicians (Jenkins & Torrisi, 1995). Abbotsford, like many nurse-managed centers, is building relationships with managed-care entities as it struggles to survive with reduced Medicare and Medicaid dollars.

The Visiting Nurse Service of New York operates a Community Nursing Organization (CNO) in Queens, New York. This is one of four pilot HCFA-funded projects and is staffed with RNs and NPs. The focus is on improving access and managing care for the elderly and for people with chronic illness in order to increase compliance and ensure positive clinical outcomes. In the CNO, NPs educate RNs in how to care for the chronically ill and are developing collaborative relationships with the patients' physicians to assure joint responsibility for primary care.

The University of Rochester Community Nursing Center is an example of a large network of NP-managed clinics linked to community agencies that shares the resources of a major university. Nurse practitioners provide primary and preventive care at all levels of health and disease to underserved individuals in urban and rural settings.

It remains to be seen if the success of such CNOs will lead to their expansion, and whether they will be aided by federal or managed-care funds. As governmental funding sources dwindle, MCO contracts with CNOs will most likely increase. This may lead to the development of multidisciplinary and NP model practices that deliver cost-effective quality care. It seems plausible that the increasing use of the interdisciplinary team approach will position NPs to provide a unique service within these collaborative models. It is incumbent upon NPs to work with MCOs in developing clinical processes that promote their own and the MCOs' goals.

CHALLENGES TO THE USE OF ADVANCED PRACTICE NURSES IN MANAGED CARE

Many nurses have sought comfort in silence, invisibility, and dependency on physicians and institutions (Joel, 1995). Within managed care, this is not a mentality that the nursing profession can afford to embrace. Opportunities lie in nurses strategically positioning themselves at the forefront of managed care. This requires a proactive mentality, one that is not so concerned with the status quo but rather with innovation and empowerment.

All indications are that health care will continue to undergo radical change. Hospitals are no longer the focal point for the delivery of care. Patients are being cared for in a variety of settings, most of them outside of the hospital, and by a mix of health care professionals. This new and changing environment presents both opportunities and challenges to NPs. Consideration needs to be given to how they can best overcome roadblocks in order to become fully integrated into managed care.

The restructuring of hospitals has left a large number of nurses unemployed. As of 1988, 85% of the nation's 2.1 million employed nurses worked in hospitals. As managed care and other system changes sweep the country, sources of employment for nurses are more varied than one could imagine just 5 years ago. By the end of 1998, it is estimated that only 50% of nurses will be working on inpatient units; hospitals are expected to lay off 200,000 nurses by the year 2000 (Manthey, 1996). Where will the other 50% of nurses work? That is the question that nurses need to ask themselves. There are unique opportunities in managed care for RNs and NPs. Nurse practitioners are particularly qualified for roles as primary care providers and health care managers as they have the clinical expertise to safely and effectively manage patients across the continuum of care with a minimum of supervision (Barter, Graves, Phoon, & Corder, 1995).

Inconsistency in the educational programs is one of the most difficult issues for MCOs as they consider according NPs provider status. Consistency and standardization on a national level is key if NPs are going to attain and maintain credibility. Because graduate nurse practitioner programs are regulated state by state, their clinical and didactic training time varies widely. While most programs require 40 credits and a minimum of 600 hours of clinical practice, inconsistencies exist in the quality of NP education. Without national standards, NP practice will continue to raise issues of credibility with physicians, institutions, managed-care organizations, and, most important, consumers. Programs that prepare NPs also need to be responsive to the changing practice sites in which they work. For example, as NPs are increasingly employed in acute care, master's programs need to expand clinical training opportunities in acute-care settings (Mezey, Dougherty, Wade, & Mersmann, 1994).

Educating consumers about the capabilities of NPs is a unique challenge. Consumers need to be made aware of the trend for hospitals to use the interdisciplinary team approach in the management of patients in order to improve care, facilitate timely discharge, and coordinate community resources. This trend has the potential to increase acceptance of NPs and other nonphysician providers.

Nursing has taken care to align itself with consumers and consumer advocacy groups both in order to market itself as the primary patient advocate, but more important to offer itself as a primary educator of managed care. These efforts are by no means cohesive. The ANA has focused on HMO regulation, most recently contributing to the eradication of the gag rule and opposing RN compensation methods linked to withholding of nursing services. At the same time, nurse entrepreneurs are CEOs of national companies that educate employers, patients, nurses, and health care executives about managed care. As a result of their employment in quality control, nurses are often seen by consumers and physicians as the provider who "denies service." Moreover, Volpe (1995) asserts that NPs will continue to have problems participating in bonus systems that operate in many IPA and Fee For Service (FFS)-type arrangements. Prepaid arrangements are used more often than IPAs in shortage areas, and so in these settings NPs are a more attractive choice.

Because NPs in many states are required to pursue primary care provider roles in collaboration with physicians, the relationship between NPs and physicians presents probably one of the biggest hurdles to NP recognition in managed care. The current health care environment that encourages role redefinition and convergence may work in favor of increased NP/ MD collaboration. Increasingly, professionals are being asked to accommodate to fluid roles. It might make sense for physicians to take on NPs as partners in private practice. As managed care matures, physicians will come to realize that they are seeing more patients, spending less time with each one (as hospital admissions and length of stay decrease), and earning less money. In such a practice environment, adding NPs is in the best interests of both the physician and the patient. Patient care outcomes that matter in a managed-care environment, such as primary health care, coordination and management of chronic illnesses and life stressors, are better achieved through the use of NPs as compared to physicians. Nurse practitioners tend to prescribe fewer drugs, order fewer tests, choose less expensive treatments, and spend more time with patients (Fitzgerald et al., 1995). The cost of a NP as compared to a physician is 50%. Clinically, NPs can do 80% of what general internists do in ambulatory practice with equally good results (Knickman et al., 1993). A collaborative NP/MD practice would enable physicians to spend more time with patients who are sicker or who have complex health needs while improving the care given to stable patients because of the emphasis NPs place on education and prevention as compared to physicians.

Health care leaders and market forces will continue to change how and by whom care is delivered in the 21st century. It is becoming increasingly apparent that future trends in health care will require greater collaboration among all medical professionals. Nurse practitioners must commit to educating themselves about opportunities in managed care and align themselves with MCOs and the integrated delivery systems in order to go forward and attain their goals as primary care providers.

REFERENCES

Berwick, D. (1996). Quality of health care, Part 5: Payment by capitation and the quality of care. *The New England Journal of Medicine, 335,* 1227–1231.

Barter, M., Graves, J., Phoon, J., & Corder, K. (1995). The changing health care delivery structure: Opportunities for nursing practice and administration. *Nursing Administration Quarterly, 19*(3), 74–80.

Bitoun Blecher, M. (1997, April 5). The nurse will see you now. *Hospitals & Health Networks,* 96–99.

Browne, R., & Biancolillo, K. (1996). The integral role of nursing in managed care. *Nursing Management, 27*(4), 22–24.

Bodenheimer, T. (1996). The HMO backlash—Righteous or reactionary? *The New England Journal of Medicine, 335,* 1601–1604.

Buerhaus, P., & Staiger, D. (1996). Managed care and the nurse workforce. *Journal of the American Medical Association, 276,* 1487–1493.

Burner, S. T., Waldo, D. R., & McKusick, D. R. (1992). National health expenditures projections through 2030. *Health Care Financing Review, 14*(1), 1–29.

Carrino, G., & Garfield, R. (1995, Fall). The substitutability of nurse practitioners for physicians. *Nursing Leadership Forum, 1*(3), 76–83.

Cintron, G., Biggs, C., Linares, E., Aranda, J. M., & Hernandez, E. (1983). The nurse practitioner role in a chronic CHF clinic: In-hospital time, costs and patient satisfaction. *Heart and Lung: Journal of Critical Care, 12,* 237–240.

Coile, R. (1995). Integration, capitation, and managed care: Transformation of nursing for 21st century health care. *Advanced Practice Nursing Quarterly, 1*(2), 77–84.

Department of Health & Human Services. (1997). *National health expenditures by type.* http://www.aoa.dhhs.gov/aoa/stats/agetrend/six2.html

Donley, R. (1995). Advanced practice nursing after health care reform. *Nursing Economics, 13*(2), 84–88.

Drake, D. (1997). Managed care: A product of market dynamics. *Journal of the American Medical Association, 277,* 560–563.

Etheridge, L., Jones, S. B., & Lewin, L. (1996). What is driving health system change? *Health Affairs, 15*(4), 93–104.

Fitzgerald, M. A., Jones, P. E., Lazar, B., McHugh, M., & Wang, C. (1995). The midlevel provider: Colleague or competitor? *Patient Care, 29*(1), 20–37.

Goldstein, D. E. (1993). *Alliances: Strategies for building integrated delivery systems* (p. 74). Alexandria, VA: Medical Alliances.

Hadley, E. (1996). Nursing in the political and economic marketplace: Challenges for the 21st century. *Nursing Outlook, 44*(1), 6–10.

Hardy Havens, D., Ronan, J. P., & Hannan, C. (1996). Maintaining the nurse practitioner identity in a world of managed care. *Journal of Pediatric Health Care, 10*(2), 87–89.

Higgins, J. M., Ponte, P. R., James, J. R., Fay, M., & Madden, M. J. (1994). Restructuring the CNS role for a managed care environment. *Clinical Nurse Specialist, 8*(3), 163–167.

Hinton Walker, P. (1994). Dollars & sense in health reform: Interdisciplinary practice and community nursing centers. *Nursing Administration Quarterly, 19*(1), 1–11.

Hoffman, C. (1996). Person with chronic conditions, their prevalence and costs. *Journal of the American Medical Association, 276,* 1473–1479.

Hooker, R. S. (1993). The Roles of Physician Assistants and Nurse Practitioners in a Managed Care Organization. In D. K. Clawson & M. Osterweis, (Eds.), *The roles of physician assistants and nurse practitioners in primary care.* Washington, DC: Association of Academic Health Care Centers.

Jenkins, M., & Torrisi, D. (1995). Marketing and management: Nurse practitioners, community nursing centers and contracting for managed care. *Journal of the American Academy of Nurse Practitioners, 7*(3), 119–124.

Joel, L. A. (1996). Entrepreneurship: A global movement. *American Journal of Nursing, 94*(12), 7.

Knickman, J. R., Lipkin, M. Jr., Finkler, S. A., Thompson, W. G., & Kiel, J. (1992). The potential for using non-physicians to compensate for the reduced availability of residents. *Academic Medicine, 67,* 429–438.

Lowe, A. (1996). Reducing variation in patient care. Nursing responds to capitation. *Journal of Nursing Administration, 26*(1), 14–20.

Loveridge, C. (1995). Preparing the workforce for managed care. *Seminars for Nurse Managers, 3*(2), 89–94.

Manthey, M. (1996). The promise of nursing in managed care. *Creative Nursing, 2*(3), 4.

Mezey, M., Dougherty, M., Wade, P., & Mersmann, C. (1994). Nurse practitioners, certified nurse-midwives, and nurse anesthetists: Changing care in acute care hospitals in New York City. *Journal of the New York State Nurses Association, 25*(4), 13–17.

Micheletti, J., & Shlala, J. (1995). Understanding and operationalizing subacute services. *Nursing Management, 26*(6), 49–56.

National Association for Home Care. (1996). *Basic statistics about home care.* Washington, DC: Author.

National Center for Health Statistics. (1997). (www) Ambulatory Care Statistics (quarterly fact sheet). Washington, DC: U.S. Government Printing Office. http://www.cdc.gov/nchswww/releases/97facts/97sheets/mhc0697.htm

Nemes, J., Barnaby, K., & Shamberger, R. C. (1992). Experience with a nurse practitioner program in the surgical department of a children's hospital. *Journal of Pediatric Surgery, 27,* 1038–1042.

Newland, J. A., & Rich, E. (1996). Nurse-managed primary care center. *Nursing Clinics of North America, 31*(3), 471–485.

Nichols, L. M. (1992). Estimating costs of underusing advanced practice nurses. *Nursing Economics, 10,* 343–351.

Office of Technology Assessment, Congress of the United States. Nurse practitioners, physicians assistants, and certified nurse midwives: A policy analysis. *Health Care Services, 37,* 106–148.

O'Neil, E., & Riley, T. (1996). Commentary: Health workforce and education issues during system transition. *Health Affairs, 15*(1), 105–112.

Parr, M. B. (1996). The changing role of advanced practice nursing in a managed care environment. *AACN Clinical Issues, 7,* 300–308.

Parsons, P. L., & McMurty, C. T. (1997). NP care/discharge planning saves money. *Nurse Practitioner, 22*(3), 238–240.

Pearson, L. (1996). Annual update of how each state stands on legislative issues affecting advanced nursing practice. *Nurse Practitioner, 21*(1), 10–70.

Riportella-Muller, R., Libby, D., & Kindig, D. (1995, Summer). The substitution of physician assistants and nurse practitioners for physician residents in teaching hospitals. *Health Affairs,* 183–191.

Scheffler, R. M., Waitzman, N. J., & Hillman, J. M. (1996). The productivity of physician assistants and nurse practitioners and health work force policy in the era of managed health care. *Journal of Allied Health, 25*(3), 241.

Simpson, R. (1993). Case-managed care in tomorrow's information network. *Nursing Management, 24*(7), 14–16.

Solovy, A. (1996, April 20). Backlash to the future. *Hospitals and Health Networks,* 42–48.

Sovie, M. (1995). Tailoring hospitals for managed care and integrated health systems. *Nursing Economics, 13*(2), 72–83.

Stutz, L. (1996). The evolution of managed care: New jobs for nurses in the 21st century. *The American Nurse, 28*(8), 6.

Torrisi, D. L. (1994). Nursing centers and managed care: Collaboration and contracting. Letter to the Editor. *Nurse Practitioner, 19*(7), 69–71.

Volpe, F. (1995). The morass of managed care: Has it a place for advanced practice nursing? *Advanced Practice Nursing Quarterly, 1*(2), 1–9.

Von Sternberg, T., Hepburn, K., Cibuzar, P., Convery, L., Dokken, B., Haefemeyer, J., Rettke, S., Ripley, J., Vosenau, V., Rothe, P., Schurle, D., & Won-Savage, R. (1997). Post-hospital sub-acute care: An example of a managed care model. *Journal of the American Geriatrics Society, 45,* 87–91.

Weil, T. P., & Jorgensen, N. E. (1995). Why market-driven forces in our health industry might eventually stumble: What could happen then? *Journal of Health Care Finance, 22*(2), 1–12.

Winslow, R. (1997, February 18). Teaching hospitals in New York State to cut doctor-training slots up to 25%. *The Wall Street Journal,* p. B6.

Yurkowski, W. (1997). The use of nonphysician providers in managed care settings. *Journal of the American Medical Association, 277,* 1095.

Chapter 14

NURSE-MIDWIFERY AND PRIMARY HEALTH CARE FOR WOMEN

Joyce E. Thompson

P RIMARY care nursing for women in an outpatient setting focuses on the promotion of health and support for the practice of healthy behaviors by women from menarche through menopause. Health care activities include health education and self-care instruction, health screening, and health supervision for women. The principal foci for primary care are contraception services, childbearing care, gynecological screening, and sexual counseling. The principal health care provider referred to in this chapter will be the certified nurse-midwife (CNM).

WOMEN AND HEALTH CARE

We live in a time when women are more actively seeking to control their own destinies. Feelings of independence, self-control, and self-determination abound as women cooperate in their health care and assume self-care activities. Until recently, society has accorded women low status and few opportunities for self-determination and control of their own destinies (Scully, 1980; Thompson & Thompson, 1981; United Nations, 1996;

Woods, 1995). Modern contraceptive means, although of some risk to the users, have given millions of women a choice in childbearing instead of almost certain motherhood (Thompson & Thompson, 1981). Though some think this choice wrong, for the majority of women the freedom to choose whether and when to bear children has opened up opportunities for greater control over their lives, including wider options in career choice, improved health with the spacing of children, and improved education without interruption for childbearing (Thompson, 1996).

Self-care is a process of education and action in which an individual learns to provide effectively for his or her own health care needs. It also includes knowing when to seek professional care. Self-care skills are learned, and this learning can be self-initiated, group-taught, or learned through an organized educational program in a health care facility with the professionals as consultants. Today the types of self-care activities gaining in importance involve nutrition, exercise, self-medication, especially with natural remedies, how to deal with violence, and stress management. All of these and other self-care activities important to the health of women serve as a model for primary health care. The practice of primary health care by CNMs is based on a cooperative, educative, and supportive relationship with women as partners in health promotion and health care (ACNM, 1993c).

If one accepts the premises that women need health care services during and after their reproductive years in order to maintain or improve their health status and that healthy women are needed for a healthy nation, it seems logical that provision of such services should be a national health priority, supported by lawmakers as well as by the people for whom the services are intended—women. Though our nation has written and monitored *Healthy People 2000* objectives, there remains evidence that these objectives are not being met—especially among the most vulnerable populations of women (*Healthy People 2000*, 1991; *Healthy People 2000: A Progress Review,* 1996). To be healthy, one needs to be responsible for one's own personal habits as well as have access to primary health care services that make good health a reality.

NURSE-MIDWIFE AS A PRIMARY HEALTH CARE PROVIDER FOR WOMEN

The primary care nurse working most closely with healthy women of childbearing age and beyond is the certified nurse-midwife (CNM). The nurse-midwife is an individual educated in the two disciplines of nursing and midwifery within an American College of Nurse-Midwives'(ACNM) accredited or pre-accredited program (ACNM, 1978). A CNM is a graduate nurse-midwife who has been certified for entry into practice by success- fully completing a national examination administered by the ACNM Certi- fication Corporation, Inc. (ACC). In 1997, there were approximately 5,000 CNMs practicing in the United States. Approximately 400 new nurse- midwives are certified annually (Thompson, 1997).

Nurse-midwifery practice as defined by the ACNM (1992b) includes the autonomous management of the care of healthy newborns and women throughout the childbearing cycle and the primary care of women seeking contraceptive and/or gynecological services (ACNM, 1992c). Nurse-mid- wifery practice occurs within a health care system that provides for medical consultation and collaborative management or referral as needed, and is in accord with the *Standards for the Practice of Nurse-Midwifery* as defined by the ACNM (1993a).

The CNM utilizes written policies and protocols as guidelines for practice, and works collaboratively with physicians when the health care needs of the woman require medical attention. The protocols speak to areas of care (antepartum, intrapartum, family planning, etc), describe procedures used by the CNM (e.g., vaginal delivery, local anesthesia, intrauterine device (IUD) insertions, newborn examinations), medication that may be used in the treatment of specific conditions such as anemia, vaginitis, or urinary tract infections, and the indications for referral to a physician, such as placenta previa, pregnancy-induced hypertension, and recurrent pelvic inflammatory disease (ACNM, 1994). Though practice protocols are helpful in providing primary care for women, the CNM must rely on current knowledge, clinical skills, and judgment (accountability) to know what to do at any given time and when to call for assistance from other professionals (ACNM, 1994; DeClerq, 1992).

Given the above definition of practice, the CNM is a *nurse and midwife* who provides *health* care to women seeking *primary care* services. In addition, nurse-midwives practice according to a philosophy whose central theme is family- and woman-centered care, supporting the woman's right to self-determination in her health care, and in which the CNM's support of client and family as "captains" of the health care team is implicit (ACNM, 1989; ACNM, 1993c). Self-determination in health care requires understandable information, fully informed consent, and responsibility for the outcomes of one's choices (Thompson & Thompson, 1981; Thompson,

Oakley, Burke, Jay, & Conklin, 1989), which in turn require learning and interest in self-care activities. Motivation for self-care is one of the primary goals of nurse-midwifery care.

EDUCATION OF NURSE-MIDWIVES FOR PRIMARY CARE

The education of nurse-midwives as providers of primary health care services was begun in the United States in 1932 at the Maternity Center Association in New York City, following the introduction of the nurse-midwife as a public health practitioner in 1925 at Frontier Nursing Service in Hyden, Kentucky. Standardization of curriculum has evolved along with a formal accreditation process administered by the ACNM since 1957, with official recognition by the U.S. Department of Education as the accrediting agency for nurse-midwives since 1982. National certification by examination for entry into practice was begun by the ACNM in 1971, and is now administered by a sister corporation, the ACNM Certification Council. There are currently two routes to basic preparation as a nurse-midwife: the 9- to 12-month certificate and the 16- to 20-month master's degree programs (ACNM, 1996a). Four- to 6-month pre-certification programs exist for foreign prepared nurse-midwives. In 1997, there were 50 ACNM accredited or pre-accredited programs preparing nurse-midwives. Of these, 37 offer midwifery within a master's degree program, 10 are certificate programs, and 3 are pre-certification programs (ACNM, 1997).

The core competencies in midwifery required in all ACNM accredited programs include theory and clinical practice in the autonomous management of women's health care, focusing particularly on preconception care, pregnancy, childbirth, the postpartum period, care of the newborn, and the family planning and gynecological needs of well women (ACNM 1992a). Knowledge of common pathological conditions of pregnancy is required, although clinical practice with high-risk pregnant women is not. Both knowledge and clinical practice with common primary care conditions of women was reintroduced into the curriculum in the 1980s (original practice in rural Kentucky, New York City, and New Mexico included primary care as practiced by public health nurses). Emphasis throughout the program is placed on health promotion activities, client/family-centered care, and development of the woman's ability to know when she should seek professional care.

The nurse-midwifery curriculum in many educational programs is based on the health model of care because nurse-midwives believe in the natural biopsychosocial phenomena of pregnancy, birth, and menopause, and direct their care efforts toward the attainment and maintenance of optimal health for the woman and for her fetus when pregnant. Perhaps nowhere else in the health care system is the truism of personal responsibility for health more obvious than during a normal pregnancy. As long as all is going well, only the pregnant woman can maintain that optimal health state through proper nutrition, exercise, sleep, and management of life's stresses. The role of the nurse-midwife is one of expectant observation, watchful screening, teaching, support, and supervision (ACNM, 1993b; Thompson et al., 1989).

Health education comprises approximately 90% of the clinical activities of nurse-midwives, including teaching self-care skills, preparation for childbearing and childrearing, and knowledge of the anatomy and physiology of women. In 1996, 90% of all visits to a CNM were for primary, preventive health care. Twenty percent were for care outside the maternity cycle, including annual gynecological care and reproductive health visits (Clarke, Martin, & Taffel, 1997; Scupholme, DeJoseph, Strobino, & Paine, 1993). These educational activities also provide women with knowledge of their bodies, contraceptive choices, pregnancy progress, and general health care needs so that informed and active participation in health care decisions result. The theoretical framework of health education builds on the woman's perception of her state of health, her view of herself as a person and as a woman, her accepted roles in society, and her particular stage of growth and development (Bermosk & Porter, 1979; Thompson, 1980; Thompson, 1990).

A concrete example of the nurse-midwife's belief in and promotion of self-determination for women is her willingness to offer care options to childbearing families. Women were encouraged to make informed decisions about the frequency of prenatal visits long before the NIH/HHS Expert Panel on the Content of Prenatal Care suggested fewer visits for healthy women (1989). Women are also asked who their support people will be during childbearing, what their birth plan is (type of delivery, place of birth, procedures to avoid, etc). Concurrent with the nurse-midwife's encouragement and support of women taking an active role in decisions about their health care is the education of women for the responsibilities inherent in self-determination. For example, if a woman plans a home birth, she must also be willing to maintain her body in optimum condition for labor, prepare herself and her family for the labor, delivery, and needs of a postpartum mother and newborn, and consent to prenatal supervision so that her appropriateness for home birth is reassessed at frequent intervals. The women-as-partners concept is often clearly delineated in the consent forms for nurse-midwifery care.

MODEL OF PRIMARY HEALTH CARE FOR WOMEN

Any model of primary health care must be based on knowledge of what determines health, what activities promote health, which type of health care provider can best support or carry out these health-promoting activities, and how that health care provider should be educated for such a crucial role in our national health care system. Each individual has a responsibility for adopting health behaviors and giving up careless, self-destructive habits. Blum (1974) noted that medical care and the provision of health services are relatively minor inputs into one's state of health. He placed greatest emphasis for the state of one's personal health on a broad range of environmental factors including the fetal and physical environment, socio-economic status, culture and level of education and, secondly, on one's personal health habits, attitudes, and behaviors. For women, consideration of gender and status must enter the health equation, for in many areas of the world, being born female means certain ill health beginning with poor nutrition and little education (Thompson, 1996). McKeown (1978), de Tornyay (1978), and *Healthy People 2000* (1991) state that the main determinant of health is the way of life an individual chooses to follow.

If one's lifestyle is the principal determinant of one's state of health, what could be a more cost-effective health program than one that promotes self-care and a healthy lifestyle? A model of primary health care for women should be based on a holistic health concept fostering maintenance and/or adoption of healthy behaviors and habits by the woman and her significant others—supported by knowing both what and how to do this.

Health, in my opinion, is a continuum from most to least healthy, with the majority of us falling along the "healthy" end and being without major illness or disease. Health is a separate condition from disease, but health and illness are not necessarily opposites of one another, as explained by Gardner and Fiske (1981).

Education for Self-Care

If health is principally determined by one's lifestyle and environment, it may be concluded that any cost-effective model of primary health care must focus on education: teaching individuals to know what constitutes health for them, how it may be achieved or maintained through alterations in their lifestyles, if necessary, and preparing each individual to assume the responsibility for self-care when appropriate. Education for self-care and assuming responsibility for one's own health are key components of the proposed primary health care model, and they are the most difficult components of the model to teach and learn, primarily because most of us, whether consumer or provider, tend to have some destructive habits. Perhaps we have all fallen into the mistaken notion often promoted by the medical world that disease can be treated and health regained no matter what we do to ourselves (McKeown, 1978; Thompson & Thompson, 1985).

Personalized, Caring Concern

A second important component of a primary health care model is a personalized, caring concern exhibited at all times by health care providers for the whole person and for that person's significant others. This *caring* concern is *not,* however, equated with a *controlling* concern by the professional (Gardner & Fiske, 1981; Garrett & Garrett, 1982; Thompson et al., 1989). All people need exposure to health care providers who are concerned enough to provide them with information and allow them the space to make informed decisions about their health and its supervision, besides encouraging them to assume health-promoting behaviors, thus maintaining control over their own bodies and lives. Health professionals need to recognize the illogical nature of their demands that clients be "good" submissive patients and yet also become responsible adults in control of their health. Such schizophrenic demands of adults often leave them with little choice but to distrust the "system" and go it alone, if at all. The health care professional must also be aware of and understand the client's need for the use of natural remedies and therapies, such as herbs, acupuncture, meditation, biofeedback, and faith healing (Bermosk & Porter, 1979). It may be difficult and unnecessary for the professional health care worker to provide all of these modalities, but it is important to know about them.

Part of the caring concern for women is knowing when to use a directive approach to health care, when to be supportive, and when mutual participation is indicated. During my own research (Thompson, 1980; Thompson et al., 1989) on the process of care used by nurse-midwives to supervise the health status of pregnant women, I concluded that even though some women responded very well to learning about pregnancy and took an active role in decisions about their care, other women seemed more responsive to being taken care of by the nurse-midwife. It seems impractical to expect all women or all people to want to and to be able to participate fully in working toward mutually agreed upon health goals, although this type of interaction is an important goal to strive toward.

Health Screening and Supervision

The other two necessary components of any model for primary health care are the activities of health screening and health supervision. The health screening component for women includes such things as routine cancer smears, breast examination, tests for sexually transmitted diseases and vaginitis, and general physical fitness exams relative to nutrition, exercise, and sleep and work patterns. The health supervision component for women includes preconception, pregnancy, contraceptive, and well-woman gynecological care for women through menopause. An integral part of health supervision is the integration of counseling activities, consultation and/or referral to other sources of care (e.g., dentist), and ongoing health education activities.

There have been several models of primary health care proposed in the literature and used in practice (ANA, 1976; Bermosk & Porter, 1979; Choi, 1981; Fagin, 1992; *Nursing's Agenda,* 1991; Welch, 1996; Young, 1993). They range from minor modifications of the medical model that include health screening activities to global ideas of holistic health care in which the provider needs expertise in both scientific and natural remedies. The shortage of health care of the type needed by women as described in this chapter led to the development of the Thompson model.

The Thompson "Women's Primary Health Care Model"

My schematic representation of a woman's primary health care model is illustrated in Figure 14.1. Most health care activities are the responsibility

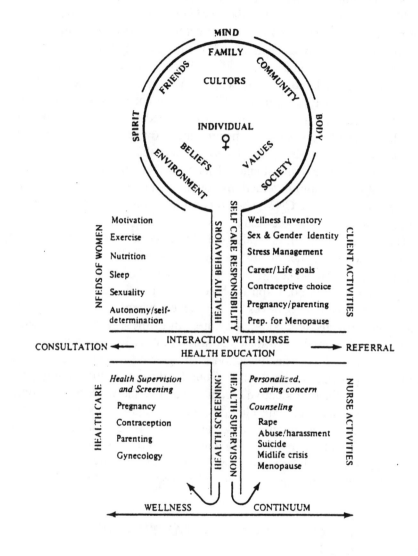

FIGURE 14.1   Women's primary health care model.

of the individual woman. Supervision and screening activities by the health care provider come after the woman makes her initial contact with the nurse-midwife and seeks out these activities. Health education is the foundation of all activities carried out by the CNM. The overlap of health activities between woman and CNM is illustrated by the appearance of certain action-needs above and below the level of interaction with the nurse-midwife, that is, the individual's point of entry into the health care system. Since there is little or no apparent need for the well woman to be taken care of by others, the health care provider (CNM) enters into the individual's mind-body-spirit system rather than providing an outside system that the woman must enter. This type of health care is represented by mutual participation/interaction providing an open system at the point of interaction with the CNM, should consultation or referral to a disease-illness system become necessary.

This model of health care also clearly indicates that it is the woman who is in control of her health and that the responsibility or decision to seek out a professional health worker is also hers. The model also attempts to portray the mind-body-spirit wholeness of the woman influenced by who she is, what she believes in and values, where she lives, and who her family, friends, and community are. All of these factors are brought to bear on an individual woman's definition of her health care needs and her motivation to take health actions. The general health needs of most women of reproductive age center around nutrition, contraception, pregnancy, care of the reproductive organs, sexuality, and work-related conditions. Educational and counseling programs center on anxiety and stress management, sexual assault, abuse, or harassment, parenting skills, role identity, accident prevention, drug abuse, and self-care skills. Specific or individualized health care needs will be determined by the woman in interaction with her health care provider (Thompson, 1990).

PRACTICE OF PRIMARY HEALTH CARE FOR WOMEN

Nurse-midwives incorporate all of the essential components of primary care for women into their practices. This "return" to primary care since the early 1980s for women throughout their lives came at the request of women who had midwifery care during childbirth and who wished to stay with the CNM as a primary care provider for gynecological needs.

The majority of a CNM's work week involves women seeking childbearing supervision. For example, an average CNM sees 140 women and attends 10 births a month. About one fifth of outpatient visits to the CNM are for care outside the maternity cycle, including family planning and annual gynecological visits. As of 1996, more than half of all CNMs work in an office/clinic environment and most list a hospital or physician practice as their place of employment. A few nurse-midwives own their own birth centers and some own their own practices, hiring an obstetrician for consultation. It is these CNMs who reported the highest level of autonomy in practice and the greatest satisfaction with their practices (Higgins, 1996)—one example of the importance of women in control of their lives. Nurse-midwifery care can be found in many settings, including HMOs, community centers, self-help collectives, as well as the newly emerging managed-care programs.

The success of CNMs as providers of primary health care services for women can be illustrated by the expansion of job opportunities for CNMs and the demand for ever-increasing numbers of new CNMs as demonstrated in the 200% increase in students enrolled in ACNM-accredited programs from 1990 to 1996. Nurse-midwives are best known for their family-centered, partnership model of health care, focusing on wellness and consumer choice. Nurse-midwives receive high marks in satisfaction from women as evidenced by the high rates of return for routine health care as well as keeping prenatal and postpartum visits (Thompson, 1997). High-quality care and the "listening to women" approach to interactions also contribute much to the popularity and success of nurse-midwifery care. If given the chance to think about it, women know what they need, if only we would listen. The midwife's long-honored tradition of being "with women" wherever they are is the hallmark of women's primary health care for the 21st century.

RECOMMENDATIONS FOR THE FUTURE

New plans for financing health-oriented services are needed for full implementation and expansion of the Women's Primary Health Care Model, or any other health model, for that matter. Nurse-midwives have benefited from years of government support of educational programs. Now it is time for government to support full reimbursement for the quality services provided by all advanced practice nurses working to improve the health of the nation, beginning with its women (Brown, 1988; Brown, 1992; Ernst, 1996). If we are to develop and expand primary health services for women that are accessible, acceptable, and affordable, we must work together with women, with lawmakers, and with other health professionals to overcome all barriers to CNM practice (ACNM, 1994). Given the current constraints in expenditures for health care, the country must carefully choose the most cost- and quality-efficient care providers using a process of caring that results in healthier women and families. Nurse-midwifery care is a premier example of such primary health care for women.

REFERENCES AND BIBLIOGRAPHY

American College of Nurse-Midwives. (1978). *Definition of a Certified Nurse-Midwife.* Washington, DC: Author.
American College of Nurse-Midwives. (1989). *Philosophy of the American College of Nurse-Midwives.* Washington, DC: Author.
American College of Nurse-Midwives. (1992a). *Core competencies for basic nurse-midwifery practice.* Washington, DC: Author.
American College of Nurse-Midwives. (1992b). *Nurse-midwifery practice.* Washington, DC: Author.
American College of Nurse-Midwives. (1992c). *Certified nurse-midwives as primary care providers.* Washington, DC: Author.
American College of Nurse-Midwives. (1993a). *Standards for the practice of nurse-midwifery.* Washington, DC: Author.
American College of Nurse-Midwives. (1993b). *Educating nurse-midwives: A strategy for achieving affordable, high-quality maternity care.* Washington, DC: Author.
American College of Nurse-Midwives. (1993c). *Summit II: Visionary planning for health care of women: Listening to the voices of women.* Washington, DC: Author.
American College of Nurse-Midwives, American College of Obstetrics and Gynecology. (1994). *Joint statement of practice relationships between Obstetricians/Gynecologists and Certified Nurse-Midwives.*
American College of Nurse-Midwives. (1994). *Today's certified nurse-midwife.* Washington, DC: Author.
American College of Nurse-Midwives. (1996a). Midwives attend more births. *Quickening,* Nov/Dec.
American College of Nurse-Midwives. (1996b). *Statement on nurse-midwifery education.* Washington, DC: Author.
American College of Nurse-Midwives. (1997). *Educational programs accredited by the ACNM Division of Accreditation as of 1/97.* Washington, DC: Author.
American Nurses Association. (1976). *Scope of primary nursing practice for adults and families.* Kansas City: Author.

Bermosk, L., & Porter, S. (1979). *Women's health and human wholeness.* New York: Appleton-Century-Crofts.

Blum, H. (1974). *Planning for change: Development and application of social change theory.* New York: Human Sciences Press.

Brown, S. (Ed.). (1988). *Prenatal care: Reaching mothers, reaching infants.* Washington, DC: National Academy Press.

Brown, S. (Ed.). (1992). *Including children and pregnant women in health care reform.* Washington, DC: National Academy Press.

Choi, M. W. (1981). Nurses and co-providers of primary health care. *Nursing Outlook, 29,* 519–521.

Clarke, S., Martin, J., & Taffel, S. (1997, January–March). Trends and characteristics of births attended by midwives. *Statistical Bulletin, 78*(1), 9–18.

DeClerq, E. (1992). The transformation of American midwifery: 1975–1988. *American Journal of Public Health, 82,* 680–684.

deTornyay, R. (1978). Primary care in a pluralistic society: Impediments to health care delivery. *American Nurses Association Publication* (G-133), 1–22.

Ernst, E. (1996). Midwifery, Birth Centers, and health care reform. *JOGNN - Journal of Obstetric, Gynecologic, and Neonatal Nursing, 25*(5), 433–439.

Fagin, C. (1992). Collaboration between nurses and physicians: No longer a choice. *Nursing and Health Care, 13,* 354–363.

Gardner, H., & Fiske, M. (1981). Pluralism and competition: A possibility for primary care. *American Journal of Nursing, 81,* 2152–2157.

Garrett, S. S., & Garrett, B. (1982). Humaneness and health. *Topics in Clinical Nursing, 3,* 7–12.

Healthy People 2000: A Report on health promotion and disease prevention. (1991). Washington, DC: U.S. Department of Health and Human Services, Pub. No. 91-55071.

Healthy People 2000: A Progress Review. (1996). Washington, DC: U.S. Department of Health and Human Services.

Higgins, K. (1996). Unpublished doctoral dissertation, University of Pennsylvania.

McKeown, T. (1978). Determinants of health. *Human Nature, 4,* 170–172.

NIH/HHS Expert Panel on the Content of Prenatal Care. (1989). *Caring for our future: The content of prenatal care.* Washington, DC: U.S. Public Health Services.

Nursing's agenda for health care reform. (1991). Washington, DC: American Nurses Association.

Scully, D. (1980). *Men who control women's health: The miseducation of obstetrician gynecologists.* Boston: Houghton Mifflin.

Scupholme, A., DeJoseph, J., Strobino, D. M., & Paine, L. L. (1993). Nurse-midwifery care to vulnerable populations. *Journal of Nurse-Midwifery 37*(5), 341–347.

Thompson, J. B. (1980). *Nurse-midwives and health promotion during pregnancy.* Unpublished doctoral dissertation, Columbia University.

Thompson, J. B., & Thompson, H. O. (1981). *Ethics in nursing.* New York: Macmillan.

Thompson, J. E. (1990). Health education during pregnancy. In I. R. Merkatz & J. E. Thompson (Eds.), *New perspectives on prenatal care.* New York: Elsevier.

Thompson, J. E. (1996). Women are dying: Midwives take action. In ICM/WHO/UNICEF, *Strengthening midwifery within safe motherhood.* Geneva: WHO.

Thompson, J. E. (1997). Midwives: Listening to women. *Nursing Spectrum, 6*(8), 8–9.

Thompson, J. E., Oakley, D., Burke, M., Jay, S., & Conklin, M. (1989). Theory building in nurse-midwifery: The care process. *Journal of Nurse-Midwifery, 34,* 3, 120.

Thompson, J. E., & Thompson, H. O. (1985). *Bioethical decision making for nurses.* Norwalk: Appleton-Century-Crofts.

United Nations. (1996). *Platform for action and the Beijing Declaration.* New York: Author.

Welch, H. (1996). Nurse-midwives as primary care providers for women. *Clinical Nurse Specialist, 10*(3), 121–124, 143.

Woods, N. F. (1995). Women's bodies. In C. I. Fogel & N. F. Woods (Eds.), *Women's health care.* CA: Sage Publications, Inc.

Young, D. (1993). Crisis in primary care: Will midwives meet the challenge? *Birth, 20*(2), 59–60.

Chapter 15

NURSE PRACTITIONERS IN THE SCHOOL-BASED HEALTH CARE ENVIRONMENT

Judith B. Igoe

SCHOOL-BASED health care offers nurse practitioners and nurses an exceptional opportunity to combine and create new forms of primary health care (population-focused programs and services), as well as primary care (personal health services). In this environment, there is support for the integration of disease prevention and health promotion services into all aspects of health care (Institute of Medicine, 1997; Marx & Wooley, 1998; Riley & Shalala, 1994).

Contrary to the opinions of some analysts, the number of nurse practitioners and nurses practicing in schools has actually increased over the last 5 years (Davis, Fryer, White, & Igoe, 1995). Their work has produced meaningful results in communities large and small throughout the country (Fryer, Igoe, & Miyoshi, 1997). As a result, the image of the school nurse has changed significantly over these years. The existence of the National Nursing Coalition for School Health and the National Center for School Nurses in Washington, DC, clearly demonstrates that primary care and primary health care nurses are committed to working together for the betterment of student health.

This chapter focuses on the education, role, functions, and accomplishments of nurse practitioners in school-based health care, and the operation and effectiveness of school-based health centers. A description of the practice of the school nurse (responsible for primary health care), and of the health needs of students as an aggregate is beyond the scope of this chapter. However, references to these aspects of school-based health care are plentiful and can be found elsewhere (Igoe, 1995; Iverson & Harp, 1994; Passarelli, 1993).

EDUCATIONAL PREPARATION OF THE SCHOOL NURSE PRACTITIONER (SNP)

Educational programs for nurse practitioners in schools had their start at the University of Colorado School of Nursing in 1969, where 4 years earlier, Ford and Silver had introduced the pediatric nurse practitioner (PNP) role and program. The PNP program at Colorado was the first primary care educational program for nurses in the United States (Ford, 1979).

In 1968, Aria Rosner, nursing supervisor for the Denver Public Schools, came to the schools of nursing and medicine at the University of Colorado with a request for an adaptation of the PNP role for improvement of school health programs in the school district (Rosner, 1973). At that time, findings from a recently released health survey concerning access to primary care for school-age youth in Denver were discouraging. Although one of the first community health centers in the country had been opened by Denver Health and Hospitals in 1965, 25% of students (approximately 15,000 children and youth) were not using these neighborhood facilities. Many of these students were poor, eligible for this care, and had serious health problems.

It was clear that the primary and secondary prevention efforts provided at the community health centers were failing to reach a large segment of Denver's public school students, and communicable disease control efforts were in jeopardy. Specifically in the 1960s, immunization laws for school entry did not exist in Colorado. Schools had only primitive surveillance systems for identifying students whose immunizations were not current. Consequently students who failed to use community health facilities were not only at risk for a contagious disease personally, but they potentially placed the entire student body at risk. Mrs. Rosner's request for assistance was compelling.

Plans to develop a school nurse practitioner (SNP) program were soon under way. Tables 15.1 and 15.2 represent the competencies and educational guidelines for the preparation of school nurse practitioners developed in 1977 by the American Nurses Association, the American School Health Association, and the Department of School Nurses/National Education Association (now the National Association of School Nurses) (1978). The American Academy of Pediatrics added its support several years later. At about the same time that these guidelines were published, the American Nurses Association established a school nurse practitioner certification program.

Between 1969 and 1989, nearly 400 school nurse practitioners were prepared at the University of Colorado. Funding to support the program came from the U.S. Department of Health and Human Services, Health Resources Services Administration, Bureau of Health Professions, Division of Nursing. Initially, nurses admitted into the program came from Colorado schools, primarily Denver public schools. Their courses, combined with closely supervised clinical practice, took place during fall and spring semesters of the academic year. By the mid-1970s, however, there was a growing demand for this program from school nurses throughout the country and the course schedule changed. A summer program was opened with distance learning arrangements so that nurses could come to Colorado for two summers for didactic and clinical work. During the months between the two summers, the nurses engaged in independent study assignments as well as an intensive year-long practicum with a physician preceptor in their own communities. Physician preceptors were especially important for nurse practitioners in schools who often were isolated from the medical community. The practicum not only enhanced the nurses' clinical skills but also provided an excellent opportunity to acquaint and recruit highly competent pediatricians into more active participation in school health. University of Colorado faculty stayed in touch with SNP participants and their preceptors with monthly phone calls and site visits.

Between 1969 and 1987, the SNP program at Colorado operated as a nondegree certificate program, offering undergraduate as well as graduate academic credit. Then it became time to integrate the program into graduate education. Today the University of Colorado School of Nursing offers

TABLE 15.1 Guidelines on Competencies of the School Nurse Practitioner

On completion of a formal course of study, the school nurse practitioners should demonstrate their competency by performing the following activities:

1. Serve as a health advocate for the child.
2. Assist parents in assuming greater responsibility for health maintenance of the child, and provide relevant health instruction, counseling, and guidance.
3. Contribute to the health education of individuals and groups, and apply methods designed to increase each person's motivation to assume responsibility for his or her own health care.
4. Assess and arrange appropriate management and referrals for children with health problems who require further evaluation and care by their personal physicians or others, and collaborate with them in decision making involving health care and services.
5. Help families who are devoid of physician services to find a personal physician or other primary care provider who will assume ongoing responsibility for health care.
6. Collaborate with teachers and other school personnel by interpreting pupil health status and provide guidance regarding adjustments and management of educational and health programs for students with special needs.
7. Identify the health status of the child by securing and evaluating a thorough health and developmental history, and record the findings succinctly and systematically.
8. Assist in obtaining an appropriate physical examination.
9. Initiate, perform, and assess appropriate preventive, developmental, and screening tests, and refer, whenever necessary, through appropriate channels.
10. Participate with other health and educational professionals in the evaluation and management of children with health, learning, and emotional problems.
11. Assist in determining the presence of significant emotional disturbances and psycho-socio-educational problems in childhood and adolescents, and in planning for referral and management of these problems.
12. Provide appropriate emergency health services.
13. Advise and counsel students concerning acute and chronic health problems, and assume responsibility for appropriate intervention, management, or referral.
14. Make home visits when indicated for effective management of health problems.
15. Participate in providing anticipatory guidance and counseling to parents concerning problems of childrearing, including those related to developmental crises, common illnesses, accidents, dental health, and nutrition.
16. Identify community resources.
17. Participate in developing and coordinating health care plans, involving family, school, and community, to enhance the quality of health care to diminish both fragmentation and duplication of services.
18. Assess and evaluate nursing practice in the school setting.

Source: Guidelines on Educational Preparation and Competencies of the School Nurse Practitioners. (1978). A Joint Statement of the American Nurses Association, the American School Health Association, the Department of School Nurses/National Education Association. *Journal of School Health, 48,* 265–266. Reprinted with permission. American School Health Association, Kent, Ohio.

TABLE 15.2   Guidelines on Educational Preparation
of the School Nurse Practitioner

The course of study of the school nurse practitioner program should add to the nurse's existing base of nursing knowledge and skills and should provide an opportunity to increase the nurse's ability to make discriminative assessments of the health status of the school child.

The following general areas should be covered in the curriculum:

Growth and Development—A comprehensive review of physical, perceptual, cognitive, and psychological growth and development and their normal variations, including the use of appropriate screening instruments.

Interviewing and Counseling—The principles of the interviewing process and basic approaches to counseling pupils and their parents, including utilization of psychotherapeutic, behavior modification, and anticipatory guidance techniques.

Family Dynamics—A study of the attitudes that affect member interactions and the critical periods in family life, including the effect of family dynamics and sociocultural patterns on health.

Positive Health Maintenance and Health Education—

a) The study of the knowledge and techniques necessary for school nurse practitioners to obtain adequate health appraisal to assess nutritional status and dental health.
b) The common emotional adjustment problems of each age group.
c) Principles of health education, including disease and accident prevention.

Childhood Illness—Review of the common pediatric illnesses, their prevention and management, and the early recognition of complications.

Exceptional Child—Study of physical, emotional, and environmental factors which influence a child's ability to function in the school setting.

Mental Health—Review of the factors that affect the emotional and psychological development of the child and his or her relationship to others.

Community Resources and Delivery of Child Health Care Services—Review of community resources, health delivery systems, and the referral process.

Family/Nurse/Physician/School Relationship—Interpretation of the goals of the team and required role changes. Review of the elements required to effect change.

Clinical Experience—Planned field experiences and practice in schools and other settings under the direction of competent instructors and practitioners that provide a transition from theory to clinical application.

Source: Guidelines on Educational Preparation and Competencies of the School Nurse Practitioners. (1978). A Joint Statement of the American Nurses' Association, the American School Health Association, the Department of School Nurses/National Education Association. *Journal of School Health, 48,* 265–266. Reprinted with permission. American School Health Association, Kent, Ohio.

one graduate degree pediatric primary care program, Primary Care of Infants, Children, and Adolescents.

ROLE, FUNCTIONS, AND EFFECTIVENESS OF THE SCHOOL NURSE PRACTITIONER

Probably the most compelling argument for differentiating the SNP from the PNP role and functions, initially, was the desire to prepare these nurses in some depth within a limited period of time. Several characteristics distinguished the SNP role and program from the PNP role and program at Colorado. First, the use of schools for the delivery of primary health care required the addition of course content related to education systems. Nurse practitioners for schools had to know how school districts operated, including their structure and organizational culture, approach to policy making, financing, capacity and resources for school health, program management models, staffing arrangements, and communication style in contrast to health systems. Second, the nurses had to learn how to set up and manage a primary care center, in a nontraditional health setting, where diagnosis and treatment would occur. They also needed to know how to obtain access to resources for simple laboratory procedures, how to expand data systems to accommodate more health information about individual students, and how to address more complicated issues of student confidentiality. Furthermore, the nurses would need to be able to bridge the gap between health and education systems for referral, follow-up, and case management of students receiving primary care in the schools. Finally, issues of role conflict between school nurses, other school and community personnel, and SNPs required additional understanding and skill.

Pediatric nurse practitioner and SNP programs also differed initially in terms of the emphasis placed on the health and developmental status of students. In its early years, the PNP program concentrated on the delivery of health care to infants, toddlers, and preschoolers. In contrast, nurses in the SNP program needed in-depth instruction and supervised clinical practice with school-aged children and adolescents.

In schools, the chief informant is often a child rather than an adult. Consequently, the child as well as his or her parents have to be informed and involved in the delivery of any health service. Acknowledgment of this fact meant that SNPs had to be extremely skilled in communicating at the child's level of understanding. This challenge has been met over the years by hiring hundreds of school-aged youth to work side by side with nurses enrolled in the SNP program. Another instructional strategy included the use of a special group of preceptors. Elementary school teachers have role-modeled and coached nurses during their interactions with young school children to enhance their ability to be more concrete in their communications.

Nurse practitioners who prepared for school-based care at Colorado received special neurodevelopment instruction and closely supervised clinical practice, so that they had a clear understanding of how students process information and learn. Eventually, all SNPs were prepared to administer and interpret a number of neurodevelopmental, mid-level assessment tools.

By the mid-1970s, the Handicapped Children's Act (now the Individuals with Disabilities Act) had passed. Nurses who were qualified to deliver primary care in schools also required the skills necessary to provide complex nursing care to students with disabilities and special health care needs. Under this legislation (reauthorized in 1997 as P.L. 105-117), students who are eligible receive related health services within the school to enable them to benefit from their individualized education plans (IEP). The key factor here is that the nurse know and be able to explain the link between the related health service to be delivered and the child's ability to learn. Interdisciplinary teams, including the school nurse, nurse practitioner, psychologist, social worker, counselor, teachers, speech pathologist, and physical and occupational therapists orchestrate this work. Therefore, school nurse practitioners also had to be familiar with developmental and educational assessment and therapeutic tools and approaches used by a wide range of professionals, and enjoy functioning as an interdisciplinary team member.

Even in the mid-70s, it was clear that emotional and behavioral disorders were as prevalent among school youth as physical health complaints. Consequently, the SNPs at Colorado also received instruction and closely supervised clinical practice in the assessment and management of children and youth experiencing emotional disorders. Although the extent of their skill was never intended to match the role of the clinical psychiatric nurse specialist, the SNP was prepared to do a mental health status exam and initiate simple interventions in school as well as to refer the children elsewhere.

The initial anecdotal studies of school nurse practitioners yielded several practice models. In one model, the SNP was responsible for the entire school health program in one or two schools. In another model, the SNP floated between several schools where assigned school nurses did the subsequent follow-up case management. The other model was one in which the SNP worked from school-based as well as mobile student health centers.

Early studies of the SNPs in the 1980s by Goodwin, DeAngeles, Oda, and Meeker indicated the nurses were capable of handling 87% of student complaints (Goodwin, 1981; Meeker, DeAngelis, & Berman, 1986). One investigation even reported a 96% problem resolution rate for SNPs. It was also this author's impression that when SNPs functioned as gatekeepers to the rest of the school and community primary care teams (thereby limiting the delivery of unnecessary services), the cost of this care in schools was probably 4 times less than the cost in traditional community health care facilities where students often failed to keep their appointments and to follow through with prescribed therapies. This estimate was based on a comparison of the average national costs of pediatric primary care per child in the community at the time versus the cost of SNP services in a school-based student health center. The assumption here was that the nurse practitioner would do the initial workup and depending upon the findings then decide if more diagnostic work was needed and by whom. This approach is in sharp contrast to the arena style of health services delivery that prevails in many school-based student health centers today, where each student sees a number of providers simultaneously (e.g., social worker, psychologist, mental health specialist, etc.).

Unfortunately during the 1990s too many school-based student health centers have been co-opted by the health care industry. Simultaneously, costs have escalated as health administrators hasten to bring these facilities into the mainstream of the community health care delivery system. Ironically, early pioneers in this field naively assumed school-based student health centers would develop as consumer health centers equally influenced and sponsored by education, health, and human service agencies, intended to deliver integrated services including health education to youth, for the purpose of improving their well-being and preparing them to function in expanded health consumer roles. The early visions of these centers had all the parties involved working hand in hand, side by side, to design and operate these centers including parents, children, and youth. This philosophy of authentic consumer participation unfortunately has been stifled and pushed to one side, in too many instances, as community health organizations compete viciously with one another to gain market share.

A CONCEPTUAL FRAMEWORK FOR THE PRACTICE OF SCHOOL NURSE PRACTITIONERS

In 1987, the conceptual framework for SNPs depicted in Figure 15.1 was developed in accordance with the competencies and educational guidelines presented in Tables 15.1 and 15.2. The framework borrows heavily from the work of nursing faculty at the University of Minnesota during the 1980s (Wold, 1981). There were three purposes for developing this framework:

1. to operationalize the role;
2. to foster uniformity of practice; and
3. to identify specific areas of practices for which new knowledge and services would need to be discovered, including the development of assessment and intervention tools.

The fact that SNPs work in settings where health and education are closely intertwined and the students, as a whole, are generally physically healthy, has always meant that their practice emerges out of nursing as well as a host of other disciplines in addition to medicine (e.g., psychology, education, speech pathology, counseling).

The perspective presented in Figure 15.1 suggests that the real and potential health problems of school-aged youth are heavily influenced

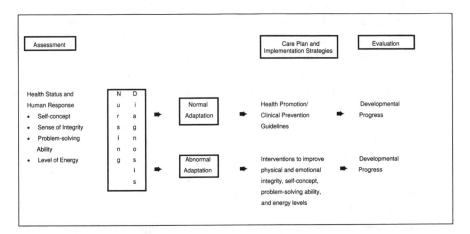

FIGURE 15.1 A conceptual framework for the practice of school nurse practitioners.

by the child/family's (1) self-concept; (2) sense of physical, emotional, academic, and social integrity; (3) problem-solving abilities; and (4) level of energy. Consequently, the subjective and objective segments of the health assessments for these children and youth target these areas. Health histories, for example, are designed to elicit in-depth information about school performance, peer relationships, and family progress with developmental tasks. Children with special health care needs, who are shuttled from one special service to the next and experience a sense of disjointedness rather than solidarity, are carefully evaluated for indications of high stress and poor coping mechanisms that interfere with their ability to learn. SNPs are also especially concerned about students who come frequently to their health office/center with vague nonspecific complaints. These symptoms often are the first signs of school adjustment problems that will eventually place these students at high risk for school failure (Lewis & Lewis, 1989).

Equally important areas of investigation for SNPs are determinations of the child's level of energy as measured subjectively and objectively by a series of questions and tests intended to identify the amount of rest, uninterrupted sleep, and exercise students receive on a regular basis as well as their physical strength and endurance levels. Although the actual biophysical relationship between health, academic performance, adequate amounts of rest, and exercise is still not well understood, an association between these variables has been documented.

Physical exams as well as health history sessions are opportunities for students to actively participate in their evaluation with their parents and the nurse. Overall and specific cerebral function are key areas of the physical examination to identify processing disorders that may slow down and/or limit the student's academic performance. Mental health status exams are indicated if the initial assessment is problematic.

For example, the ability to problem solve is a critical life skill. School years offer girls and boys numerous opportunities for practice. How well students have mastered each of the steps of problem solving, especially in relation to their developmental stage and their own health matters, is another assessment area for SNPs.

Finally, other developmental assessments are often conducted, depending on the need. The child/family strengths and functional abilities as well as real or potential limitations are incorporated into the diagnosis.

Interventions are designed to manage acute and chronic physical and mental health complaints as well as difficulties associated with poor self-concept, a diminished sense of integrity, dilemmas with problem-solving, and low levels of energy. For students who are uninsured, poor, and struggling with chronic diseases that require medications and special therapeutic services, the case management work is complex and time consuming. While some of these students are eligible for related health services in schools, others are not. Since the insurance benefit plans of these students who are insured vary a great deal, negotiation and conflict management skills are also essential as is teamwork with the interdisciplinary staff at school and community agencies. Making the link between school, family, and community agencies is frequently a challenge that SNPs and school nurses share.

Perhaps the best overall indicator of the impact of the evidence-based practice of SNPs as reflected in Figure 15.1 is the developmental progress of the students academically, psychologically, and physically. While problem-resolution rates and documentation of the cost-effectiveness of this role have special appeal to policy makers, what really matters in the end is whether children and youth grow and develop into healthy well-adjusted adults.

School nurse practitioners need a variety of data-based assessment and intervention tools to operationalize the framework presented in Figure 15.1. Health history techniques for youth, who view such activities as interrogations, need to be designed to increase the reliability of the informant. Validated stress-management services for students who frequently seek assistance from SNPs are also needed. Even the centuries-old problem of head lice continues to consume an enormous amount of time, and benchmarking of the best practice must be done. Strategies to address nonadherence to care plans also deserve a great deal more attention.

HEALTH EDUCATION AND SCHOOL NURSE PRACTITIONERS

Health education in schools is a major component of school health programming. While nurse practitioners could be taught classroom teaching skills, it seemed unlikely that they would be free from clinic responsibilities for this type of health teaching. Furthermore, their school nurse colleagues, in many instances, have already been well prepared and are working closely with school health educators and teachers to manage the classroom-based health education component of school health. Therefore, a new consumer health education program was designed in the 1970s for SNPs and other primary care providers at school to fill an existing void in the health education curriculum for schools. Known as HealthPACT, the consumer health education lessons taught by primary care providers focus on the development of a more participatory and informed consumer role beginning in early childhood (Igoe, 1991). Specifically, students, their families, teachers, and community health providers are introduced to a new set of social skills or norms for students to strengthen and enhance their consumer behavior during visits for health care. An acronym for this skill set, TLADD, helps them to remember and use the code: talk, listen and learn, ask, decide, do. Subsequently other HealthPACT lessons help students learn developmentally appropriate self-help measures. Finally, the topic "What is the health system and how does it work?" is being introduced into social studies classes at the elementary and middle school grade levels and into consumer studies in secondary schools.

THE FUTURE OF SCHOOL NURSE PRACTITIONERS

From the late 1980s to the present, numerous graduate-level pediatric and family nurse practitioner programs have incorporated student learning experiences in the school setting, including school-based student health centers. Anecdotal reports raise questions as to whether the content areas and supervised practice guidelines listed in Tables 15.1 and 15.2 have actually been integrated into these degree programs. Today, instruction time is limited and there is pressure to limit rather than expand these graduate nurse practitioner programs. Consequently, postgraduate certificate programs for primary care providers who wish to subspecialize is a sensible option.

The complexity of student health problems has intensified. The design and operation of school-based health centers (including the linkage of data management systems between the community health system and the school for case management purposes) has also become more complicated. In addition, new morbidities like substance abuse, adolescent pregnancy, and depression demand additional skill from nurse practitioners as does the challenge of introducing the clinical prevention guidelines into school-based student health centers.

Consequently, nurse practitioners working in school-based centers without experience in school health, primary health care, and educational systems, and in need of more advanced skills in mental health, neurodevelopment, adolescent health, consumer health education, and care of students with special health care needs, are entitled to postgraduate education. Some will choose to pursue an SNP certificate from ANA, others will not. In time the National Nursing Coalition for School Health will, hopefully, clarify this issue.

Following an invitational conference on school nursing roles sponsored by the Centers for Disease Control and Prevention, Division of Adolescent and School Health, the publication of an Institute of Medicine report on school health, and the start of a cooperative agreement between the Maternal and Child Health Bureau, Health and Resource Services Administration, the American Academy of Pediatrics, and the National Association of School Nurses to develop national health and safety standards for schools, a consensus has been reached to develop and operationalize a comprehensive research agenda for school nursing roles and functions (Bradley, 1998; Constante & Wessel, 1997). School nurse practitioners must and will play a leadership role in these endeavors.

SCHOOL-BASED STUDENT HEALTH CENTERS

School-based student health centers (SBHCs) have grown rapidly in the United States since the first centers appeared in 1970. In the fall of 1994, 623 sites were reported, operating in middle schools and high schools. In 1997, 900 sites were in existence. School-based health centers still reach only a small fraction of U.S. students, however. For example, in 1991–1992, the 330 SBHCs were operating in high schools, providing services to 270,000 students, but these students comprised only 2% of students enrolled in grades 9–12 (Santelli, Morreale, Wigton, & Grason, 1996). While more school-based student health centers are being located in pre-school, elementary, and middle schools, this discussion focuses on high school centers. Descriptions of these centers for younger students may be found elsewhere (Shearer, 1995; Shearer & Holschneider, 1995).

School-based health care centers are typically located in low-income communities which are underserved by other health providers. A wide range of free or minimum-cost services are commonly offered, including treatment/referral for acute illnesses, injuries, pregnancy, and sexually transmitted diseases; routine screenings (vision, hearing); preventive care (physical examinations, immunizations); birth control services (prescribing/dispensing contraceptives); management of chronic diseases and disorders; and care and consultation for psychosocial problems (Kisker & Brown, 1996).

Many centers are not able to offer a full range of reproductive health care services due to community or political opposition. A 1994 report on school health centers noted that while over 75% offered counseling for birth control, only 37% offered prescriptions for oral contraceptives, 30% offered condoms, 20% offered oral contraceptives, and 3% offered Norplant (Santelli, Morreale, et al., 1996).

Staffing for SBHCs varies, depending on the facility. Typically, the full-time staff consists of a nurse practitioner or physician assistant, a school nurse or licensed practical nurse, a medical aide, and a receptionist. Part-time staff may include a physician, a licensed clinical social worker, nutrition and drug abuse specialists, and a health educator (Kisker & Brown, 1996).

The Clinton Administration looked to SBHCs in 1994 as one vehicle of health care reform, whereby an improved system of personal health services for children and adolescents could be delivered on a national scale. Although federal health care reform legislation was never enacted, the Federal Bureau of Primary Care and the Maternal Child Health (MCH) Bureau of the Health Resources and Services Administration (HRSA) joined together in 1994 to provide the first direct federal funding, $11.9 million, for 27 SBHC demonstration projects (Santelli, Kouzis, et al., 1996; Santelli, Morreale et al., 1996).

These projects, in most instances, linked community health centers funded under HRSA (Bureau of Primary Care) with schools. Nationally there are approximately 600 community health centers. In that same year, states spent $25.2 million in support of SBHCs and the Robert Wood Johnson Foundation provided initial funding to 12 states to create new state-level SBHCs (Santelli, Kouzis, & Newcomer, 1996; Santelli, Morreale, et al., 1996). Local funds have also been raised by communities to develop SBHCs.

Community Support for SBHCs

Most school-based health centers face considerable community scrutiny during the planning and implementation phases and are established with strong community support, but with varying degrees of support for provision of reproductive health services. The goals stated for most school clinics are to improve adolescent access to primary care and adolescent health or educational status, including reduction of teenage pregnancy. Most decisions about the scope of clinic services are made on the local level, although 8 states have passed laws limiting school-based reproductive health care (Santelli et al., 1992).

Support from the parents of student enrollees at Baltimore's 10 SBHCs was strong in 1990, when they were polled regarding whether the centers, which had been in existence for 5 years, should dispense contraceptives directly to students. Sixty-three percent of the parents supported providing contraceptives in general, 76% supported dispensing contraceptives to sexually active adolescents, and 93% supported providing contraceptives with parental permission. The parents also highly endorsed the services currently provided by the clinics, including family planning for sexually active teens, annual physicals, and drug and alcohol counseling. Most parents rated the SBHC as excellent (25%) or very good (36%). Parental support was key to Baltimore's SBHCs' initiating contraceptive dispensing, and parent/community response has been supportive (Santelli et al., 1992).

Access to Care

Many researchers and government studies have confirmed that school-based health centers have improved students' access to primary care health services, especially for low-income, medically underserved, and high-risk students (Santelli et al., 1996). Barriers to health care for adolescents include lack of health insurance, lack of providers who accept Medicaid; inability to obtain care on their own because of their age and limited financial resources; confidentiality concerns; lack of transportation to doctors' facilities; and school schedules that conflict with doctors' hours. SBHCs remove these barriers by offering free health care on the school premises, where most youth spend a significant portion of their day (Kisker & Brown, 1996).

A study of 24 Robert Wood Johnson Foundation-funded SBHCs found that for a small, but significant, number of students, the student health center became their usual place for receiving health care. These students were those with less access to other health care providers and those with greater health care needs. As a rule, however, the student health center did not replace students' usual place for health care (Kisker & Brown, 1996).

Part of the reason student health centers have not become the usual place for student care lies in the fact that SBHCs do not provide 24-hour service. Tight budgets and lack of staff and resources limit most centers to operation only during school hours. Most centers must also limit their services to only their student population, and do not provide services to adolescents in the broader community, nor to children of students or other members of a student's family. These limitations may be reduced if SBHCs become integrated into community systems of care (Santelli, Morreale, et al., 1996). The other option would be to increase the number of states that provide Medicaid reimbursement for school-based student health services as well as other existing reimbursements.

Student Usage Patterns

Studies of student enrollment and use of SBHCs correlate with several factors, including race, gender, insurance coverage, and existing health problems.

In a 1991 study of nine Baltimore schools with SBHCs, Santelli et al. found SBHC enrollees more likely than nonenrollees to be African-American, female, attending one or more special education classes, or to have Medicaid. Enrollee percentages, however, were influenced by the fact that these nine schools had an overall higher proportion of Blacks and females. Other predictors of enrollment were: one or more self-reported health problem, enrollment of close peers, and membership in a school club, sports team, or church organization. The most common reason for not enrolling was satisfaction with the current health provider (Santelli, Kouzis, & Newcomer, 1996). Another study showed that students with no health insurance coverage were 5 percentage points more likely to visit their SBHC than students with private insurance or HMO coverage (Kisker & Brown, 1996).

Student use of a health center presumably increases as trust is developed through positive experiences. The enrollees in the nine Baltimore schools discussed above said they would be *most* supportive of using their SBHC for first aid, treatment for colds, and sports physical examinations and least supportive of using it for counseling services. Studies of SBHC use, however, show heavy use of counseling services, much of which may come from frequent SBHC users (Santelli, Kouzis, & Newcomer, 1996, citing their references #17 and #20). In the nine schools, the students who reported the most favorable attitudes and trust were those who used their health centers the most. Santelli concludes that "treatment for minor problems probably increases adolescent willingness to use the health center for more serious problems" (Santelli, Kouzis, & Newcomer, 1996).

Twenty-four SBHCs located in major U.S. cities, funded by the Robert Wood Johnson Foundation, showed the following overall usage patterns in 1991–1992: 29% of student visits were for acute illness or injury; 18% were for mental health problems; 18% were for immunizations, nutrition counseling, and dental care; 15% were for physical examinations; 10% were for reproductive health, sexually transmitted diseases, and family planning; 6% were for chronic disease management; and 4% were for skin problems (Santelli, Morreale et al., 1996).

Other studies generally support the above usage patterns, although age seems to be a factor in the type of services needed by students. For instance, among New York City school health centers in 1992, 44% of visits were for acute or chronic medical problems; 17% were for gynecological or sexuality related issues (Santelli, Morreale et al., 1996). Among Baltimore middle school SBHCs, 30% of all diagnoses were for mental health problems and 11% were for reproductive health problems; among Baltimore high-school SBHCs, the most common diagnoses for visiting students were reproductive health (28%) and mental health issues (11%) (Santelli, Morreale et al., 1996).

Evaluation of SBHC Outcomes

A 1996 review of the SBHC literature by Santelli, Morreale, et al. concluded that the outcomes produced by school-based health centers have yet to be thoroughly evaluated. Evaluations in general have suffered from methodologic limitations, lack of outcome data, and an unclear vision of the outcomes to be expected. School-based health centers have diverse functions, including primary medical health care, mental health care, counseling, and other social services; health education; health promotion interventions; and delinquency prevention. Because of this, researchers have had difficulty designing research models that will reveal the real effects of school-based health centers. Santelli suggests that several different frameworks are needed to analyze school-based health centers for their health, social, educational, and economic outcomes (Santelli, Morreale et al., 1996).

Health Outcomes

Generally speaking, the health outcomes that could be expected of school-based health centers would include improvement of student overall health status, increase in health knowledge, increase in student preventive health practices, and reduction of student risk-taking behaviors (Kisker & Brown, 1996). Studies so far have yielded mixed findings on these expected outcomes. Some studies have shown that SBHCs have influenced reductions in school absenteeism, alcohol consumption, smoking, sexual activity, and pregnancy, but findings have been inconsistent (Santelli, Morreale et al., 1996).

For example, a study of 24 SBHCs, begun in 1989 by Kisker and Brown, followed students from their 9th or 10th grade in school through graduation age. Findings indicated that school-based health centers can increase students' access to health care and their health knowledge, but that centers are not effective in significantly reducing risk-taking behaviors, such as smoking, use of alcohol, and unprotected sexual activity. Kisker reported the findings to be consistent with those of previous studies on student pregnancy and birth rates, smoking, alcohol use, and marijuana use. She concluded that "the nature or intensity of the intervention [at these centers] was inadequate to prevent these behaviors" and recommended that student health centers institute more intense, consistent interventions earlier, before students engage in risk-taking behavior. Another explanation for this outcome might be the disconnect between the school-based student health center and the rest of the school health and prevention programs. It is also quite possible that many primary care providers in schools now are not well prepared for these types of interventions.

School Performance Outcomes

Because good health is essential to effective learning, school performance outcomes occur after one or more health outcomes are observed. These could be expected to include consistent attendance, involvement in school activities, positive feelings about school and self, adequate progress in school, and high school graduation. The influence of the student health center in student education outcomes may be even more indirect, as the research by McCord (below) seems to indicate.

McCord and colleagues studied student use of a school-based clinic and student absence, suspension, withdrawal, and grade promotion/graduation status over one academic year (McCord, Klein, Foy, & Fothergill, 1993). Study subjects were high-risk adolescents attending an alternative high school in Greensboro, North Carolina. On average, the student body attended school only 56% of the time, 24% were suspended, and 26% were promoted. McCord found that the students who used the school health clinic (49% of the student body) were just as likely to miss school or be suspended as were students not enrolled in the clinic; however, clinic users were twice as likely to stay in school and graduate or be promoted than nonclinic students. Black males showed the strongest relationship. They were nearly three times more likely to stay in school if they were enrolled in the clinic. The greater the students' exposure to the clinic, the stronger the relationship between clinic use and graduation or promotion became.

McCord was unable to study the ways in which clinic-registered students differed from those who were not registered. Several postulations were made, including that clinic students had more health problems than nonclinic students, and clinic students had parents who were more involved with them. The research concluded that clinic personnel had provided students with positive role models and social support, which helped students identify with these role models and function better in school.

Another study compared students in 19 regular high schools, who were enrolled in their school health center, against a national sample of urban youths. In that study, the levels of absences because of illness were not significantly different between the two groups, but the percentage of students who progressed through school at the expected pace was slightly higher than the national urban sample. The difference was small, but statistically significant: 78% vs. 75% (Kisker & Brown, 1996).

FUTURE OF SBHCs AND PRIMARY CARE IN SCHOOLS

While SBHCs have gained a foothold as providers of primary health care over the past 25 years, trends toward ever more competitive, managed care raises questions regarding their viability in the future, including how they will be funded and integrated into new systems of care. Nevertheless, interest in SBHCs continues. This is not only because of the potential of SBHCs to improve youth and adolescent health in general., but also because of their potential to improve the country's social and economic conditions. For example, if school-based health centers were to become effective in reducing teen pregnancy and high-school dropout rates, there could be a corresponding reduction in the multiple health problems, unemployment, welfare dependency, and homelessness for which adolescents who do not finish high school are at increased risk (McCord et al., 1993).

Fortunately, the Assembly for School-Based Student Health Centers has invested hundreds of hours in the development of standards and guidelines for primary care centers in schools (Brellochs & Fothergill, 1995). These efforts should be very useful for health and education planners who wish to establish a school-based student health center.

An indication of the sustained national interest in school-based health centers is shown in Table 15.3: Recent Topics in School-Based Health Care. The table shows a range of SBHC-related topics that have appeared in the literature since 1985 and, as important, shows the groups that are interested in SBHCs. The table includes references in addition to the ones cited in this school-based student health center discussion.

SUMMARY

Primary care providers in school settings and school-based student health centers are effective in their efforts to improve student health. Schools as nontraditional health settings are newcomers to the primary care delivery system. Therefore, it will be important in the years to come to recognize and take into account certain dilemmas that are somewhat unique to schools and to intensify our efforts to investigate these issues.

For example, the majority of America's school systems (79%), urban, suburban, and rural, each have a total enrollment of 2,500 students or less. Hence, a challenge arises in terms of effective and economical staffing arrangements. Should there be a school-based student health center in all 15,000 school districts?

As school nurse supervisors struggle to design safe and sensible staffing arrangements, the issue of differentiated practice will also have to be addressed. An estimated 500,000 paraprofessionals are now engaged in health-related activities in schools as well as the 40,000 school nurses. What relationships need to exist here to ensure that the health services provided at school are of the highest quality?

Finally for some community organizations, school-based student health centers represent too much of a competitive threat with the student body being literally a captive audience. Yet others worry about the type of services being delivered and whether parental rights are being ignored. The point here is that advanced practice nurses have a great deal of knowledge and skill to contribute to these discussions. In the decades to come, this author believes school health care will rise or fall depending upon the talent, creativity, and leadership of the nurses on its team. This chapter has provided a historical perspective of the SNP role, educational guidelines, and conceptual framework for practice. Some of the key literature concerning school-based student health centers has also been reviewed. It is hoped that readers will be stimulated by this information to explore the opportunities and challenges the field of school health has to offer.

TABLE 15.3 Recent Topics in School-Based Health Care*

Year	Topic	Journal/Organization	Author
	The School-Based Adolescent Health Care Program: The answer is at school: Bringing health care to our students	School-Based Adolescent Health Care Program	
1985	Health clinics in high schools	*Journal of the American Medical Women's Association*	Lisoske
1985	School-Based Health Clinics: An Emerging Approach to Improving Adolescent Health and Addressing Teenage Pregnancy	Center for Population Options	Kirby, Lovick, Levin-Epstein, & Hadley
1985	School-based health clinics: A new approach to preventing adolescent pregnancy?	*Family Planning Perspectives*	Dryfoos
1985	Adolescent health care: Improving access by school-based services	*Journal of Family Practice*	Gonzales, Mulligan, & Kaufman
1986	The School-Based Adolescent Health Care Program	Robert Wood Johnson Foundation	
1986	School-based adolescent health care programs	*Pediatric Nursing*	Keenan

(continued)

TABLE 15.3 *(continued)*

Year	Topic	Journal/Organization	Author
1986	A Comprehensive School Health Initiative	*Journal of Nursing Scholarship*	Meeker, DeAngelis, & Berman
1986	Comprehensive school-based health clinics: A growing movement to improve adolescent health and reduce teenage pregnancy	*Journal of School Health*	Kirby
1986	School clinics help kids and hospitals, too	Hospitals	Cherskov
1986	Comprehensive school-based teen centers	*Western Journal of Medicine*	Davis & Devaney
1986	Evaluation of New York State school health demonstration program	Welfare Research, Inc.	Farrell, Simkin, & Ross
1986	Parental response to the initiation of school-based clinic	Annual Meeting, American Public Health Association	Brindis & Coray
1987	Poll shows support for teen health clinics	The Oregonian	Hill
1987	Health services for high-school students: Short-term assessment of New York City high-school-based clinics	Welfare Research, Inc.	
1988	Testimony on the Year 2000 Objectives for the Nation: Recommendations for the School Health Program	American School Health Association	
1988	Evaluation of pregnancy prevention programs in the school context	Book	Zabin & Hirsch
1988	Evaluation of Pregnancy Programs in the School Context	Book	Zabin & Hirsch
1988	School-based health clinics: Three years of experience	*Family Planning Perspectives*	Dryfoos
1988	Adolescents willingness to use a school-based clinic in view of expressed health concerns	*Journal of Adolescent Health*	Riggs & Cheng
1988	The Potential of School-Linked Centers to Promote Adolescent Health and Development	Carnegie Council on Adolescent Development	Millstein

TABLE 15.3 *(continued)*

Year	Topic	Journal/Organization	Author
1988	School-based clinics: their role in helping students meet the 1990 objectives	*Health Education Quarterly*	Dryfoos & Klerman
1988	School-Based Health Clinics: Legal Issues	Center for Population Options	English & Tereszkiewicz
1988	Role and success of school-based clinics	*Henry Ford Hospital Medical Journal*	Joiner
1989	Providing medical services through school-based health programs	*Journal of the American Medical Association*	Council on Scientific Affairs
1989	School-based clinics enter the 90s: Update evaluation and future challenges	Center for Population Options	Donovan & Waszak
1990	An assessment of six school-based clinics: Services, impact and potential	Center for Population Options	Kirby, Waszak, & Ziegler
1990	School-based clinic update	Center for Population Options	Hyche-Williams & Waszak
1991	School-Based and School-Linked Clinics: Update 1991	Center for Population Options	Waszak & Neidell
1991	Code Blue: Uniting for Healthier Youth	National Association of State Boards of Education & The American Medical Association	National Commission on Role of School/Community in Improving Adolescent Health
1991	Six school-based clinics: Their reproductive health services and impact on sexual behavior	*Family Planning Perspectives*	Kirby, Waszak, & Ziegler
1991	Reorganizing health care for adolescents: The experience of the school-based adolescent health care program	*Journal of Adolescent Health Care*	Lear, Gleicher, & St. Germaine
1991	A comparison of users and non-users of a school-based health and mental health clinic	*Journal of Adolescent Health Care*	Balassone, Bell, & Peterfreund
1991	Evaluation of school-based health centers in California, 1990–1991	Center for Reproductive Health Policy Research	Brindis, McCarter, & Morales

(continued)

TABLE 15.3 *(continued)*

Year	Topic	Journal/Organization	Author
1991	*Adolescent health, Vols. 1 and III*	U.S. Congress	Office of Technology Assessment
1991	Reorganizing health care for adolescents: The experience of the School-Based Adolescent Health Care Program	*Journal of Adolescent Health Care*	Lear, Gleicher, & St. Germaine
1992	Bringing parents into school clinics: Parent attitudes toward school clinics and contraception	*Journal of Adolescent Health*	Santelli, Alexander, & Farmer
1992	Involving parents in their adolescents' health: A role for school clinics	*Journal of Adolescent Health*	Dryfoos & Santelli
1992	Program evaluation of a school-based clinic: One method of demonstrating effectiveness	*Journal of Nursing Care Quality*	Graham, Uphold, & Blakeslee
1992	School-based adolescent health care: Review of a clinical service	*American Journal of Disabled Children*	Fisher, Juszczak, & Friedman
1992	Access to health care for adolescents	Position Paper, Society of Adolescent Medicine	Klein, Slap, & Elster
1993	School-based clinic use and school performance	*Journal of Adolescent Health*	McCord, Klein, Foy, & Fothergill
1993	School-based clinics that work	U.S. Dept. of Health and Human Services	Bureau of Primary Health Care
1993	The politics of school-based clinics	*Journal of School Health*	Rienzo & Button
1993	Frequent school-based clinic utilization: a comparative profile of problems and service needs	*Journal of Adolescent Health*	Wolk & Kaplan
1993	Confidentiality in health care: A survey of knowledge, perceptions, and attitudes among high-school students	*Journal of the American Medical Association*	Cheng, Savageau, Sattler, & DeWitt
1993	Confidential health services for adolescents	*Journal of the American Medical Association*	Council on Scientific Affairs

TABLE 15.3 *(continued)*

Year	Topic	Journal/Organization	Author
1993	A guide to school-based and school-linked health centers: Vol. II: Designing and implementing school-based and school-linked health centers	Center for Population Options	Hauser
1993	Healthy caring: A process evaluation of the Robert Wood Johnson Foundation's School-Based Adolescent Health Care Program	Book	Marks & Marzke
1993	AIDS risk reduction among a multi-ethnic sample of urban high-school students	*Journal of the American Medical Association*	Walter & Vaughn
1993	The effects of school-based health clinics in St. Paul on school-wide birthrates	Family Planning Perspectives	Kirby, Resnick, & Downes
1993	Opportunities for enhancing preventive and primary care through school-based health centers: Three states' Title V program experiences	Association of Maternal and Child Health Programs, Washington, DC	
1993	School-based health centers and managed care	U.S. Dept. of Health and Human Services	Office of Inspector General
1994	Full Service Schools: A revolution in health and social services for children, youth, and families	Book	Dryfoos
1994	School-based programs to reduce risk-taking behaviors: Sexuality and HIV/AIDS education, health clinics, and condom availability programs	American Enterprise Institute for Public Policy Research	Kirby
1994	School-based and school-linked health centers: Update 1993	Center for Population Options	McKinney & Peak
1994	Health care reform: School-based health centers can promote access to care	General Accounting Office, Washington, DC	
1994	School (health) nursing in the era of health care reform: What is the outlook?	*Journal of School Health*	Salmon

(continued)

TABLE 15.3 *(continued)*

Year	Topic	Journal/Organization	Author
1994	Current issues of comprehensive school-based health centers: Defining services, financing in a managed care environment, and staffing	Center of Population and Family Health & Columbia University School of Public Health	Brellochs & Fothergill
1995	State initiatives to support school-based health centers: A national survey	*Journal of Adolescent Health*	Schlitt, Rickett, & Montgomery
1995	School-based health centers and managed care health plans: Partners in primary care	*Journal of Public Health Management Practice*	Zimmerman & Reif
1996	Student attitudes toward school-based health centers	*Journal of Adolescent Health*	Santelli, Kouzis, & Newcomer
1996	Patterns of ICD-9 diagnosis among adolescents using school-based clinics: Diagnostic categories by school level and gender	*Journal of Adolescent Health*	Borenstein
1996	School health centers and primary care for adolescents: A review of the literature	*Journal of Adolescent Health*	Santelli
1996	Do school-based health centers improve adolescents' access to health care, health status, and risk-taking behavior?	*Journal of Adolescent Health*	Kisker & Brown
1997	Cost of Interdisciplinary Practice in a School-Based Health Center	Outcomes Management for Nursing Practice	Walker, Baker, & Chiverton
1997	School Clinics and Socialized Medicine	*Education Reporter*	Young
1998	School-Based Health Care: Adolescent Health Services in School	Book	Lear

*Citations are located in the reference list at the end of the chapter.

REFERENCES

American Medical Association, Council on Scientific Affairs. (1989). Providing medical services through school-based health programs. *Journal of the American Medical Association, 261,* 1939–1942.

American Nurses Association. (1992). *Expanding school health services to serve families in the 21st century.* Washington, DC: American Nurses Association. Available from the Office of School Health, University of Colorado Health Sciences Center, Denver, CO.

American Nurses Association, American School Health Association, National Education Association, Department of School Nurses. (1978). Guidelines on educational preparation and competencies of school nurse practitioners: A joint statement. *Journal of School Health, 48,* 265–266.

American School Health Association. (1988, April). *Testimony on the Year 2000 objectives for the nation: Recommendations for the School Health Program.* Dayton, OH.

Association of Maternal and Child Health Programs. (1993). *Opportunities for enhancing preventive and primary care through school-based health centers: Three states' Title V program experiences.* Washington, DC: Association of Maternal and Child Health Programs.

Balassone, M. L., Bell, M., & Peterfreund, N. (1991). A comparison of users and nonusers of a school-based health and mental health clinic. *Journal of Adolescent Health, 12,* 240–246.

Borenstein, P. E. (1996). Patterns of ICD-9 diagnoses among adolescents using school-based clinics: Diagnostic categories by school level and gender. *Journal of Adolescent Health, 18,* 203–210.

Bradley, B. (1998). Establishing a research agenda for school nursing. *Journal of School Nursing, 14,* 4–13.

Brellochs, C., & Fothergill, K. (1995). *Ingredients for success: Comprehensive school-based centers.* A special report on the 1993 national work group meetings. Bronx, NY: The School Health Policy Initiative, Montefiore Medical Center, Albert Einstein College of Medicine.

Brindis, C. D., & Coray, G. (1986, Oct. 1). *Parental response to the initiation of school-based clinics.* Paper presented at the Annual Meeting of the American Public Health Association, Population and Family Planning Section.

Brindis, C. D., McCarter, V., Morales, S., Dobrin, C., Wolfe, A., & Kidd, Z. (1991). *Evaluation of school-based health centers in California, 1990–1991: Annual Report to the Carnegie Corporation of New York and The Stuart Foundations.* San Francisco: Center for Reproductive Health Policy Research.

Bureau of Primary Health Care. (1993). *School-based clinics that work.* Washington, DC: United States Department of Health and Human Services, Public Health Service, Health Resources and Services Administration, Division of Programs for Special Populations.

Cheng, T. L., Savageau, J. A., Sattler, A. L., & DeWitt, T. G. (1993). Confidentiality in health care: A survey of knowledge, perceptions, and attitudes among high school students. *Journal of the American Medical Association, 269,* 1404–1407.

Cherskov, M. (1986). School clinics help kids and hospitals, too. *Hospitals, 60,* 95.

Constante, C., & Wessel, G. (1997). School Nursing Research: Are you ready to get involved? *Journal of School Health, 67,* 315.

Council on Scientific Affairs, American Medical Association. (1989). Providing medical services through school-based health programs. *Journal of the American Medical Association, 13,* 1939–1942.

Council on Scientific Affairs, American Medical Association. (1993). Confidential health services for adolescents. *Journal of the American Medical Association, 269,* 1420–1424.

Davis, J. M., & Devaney, J. M. (1986). Comprehensive school-based teen centers. *Western Journal of Medicine, 144,* 625–626.

Davis, M., Fryer, G., White, S., & Igoe, J. (1995). *A closer look: A report of select findings from the National School Health Survey 1993–94.* Denver, CO: Office of School Health, University of Colorado Health Sciences Center.

Donovan, P., & Waszak, C. (1989). *School-based clinics enter the '90s: Update evaluation and future challenges.* Washington, DC: Support Center for School-based clinics, Center for Population Options.

Dryfoos, J. (1994). *Full service schools.* San Francisco: Jossey-Bass.

Dryfoos, J. (1988). School-based health clinics: Three years of experience. *Family Planning Perspective, 20,* 193–200.

Dryfoos, J. G. (1985). School-based health clinics: A new approach to preventing adolescent pregnancy?. *Family Planning Perspective, 17,* 70–75.

Dryfoos, J. G., & Klerman, L. V. (1988). School-based clinics: Their role in helping students meet the 1990 objectives. *Health Education Quarterly, 15,* 71–80.

Dryfoos, J., & Santelli, J. (1992). Involving parents in their adolescents' health: A role for school clinics. *Journal of Adolescent Health, 13,* 259–260.

Edwards, L. E., Steinman, M. E., Arnold, K. A., & Hakanson, Y. E. (1980). Adolescent pregnancy prevention services in high school clinics. *Family Planning Perspective, 12,* 6–14.

English, A., & Tereszkiewicz, L. (1988). *School-based health clinics: Legal issues.* Washington, DC: Center for Population Options.

Farrell, G., Simkin, L. S., & Ross, T. (1986). *Evaluation of the New York state school health demonstration program: Final report.* Albany, NY: Welfare Research, Inc.

Fisher, M., Juszczak, L., Friedman, S. B., Schneider, M., & Chapar, G. (1992). School-based adolescent health care: Review of a clinical service. *American Journal of Diseases in Children, 146,* 615–621.

Ford, L. (1979). The future of pediatric nurse practitioners. Commentary. *Pediatrics, 64,* 113–114.

Fox, H. B., Wicks, L. B., & Lipson, D. J. (1992). *Improving access to comprehensive health care through school-based programs.* Washington, DC: Fox Health Policy Consultants, Inc.

Fryer, G., Igoe, J., & Miyoshi, T. (1997). Considering school health program screening services as a cost offset: A comparison of existing reimbursements in one state. *Journal of School Nursing, 13,* 18–21.

General Accounting Office. (1994). *Health care reform: School-based health centers can promote access to care.* Washington, DC: General Accounting Office.

Gonzales, C., Mulligan, D., & Kaufman, A. (1985). Adolescent health care: Improving access by school-based services. *Journal of Family Practice, 21,* 263–270.

Goodwin, L. D. (1981). The effectiveness of nurse practitioners: A review of the literature. *Journal of School Health, 51,* 623–624.

Graham, M. V., Uphold, C. R., Blakeslee, D. J., Gibbons, R. B., & Barnes, M. M. (1992). Program evaluation of a school-based clinic: One method of demonstrating effectiveness. *Journal of Nursing Care Quality, 7,* 70–79.

Hauser, D. (1993). *A guide to school-based and school-linked health centers: Vol. III: Designing and implementing school-based and school-linked health centers.* Washington, DC: Center for Population Options.

Hill, A. (1987, March 1). *Poll shows support for teen health clinics.* Portland, OR, The Oregonian.

Hyche-Williams, H., & Waszak, C. (1990). *School-based clinic update 1990.* Washington, DC: Center for Population Options.

Igoe, J. B. (1991). Empowerment of children and youth for consumer self-care. *American Journal of Health Promotion, 6,* 55–64.

Igoe, J. B. (1995). School health: Designing the policy environment through understanding. *Nursing Policy Forum,* 13–36.

Institute of Medicine. (1997). *Schools and health: Our nation's investment.* Washington, DC: National Academy Press.

Iverson, C. J., & Harp, B. (1994). School nursing in the 21st century: Prediction and readiness. *Journal of School Nursing, 10,* 19–24.

Jemmott, J. J., Jemmott, L. S., & Fong, G. T. (1992). Reductions in HIV risk-associated sexual behaviors among black male adolescents: Effect of AIDS prevention intervention. *American Journal of Public Health, 82,* 372–377.

Joiner, T. (1988). The role and success of school-based clinics. *Henry Ford Hospital Medical Journal, 36,* 230–231.

Keenan, T. (1986). School-based adolescent health care programs. *Pediatric Nursing, 12,* 365–369.

Kirby, D. (1994, January 24). *School-based programs to reduce sexual risk-taking behaviors: Sexuality and HIV/AIDS education, health clinics, and condom availability programs.* Paper prepared for the American Enterprise Institute for Public Policy Research Seminar on Sex Education and Condom Distribution Programs in the Schools.

Kirby, D. (1990). Comprehensive school health and the larger community: Issues and a possible scenario. *Journal of School Health, 60,* 170–177.

Kirby, D. (1986). Comprehensive school-based health clinics: A growing movement to improve adolescent health and reduce teenage pregnancy. *Journal of School Health, 56,* 289–291.

Kirby, D., Lovick, S., Levin-Epstein, J., & Hadley, E. (1985). *School-based health clinics: An emerging approach to improving adolescent health and addressing teenage pregnancy.* Washington, DC: Center for Population Options.

Kirby, D., Resnick, M. D., Downes, B., Kocher, T., Gunderson, P., Potthoff, S., Zelterman, D., & Blum, R. W. (1993). The effects of school-based health clinics in St. Paul on school-wide birthrates. *Family Planning Perspective, 25,* 12–16.

Kirby, D., Waszak, C., & Ziegler, J. (1990). *An assessment of six school-based clinics: Services, impact and potential.* Washington, DC: Center for Population Options.

Kirby, D., Waszak, C., & Ziegler, J. (1991). Six school-based clinics: Their reproductive health services and impact on sexual behavior. *Family Planning Perspective, 23,* 6–16.

Kisker, E. E., & Brown, R. S. (1996). Do school-based health centers improve adolescents' access to health care, health status, & risk-taking behavior. *Journal of Adolescent Health, 18,* 335–343.

Klein, J. D., Slap, G. B., Elster, A. B., & Cohen, S. E. (1992). Access to health care for adolescents: A position paper for the Society of Adolescent Medicine. *Journal of Adolescent Health, 13,* 162–170.

Lear, J. (1998). *School-Based Health Care.* in Friedman, S. B., Fisher, M., Schonberg, D. K., & Alderman, E. (Eds.), *Comprehensive adolescent health.* St. Louis: Mosby.

Lear, J. G., Gleicher, H. B., St. Germaine, A., & Porter, P. J. (1991). Reorganizing health care for adolescents: The experience of the School-Based Adolescent Health Care Program. *Journal of Adolescent Health, 12,* 450–458.

Lewis, C., & Lewis, M. A. (1989). Educational outcomes and illness behaviors of participants in a child-initiated care system: A 12-year follow-up study. *Pediatrics, 84,* 845–850.

Lioske, S. (1985). Health clinics in high schools. *Journal of American Medical Women's Association, 41,* 106–126.

Marks, E. L., & Marzke, C. H. (1993). *Healthy caring: A process evaluation of the Robert Wood Johnson Foundation's School-Based Adolescent Health Care Program.* Princeton, NJ: Mathtech, Inc.

Marx, E., & Wooley, S. F., with D. Northrop (Ed.). (1998). *Health is academic.* New York: Teachers College Press.

McCord, M. T., Klein, J. D., Foy, J. M., & Fothergill, K. (1993). School-based clinic use and school performance. *Journal of Adolescent Health, 14,* 91–98.

McKinney, D. H., & Peak, G. L. (1994). *School-based and school-linked health centers: Update 1993.* Washington, DC: Center for Population Options.

Meeker, R. J., DeAngelis, C., Berman, B., Freeman, H. E., & Oda, D. (1986). A comprehensive school health initiative. *Image: Journal of Nursing Scholarship, 18,* 86–91.

Millstein, S. (1988). *The potential of school-linked centers to promote adolescent health and development.* Washington, DC: Carnegie Council on Adolescent Development, Carnegie Corporation of New York.

National Center for Youth Law, and the Center for Population Options. (1989). *School-based health clinics: Legal issues.* San Francisco, CA: National Center for Youth Law.

National Commission on the Role of the School and the Community in Improving Adolescent Health. (1991). *Code Blue: Uniting for healthier youth.* National Association of State Boards of Education and American Medical Association.

National Health Policy Forum. (1992). *Creating a vision for child health: School-based clinics confront access, training, coordinating, and funding issues. Issue Brief No. 598.* Washington, DC: George Washington University.

National Nursing Coalition for School Health. (1995). Issues, priority actions, and possible means to implement priority actions. *Journal of School Health, 65,* 370–385.

Office of Inspector General. (1993). *School-based health centers and managed care.* Washington, DC: United States Department of Health and Human Services.

Passarelli, C. (1993). *School nursing: Trends for the future.* Washington, DC: National Health and Education Consortium.

Rienzo, B. A., & Button, J. W. (1993). The politics of school-based clinics: A community-level analysis. *Journal of School Health, 63,* 266–272.

Riggs, S., & Cheng, T. (1988). Adolescents willingness to use a school-based clinic in view of expressed health concerns. *Journal of Adolescent Health Care, 9,* 208–213.

Riley, R., & Shalala, D. (1994). Joint statement on school health by the Secretaries of Education and Health and Human Services. *Journal of School Health, 64,* 135–136.

Robert Wood Johnson Foundation. (1986, April). *The school-based adolescent health care program.* Washington, DC: Author.

Rosner, A. (1973). Cooperation and change in child health care. *Journal of School Health, 43,* 83–84.

Salmon, M. E. (1994). School (health) nursing in the era of health care reform: What is the outlook? *Journal of School Health, 64,* 137–149.

Santelli, J., Alexander, M., Farmer, M., Papa, P., Johnson, T., Rosenthal, B., & Hotra, D. (1992). Bringing parents into school clinics: Parent attitudes toward school clinics and contraception. *Journal of Adolescent Health, 13,* 269–274.

Santelli, J., Kouzis, A., & Newcomer, S. (1996). Students' attitudes toward school-based health centers. *Journal of Adolescent Health, 18,* 339–346.

Santelli, J., Morreale, M., Wigton, A., & Grayson, H. (1996, May). School health centers and primary care for adolescents: A review of the literature. *Journal of Adolescent Health, 18*(5), 357–366.

Schlitt, J. J., Rickett, K. D., Montgomery, L. L., & Lear, J. G. (1995). State initiatives to support school-based health: A national survey. *Journal of Adolescent Health, 17,* 68–76.

School Health Policy Initiative, Division of Adolescent Medicine, Department of Pediatrics, Montefiore Medical Center. (1996). *A partnership for quality and access to school-based health centers and health plans.* Bronx, NY: Author.

School-Based Adolescent Health Care Program, The. (1993). *The answer is at school: Bringing health care to our students.* Washington, DC: Robert Wood Johnson Foundation.

Shearer, C. A. (1995). *Where the kids are: How to work with schools to create elementary-school-based health centers, a primer for health professionals.* Washington, DC: National Health and Education Consortium.

Shearer, C. A., & Holschneider, S. O. M. (1995). *Starting young: School-based health centers at the elementary level.* Washington, DC: National Health and Education Consortium.

Silver, H. K., Igoe, J. B., & McAtee, P. (1976). The school nurse practitioner: Providing improved health care to children. *Pediatrics, 58,* 580–584.

U.S. Congress, Office of Technology Assessment. (1991). *Adolescent health, Vols. I and III (OTA-H-467 and OTA-H-468).* Washington, DC: U.S. Government Printing Office.

Walker, P. H., Baker, J. J., & Civerton, P. (1997). Costs of interdisciplinary practice in a school-based health center. *Outcomes Management for Nursing Practice, 2,* 37–44.

Walker, P., Bowllan, N., Chevalier, N., Gallo, S., & Lawrence, L. (1996). School-based care: Clinical challenges and research opportunities. *Journal of the Society of Pediatric Nursing, 1,* 64–74.

Walter, J., & Vaughn, R. D. (1993). AIDS risk reduction among a multiple-ethnic sample of urban high school students. *Journal of the American Medical Association, 270,* 725–730.

Waszak, C., & Neidell, S. (1991). *School-based and school-linked clinics: Update 1991.* Washington, DC: Center for Population Options.

Welfare Research, Inc. (1987, June 3). *Health services for high school students: Short-term assessment of New York City high-school-based clinics.* New York: Welfare Research, Inc.

Wold, S. (1981). *Assessing and promoting adaptation in school populations in school nursing: A framework for practice* (pp. 77–82). North Branch, MN: Sunrise River Press.

Wolk, L. I., & Kaplan, D. W. (1993). Frequent school-based clinic utilization: A comparative profile of problems and service needs. *Journal of Adolescent Health, 14,* 458–463.

Young, G. (1997). School clinics and socialized medicine. *Education Reporter,* 7–11.

Zabin, L. S., & Hirsch, M. B. (1988). *Evaluation of pregnancy prevention programs in the school context.* Lexington, MA: Lexington Books.

Zabin, L. S., Hirsch, M. B., Smith, E. A., Streett, R., & Hardy, J. B. (1986). Evaluation of a pregnancy-prevention program for urban teenagers. *Family Planning Perspective, 18,* 119–126.

Zimmerman, D. J., & Reif, C. J. (1995). School-based health centers and managed care health plans: Partners in primary care. *Journal of Public Health Management Practice, 1,* 33–39.

Chapter 16

MEETING THE NEEDS
OF OLDER ADULTS
FOR PRIMARY HEALTH CARE

Geraldine S. Paier and Neville E. Strumpf

> "Compassion, patience, and a sense of proportion, humor, and
> adequate awareness of the dynamics of human behavior are
> a circle of safety in which to gather strength; the elderly person
> needs a health care worker who is an advocate and a friend."
> Doris Schwartz (1981, p. 104)

HEALTH care services in the United States are undergoing more rapid change than at any other time in recent history. Professionals and consumers alike are made uneasy by an evolving system preoccupied with acquisition and consolidation of health care institutions, care delivered in a managed-care environment, and a blurring of lines between traditional nonprofit, community-based health care and for-profit, national corporations in the "business" of health care. These changes are being driven by multiple factors including cost containment demands from both the public and private sector, the demographic imperative of a burgeoning population of elders, morbidity and mortality increasingly caused by chronic disease and lifestyle factors, and continuing advances in medical and communication technology. Some health professionals decry the movement to managed care as a loss of autonomy for both practitioner and patient, a "bottom-line" approach to the delivery of care with emphasis on denial of services. Others envision the positive potential of a new health care environment focused on the health outcomes of a targeted population as the first real opportunity to invest in the provision of primary care in an integrated system of longitudinal care coordination. Restructuring of health care from traditional fee-for-service to managed care will affect virtually everyone, but older Americans, because they experience more medical problems and a concomitant threat of functional loss as they age, will be one of the first groups to be affected. Of particular concern in the midst of this transition is the direction and role of primary care in health services that are aimed at serving the population of older adults.

The purpose of this chapter is to review the factors that influence the delivery of primary health care services to older Americans, to discuss the impact of managed care on older people, to articulate the evidence-based principles of comprehensive geriatric assessment, health promotion, and disease prevention that are the foundation of primary care, and to describe the central role that gerontologic advanced practice nurses have in current and emergent models of primary care.

DEMOGRAPHICS, COST, AND HEALTH SERVICES UTILIZATION

Demographic features are well known to gerontologists and providers of care, but bear repetition as we examine the impact older individuals will have on national needs for primary care now and in the future. Over the next 50 years, the United States will undergo a profound transformation, becoming a mature nation where 1 in 5 citizens is 65 or older (Waite, 1996). In 1900, persons over the age of 65 comprised only 1 in 25 and in 1994, 1 in 8. The most dramatic increase will occur among the "oldest-old," those age 85 and over. Between 1960 and 1994, their numbers rose 274%. In 1994, the oldest-old numbered 3 million, 1% of the total population. It is expected that this population will soar to 19 million in 2050, comprising 24% of elderly Americans and 5% of all Americans (Bureau of the Census, 1995). This aging process applies worldwide as well, and the result will be a global society that is by far the oldest in the history of the world (New York Times, Sept. 26, 1996).

Three out of four noninstitutionalized persons aged 65 to 74 consider their health to be good. Two in three aged 75 or older report similar feelings of good health. Nevertheless, with age comes increasing risk of poor health and dependency. For example, while 1% of those aged 65 to 74 years lived in a nursing home in 1990, nearly 25% aged 85 or older did. Among the community-dwelling population in 1990, 9% aged 65 to 74 years, but 50% aged 85 or older, needed assistance with everyday activities such as bathing, getting around inside the home, and preparing meals (Bureau of the Census, 1995).

Older Americans utilize acute health care services extensively, accounting for 28% of all hospital and 20% of all physician payments (National Academy on Aging, 1995). Rates of hospitalization and lengths of stay are greater for the elderly when compared to younger persons. The average length of a hospital stay was 8.7 days for older persons, compared with 5.3 days for people under age 65 (AARP, 1995). Average annual health care costs per person rise substantially with age, from $3,649 for individuals aged 65 to 74 years to $8,979 for those aged 85 and above (Health Care Financing Administration, 1995).

In addition to acute illness requiring care in hospitals or by physicians, older Americans suffer from chronic conditions that require long-term care either at home or in nursing homes. The costs of nursing home and home care are not covered to any significant extent either by Medicare or private insurance. Instead, the elderly must rely on their own resources and when these are exhausted, turn to welfare in the form of Medicaid (Wiener & Illiston, 1994). At an average of more than $37,000 a year for nursing home care, along with expenditures for prescription drugs, long-term care is the leading cause of out-of-pocket catastrophic health care costs among the elderly (Coughlin, Liu, & McBride, 1992; Liu, Perozek, & Manton, 1993). In the case of nursing home care, high costs are no guarantee of good or even adequate care. It is thus not surprising that home health care, as the alternative preferred by most older people and their families, is one of the fastest growing sectors in the provision of services to the elderly. The home care industry more than doubled its revenues from 1990 to 1995 from $13.1 billion to $28.6 billion, respectively. The Health Care Financing Administration (HCFA) projects that national home health care expenditures will grow to $45.9 billion by 2000 and $68 billion by 2005 (Provider, 1997). It is further predicted that by 2050, the costs of all long-term care could reach 150 billion dollars (U.S. Senate Special Committee on Aging, 1986; Wilensky, 1987).

These figures leave no one doubting the significant challenges before us as we enter the 21st century. At a minimum, we will need to emphasize the efficacy of models shaped by a philosophy of primary health care; ones where health promotion and disease prevention strategies are thoroughly understood and integrated, principles of interdisciplinary comprehensive geriatric assessment and collaborative practice are incorporated, and quality of life emphasized. This will require achievement of the essential components and ideals of primary care—comprehensiveness, continuity, and accessibility. Although the current health care system remains in a state of flux, opportunities exist in evolving systems of care to achieve a full realization of a seamless complex of primary health care services for older people.

PRIMARY CARE AND EMERGENT MANAGED-CARE SYSTEMS

The Institute of Medicine defines primary care as "the provision of integrated accessible health care services by clinicians who are accountable for addressing a large majority of personal health care needs, developing a sustained partnership with patients and practicing in the context of family and community" (Vaneslow, Donaldson, & Yurdy, 1995, p. 8192). In a similar vein, the American Academy of Nursing states, "Nurse practitioners are primary care providers . . . they provide nursing and medical services to individuals, families, and groups . . . emphasis is placed on health promotion and disease prevention as well as diagnosis and management of acute and chronic diseases. . . . Teaching and counseling are a major part of nurse practitioners' activities" (American Academy of Nursing, 1993, p. 1). In many ways, primary care exemplifies a nursing model where success is determined by physical, mental, and social function, with the focus on holistic approaches, and participatory roles for patients and families (American Nurses' Association, 1995). It appears that the realization of effective primary care for older people can be achieved by gerontologic advanced practice nurses who, by philosophy and education, are best suited to the role. In contrast to the fee-for-service-based health care system that dominated the last few decades with its emphasis on physician-centered, disease-focused care, managed-care systems are part of an evolutionary change in the redefinition of heath care in the United States. What we know today as managed care is in a transitional stage. In its essence, however, managed care refers to "the assumption of responsibility and accountability for the health of a defined population, and the simultaneous acceptance of the financial risks inherent in assuming that responsibility. Managed care promotes the effective, responsible, and efficient overseeing of the health of an individual within a given population" (Pew Health Commissions Report, 1995, p. 4).

Emerging systems of managed care will play a larger role in the health care of older Americans well into the next century. In 1991, 1.3 million older people were enrolled in Health Maintenance Organizations (HMO) and other competitive medical plans and that number is expected to grow (HCFA, 1995). It remains to be seen if systems of managed care will achieve a true model of primary care for the elderly; nevertheless, they make extensive use of gerontologic advanced practice nurses as primary care providers (Kramer, Fox, & Morgenstern, 1992), an indication that they have enormous potential for the achievement of care focused on prevention as well as cure, populations as well as individuals, and management of chronic illness as well as acute treatment (Pew Health Professions Commission, August, 1995).

COMPREHENSIVE GERIATRIC ASSESSMENT, HEALTH PROMOTION, AND DISEASE PREVENTION

Healthy aging has been the major goal of United States health policy since the publication of *Healthy People: The Surgeon General's Report on Health Promotion and Disease Prevention* (U.S. Department of Health, Education, and Welfare, 1979). The role of healthy aging was further emphasized with the release of *Healthy People 2000: National Health Promotion and Disease Prevention Objectives* (U.S. Department of Health and Human Services, 1990). This document lists three goals to be achieved by the year 2000: (1) increase the span of healthy life for Americans; (2) reduce health disparities among Americans; and (3) achieve access to preventive services for all Americans.

The provision of primary care for older adults is essential to the accomplishment of these goals. Central to primary care are the concepts of Comprehensive Geriatric Assessment (CGA). CGA was defined by the National Institutes of Health Consensus Development panel (1987) as a "multidisciplinary evaluation in which the multiple problems of older persons are uncovered, described, and explained, if possible, and in which the resources and strengths of the person are catalogued, need for services assessed, and a coordinated care plan developed to focus interventions on the person's problems" (p. 342). Basic elements include physical and mental health, social and economic status, environmental characteristics, and functional status. The principles of comprehensive assessment and functionally oriented care were first applied as part of the National Health Service in the United Kingdom 50 years ago (Barker, 1987). In the United States, CGA is found mainly in academic health centers, and in a growing number of managed-care networks utilizing some form of CGA for risk assessment of older clients (Kramer, Fox, & Morgenstern, 1992). The results of CGA studies have thus far been inconsistent and inconclusive, particularly with regard to geriatric consultation teams and outpatient geriatric evaluation programs. Nevertheless, research suggests that efficacy of CGA can be improved by targeting patients that are at greatest risk for poor outcomes and can benefit from the program, by enabling the geriatric assessment team to directly modify patient care, and by following patients beyond the initial assessment with ongoing assessment and intervention where necessary (Kramer et al., 1992). It may be that CGA's utility will be best demonstrated in managed care models.

Health promotion is the second principle of primary care and the first phase of primary prevention (Lauzon, 1977). Broadly defined, health promotion is "any combination of health education and related organizational, political and economic interventions designed to facilitate behavioral and environmental changes conducive to health" (Green, 1980, p. 7). At a systems level, it may involve increasing problem solving capacity of older persons or the community, providing a comprehensive continuum of community and social services conducive to health and self-reliance, and helping older persons gain access to knowledge, skills, and other resources needed to meet personal health objectives (Minkler & Pasick, 1986). Activities are aimed at persons without evidence of overt disease; emphasis is on facilitation or reinforcement of healthful living. In assessing the needs for health promotion in a program of primary care for older persons, the focus should be on determining those practices that have enabled the person to reach a particular age and incorporating practices that might make a significant difference in delaying or deterring health-related problems associated with aging.

Haber (1994) identifies health-related problems associated with aging and amenable to health promotion as nutrition, smoking, stress control, misuse of alcohol and drugs, accident prevention, and exercise and fitness. Prevailing notions that health promotion isn't "worth it" for older people are gradually disappearing. In the case of smoking cessation, for example, research has demonstrated that within 5 years of smoking cessation, the relative risk of mortality was lower in a population of community-dwelling adults 65 years of age or older (Scheitel, Fleming, Chutka, & Evans, 1996). There are similar findings for exercise and nutrition as critical health promotion activities associated with function (Duffy & MacDonald, 1990; Sullivan, 1995). These developments draw further attention not only to the efficacy of health promotion, but to the need to support it in practice, policy decisions, allocation of resources, continued research, and education of providers and the public. Success will depend greatly on ability to entice those most needing to participate: older individuals who smoke, are sedentary, isolated, multiply medicated and depressed, have low incomes, and suffer from sensory impairment (Omenn, 1990).

Beyond basic efforts directed toward health promotion is the sizable and complex challenge of disease prevention, aimed at early detection of potential factors such as genetic history, age, weight, certain health habits, or environmental exposure. Surveillance for the onset of acute illness or the worsening of a chronic disease involves the identification of these risk factors. Nevertheless, despite considerable support, medical screenings are neither systematically nor uniformly implemented by clinicians. Inconsistent screening recommendations, argument over the clinical effectiveness of screenings, and lack of reimbursement for preventive services have hampered their widespread use in practice (Haber, 1994). Routine annual medical screening is no longer recommended. Rather, the clinician has the responsibility to assess patients' relative risks for disease and utilize screening recommendations on an individualized basis.

The U.S. Preventive Services Task Force (1989) developed recommendations for clinicians on the basis of a comprehensive review of the evidence of clinical effectiveness. The conclusions were published in the *Guide to Clinical Preventive Services*, which documents more than 100 interventions for 60 potentially preventable diseases and conditions and provides guides to help professionals select primary, secondary, or tertiary prevention. Primary prevention is aimed at asymptomatic persons who lack clinical evidence of the targeted conditions, such as counseling about behavioral risk factors, immunizations, and chemoprophylaxis. Secondary prevention is also practiced when an individual is asymptomatic but when actual health risks have been identified. Blood pressure, cholesterol, and diabetic screening are the most widely implemented form of secondary prevention. Tertiary prevention takes place after a disease or disability becomes symptomatic and focuses on the restoration or maintenance of function through rehabilitation (Haber, 1994).

Medical screenings and immunizations are undeniably important tools for disease prevention but the data collected by the U.S. Preventive Services Task Force (1989) state the "conventional clinical activities (e.g., diagnostic testing) may be of less value to patients than activities once considered outside the traditional role of the clinician—counseling and patient education" (p. xxii). Indeed, the advantage of the use of the term health promotion, according to Haber (1994), is "its likelihood of encompassing mental and spiritual health concerns" (p. 14). It is in these domains that advanced practice nursing has demonstrated its fundamentally different approach to care from that of the traditional medical model (Eccard & Gainor, 1993). The health needs of people encompass lifestyle adjustments, health education, and self-care, elements that are definitive of both primary care and the abilities of advanced practice nurses to provide them (Brush & Capezuti, 1996).

DEVELOPMENT OF SPECIALIZED PRACTICE IN GERONTOLOGIC NURSING

As will be discussed further in this chapter, research over the last 10 years has identified the pivotal role that gerontologic nurse specialists have in the design and provision of primary care services to older adults. Nursing has a long history of caring for older people. A 1925 editorial in the *American Journal of Nursing* alerted nurses to the growing need for care of the elderly (Editorial, 1925), but the first text in geriatric nursing was not published until 1950. It described in detail the care of older persons, including constructive health practice and prevention of disease (Newton, 1950). Geriatric Practice was established as one of the five divisions of the American Nurses' Association (ANA) in 1966. The first Standards for Geriatric Nursing Practice were published in 1970; the latest evolution of these initial guidelines appeared in 1995 as *Standards and Scope of Gerontological Nursing Practice* (American Nurses Association, 1995). The current standards are congruent with the basic tenets of primary health care, with particular emphasis on data collection, planning and continuity of care, and interdisciplinary collaboration. Paralleling similar developments in advanced practice in the United States, gerontologic clinical specialists and nurse practitioners emerged in the late 1960s. Advanced practice nurses now can be found in most care settings that serve an older population; however, the present percentage of those with master's preparation in gerontology and skill in primary care covers a fraction of the actual need.

Practice characteristics of gerontologic advanced practice nurses (GANPs) in acute care, ambulatory care, home care, and nursing homes illustrate the implementation of the principles of primary care as identified by the ANA. Ruiz and her colleagues (1995) identified objectives in GANP practice that incorporate improvement of functional ability of older persons, emphasis on diagnosis and treatment of human responses to health and illness, patient and family education and interaction, and interdisciplinary collaboration to ensure quality of care. Other research over the last decade identified positive outcomes of GANP practice including decreased hospitalization rates for nursing home residents (Wieland, Rubenstein, & Ouslander, 1986), reduction in the use of physical restraints in nursing homes (Evans et al., 1997), timely discharge and prevention of readmission in acute care (Naylor et al., 1994), and maintenance of overall function and health of patients in ambulatory care settings through early detection and assessment of memory loss, depression and altered mental status, nutritional deficits, or other symptomatology that requires careful evaluation (Rubenstein, Bernabel, & Wieland, 1994). A growing literature on the impact of interventions carried out by GANPs provides clearest support for more widespread implementation of models of primary care.

MODELS OF PRIMARY CARE OF OLDER ADULTS

As mentioned earlier, health care services provided to older adults are evolving at an unprecedented rate. Innovative models in the delivery of primary care health services to older adults can now be found across all settings that serve a population of older adults, from acute hospital settings to care in the community including adult day care centers, day hospitals, geriatric evaluation clinics, nurse-managed community clinics, home care, hospice, continuing-care retirement communities, and traditional nursing home care. Central to the provision of high-quality, cost-effective care in these various settings is utilization of clinical expertise of gerontologic advanced practice nurses.

Hospital-Based Primary Care

Models of care for acutely ill elders in the hospital have evolved over the last 10 years to include geriatric consultation teams, geriatric evaluation and management (GEM) units, and a cluster of models that have been examined in the John A. Hartford Foundation's Hospital Outcomes Project for the Elderly (HOPE) (Fulmer & Mezey, 1993; Margitic et al., 1993; Nurses Improving Care to the Hospitalized Elderly (NICHE), 1994). Geriatric consultation teams consisting, usually, of specialists from medicine, nursing, social work, and psychiatry, function in a variety of ways, e.g., evaluation of all hospital patients above a certain age, response to specific consultation requests, follow-up of all patients admitted from other geriatric services in the system (i.e., home care or ambulatory geriatric clinic), or care of patients in a dedicated GEM unit. Typically a consultation team focuses on problems related to functional status, mental status, drug therapy, potential for rehabilitation, and discharge planning (Strumpf, 1994). Improved outcomes for hospitalized patients receiving geriatric consultation have been reported (Rubenstein, Josephson, Harker, Miller, & Weiland, 1995), including better utilization of resources (Germain, Knoeffel, Weiland, & Rubenstein, 1995); reduced medications; improved physical and mental status (McVey, Becker, Salz, Feussner, & Cohen, 1989; Wanich, Sullivan-Marx, Gottlieb, & Johnson, 1992); and higher survival rates (Applegate et al., 1990; Hogan & Fox, 1990; Rubenstein et al., 1995). The best results have been documented in combined geriatric assessment and rehabilitation settings, or in inpatient units focused on individuals with a good potential to reverse disabilities. Assessment and rehabilitation without adequate postdischarge follow-up may be of little benefit (Epstein et al., 1990; Stuck, Siu, Wieland, Adams, & Rubenstein, 1993).

A cluster of models developed to improve geriatric care in hospitals, the Hospital Outcomes Project for the Elderly (HOPE), focuses primarily on nursing care, specifically on the gerontologic nurse specialist whose expertise is an essential component of these models. These models include the Geriatric Resource Nurse (GRN), Acute Care of the Elderly (ACE) unit, Geriatric Nurse Specialist (GNS), Comprehensive Discharge Planning (CDP), and Case Management (CM).

In the GRN model, specifically trained geriatric resource nurses, gerontologic nurse specialists, and geriatric physician specialists provide support and expertise for staff throughout the hospital in the management of specific conditions common to geriatric patients, such as incontinence, functional and mental status changes, delirium, and the development of pressure ulcers (Fulmer & Mezey, 1993; Inouye et al., 1993).

The Acute Care of the Elderly (ACE) model utilizes specialty units to provide care to a targeted group of acutely ill older patients. Collaborative team building with significant roles for geriatric medicine specialists, clinical nurse specialists, and the use of clinical protocols are the special features of the model. In addition, the physical environment of the unit is designed specifically to meet the needs of older patients and to prevent functional decline, including use of low beds, an activity room, reclining chairs, and levered doors (Strumpf, 1994).

The Geriatric Nurse Specialist (GNS) model provides advanced practice nurses for ongoing consultation and education to assist staff nurses to define and implement strategies for specific geriatric problems.

The Comprehensive Discharge Planning (CDP) model was tested at the University of Pennsylvania specifically for the elderly. In the CDP protocol, a nurse specialist enrolls the patient within 24–48 hours of admission, assesses both patient and caregiver, makes interim hospital visits at least every 48 hours until discharge, and maintains contact with the patient for 2 weeks after discharge through follow-up telephone calls. For those patients receiving the CDP protocol, as compared to the control group, there were fewer readmissions, fewer rehospitalized days, lower readmission charges, and lower charges for health care services after discharge (Naylor et al., 1994).

The multidisciplinary Case Management (CM) model, developed at Beth Israel Medical Center in New York City, is designed to provide outcome-oriented patient care and appropriate use of resources. Targeted patients are those having complex conditions and comorbidities, high acuity and increased risk for complication, frailty, noncompliance, and absence of a support system. The goals of CM include integration and coordination of clinical services, collaborative practice and continuity of care, and patient and provider satisfaction. Success of this model is dependent on the clinical expertise of the nurse specialist selected as case manager (Strumpf, 1994).

It must be noted here that all of these models to provide primary care for the elderly in hospitals emphasize the importance of the geriatric nurse specialist or APN in the attainment of positive outcomes for patients. Indeed, many of these innovative approaches arose from nurses' recognition of the complexities of acute-care treatment of older persons that, often, can complicate or diminish physical and mental function and contribute to loss of independence.

Community-Based Primary Care

Cost-containment initiatives continue to shift care from hospitals to the community. Several successful programs have been described over the years including the multiple-state National Long-Term Care Demonstration, On Lok Senior Health Services Community Organization for Older Adults in San Francisco, Access in New York, South Carolina Long-Term Care Demonstration, and a national demonstration sponsored by the HCFA, The Social/Health Maintenance Organization (SHMO) (Fanale, Kennan, Hepburn, & Von Sternberg, 1991). As summarized by Fanale et al., these projects, in general, have shown that care management may improve clients' independence and reduce social isolation, may enhance quality of life, and may reduce nursing home utilization and retard entry to a nursing home.

Utilizing approaches developed in these early programs, a variety of services that emphasize primary care and case management have evolved. In the Beth Israel Home Care Program in Boston, geriatric nurse practitioners provide "medical" aspects of care and serve as case managers, providing linkages to the health care system, assurance of adequate follow-up, and delivery of necessary services (Burns-Tisdale & Goff, 1989). The nurse practitioner's ability to provide comprehensive physical examinations and make assessments allows quick identification of changes affecting treatment plans or requiring emergency care. Collaboration with the physician enables prompt resolution of potentially critical declines in the patient's condition.

The Community Nursing Organization (CNO) is another innovative model that utilizes advanced practice nurses to provide health promotion, screening, and early intervention to patients in the community. There are currently four demonstration practice sites funded by HCFA: the Visiting Nurse Service of New York (VNSNY), serving 4 boroughs of New York City and comprising the largest nonprofit Medicare-certified home health agency in the city; Carle Clinic Association in Urbana, Illinois, a multispecialty physician group practice; Carondelet Health Services in Tucson, Arizona, a health system using nurse-managed clinics as a primary component; and the Living at Home/Block Nurse program in St. Paul, Minnesota, a community-based program of health care and supportive services to elderly persons in their homes, delivered primarily by volunteers (Daley & Mitchell, 1996).

The CNO uses a model of community-focused nursing which includes patient services, aggregate needs identification, and aggregate planning and intervention (Storfjell & Cruise, 1984). Each nurse's practice includes the family, the environment, and the community. CNO practice sites include senior centers, churches, senior clubs, apartment complexes, storefront offices, and patients' homes. The nurses provide assessments and screening, ongoing monitoring of acute and chronic conditions, patient education, and health promotion and illness prevention classes to groups of CNO members (Daley & Mitchell, 1996).

The Collaborative Assessment and Rehabilitation for Elders (CARE) program established by the School of Nursing at the University of Pennsylvania in Philadelphia, utilized the British Day Hospital model to provide a comprehensive approach to care of frail older adults that bridges the gap between acute home-based, and institutional long-term care. With a gerontologic nurse practitioner as care manager, clients receive an intensive, individualized, time-limited program of nursing, rehabilitation, mental health, social, and medical services in one setting several times a week. The targeted population is persons over 65 who have complex medical problems and are living at home. Individuals must need multiple services, including at least one rehabilitation therapy, and they must be unsuitable for inpatient rehabilitation. Preliminary data support the beneficial effects as well as the economic feasibility of this approach (Evans, Yurkow, & Seigler, 1995).

These models of primary care in the community demonstrate the effectiveness of gerontologic nursing expertise and advanced practice nursing in these settings. It is conceivable that, in the future, only very sick patients requiring highly complex care will be seen in the hospital and nursing homes will serve persons with serious disabilities or with rehabilitative and subacute care needs. The rest of the population will increasingly receive care in outpatient, home, and community-based settings (Institute of Medicine, 1994). There is no doubt that GANPs will be an essential element in the design and implementation of programs to meet the needs for quality, community-based care.

Nursing Home Care

Although provision of adequate health care for older people must be considered from the standpoint of a continuum of services ranging across settings from home to hospital to long-stay institutions, nursing homes dominate and symbolize the problems and dilemmas of long-term care. Earlier hospital discharge to long-term-care settings has substantially increased the needs and acuity of residents in nursing homes (Kanda & Mezey, 1991; Shaughnessey, Kramer, Hittle, & Steiner, 1995). A persistent lack of funds has affected quality of care and the ability to attract and pay professional staff. The average 100-bed nursing home has only one registered nurse and 1.5

licensed practical nurses per shift, and delivers to each resident less than 12 minutes of care per day by the registered nurse (Mezey & Fulmer, 1991). Here lies the greatest challenge of all: getting primary care services to these elders in greatest need.

Perhaps the most significant experiment toward improving nursing home care was the Robert Wood Johnson Foundation Teaching Nursing Home Program (Mezey & Lynaugh, 1991). This experiment in social change was conceived as a model for restructuring and enhancing clinical care. Its purposes were to upgrade care of residents using a cadre of nurse specialists; to create an environment supportive of education, and to promote research. The 5-year national demonstration project involved 11 schools of nursing and 12 nursing homes with established joint appointments. Two other demonstrations, the Kellog Foundation's project with the Mountain States Health Corporation and the Nursing Home Connection, also used advanced practice nurses to deliver care to nursing home residents (Mezey, 1990). Findings from all three projects consistently supported the effectiveness of these nurses as providers of care: They responded to changes in resident status, conducted assessments, monitored medication, provided direct care or supervision for the more complex problems, and counseled patients and families.

There is substantial evidence that geriatric nurse practitioners in all three demonstration projects significantly lowered hospitalization rates of nursing home residents (Shaugnessey & Kramer, 1994). In addition, residents had better functional outcomes, fewer urinary catheters, less incontinence, fewer nosocomial infections, and more appropriate use of medications. Reductions in psychotropic medications and use of physical restraints also occurred, along with better management of wandering and disruptive behavior. Presence of a gerontologic nurse practitioner assured the transmittal of timely and accurate information to physicians and reduction in unnecessary trips to the hospital emergency room. Evaluation to date supports a significant role for geriatric nurse practitioners in nursing homes (Kane et al., 1988; Kane et al., 1989; Kane et al., 1991). Furthermore, employment of nurse practitioners does not adversely affect profits (Buchanan et al., 1990). The effectiveness of models using APNs is a given; it remains now to find mechanisms making possible its wide establishment in long-term care.

This brief description of health service delivery and evolving models of primary care demonstrates the pivotal roles that gerontologic nurses play not only in the provision of evidence-based practice, but also in the design and implementation of primary care services appropriate for older adults and their families. In 1997, we have "an impressive array of innovative gerontologic practices using nurses, nursing interventions, and the interdisciplinary care team in a variety of settings and across the continuum of care" (Strumpf, 1994, p. 38). Nursing must continue in its efforts to redefine how America cares for the elderly, utilizing its expertise in coordinated, comprehensive approaches that maintain the health, well-being, and independent living of older adults.

CONCLUSIONS

This chapter differs markedly from its previous iterations. No one could have predicted the rapid transformation of the American health care system from fee-for-service to managed care and, in its current transitional phase, it is difficult to determine what effect managed care will have on primary care services for the elderly. Elder care in the 21st century will require individualized approaches for large numbers of older persons and their families and accelerate the move to community-based primary and long-term care. The foundation is being laid by gerontologic advanced practice nurses for the implementation of models of primary care that best serve the needs of these older persons and their families and the positive outcomes of a nursing-centered approach with the elderly are increasingly documented. As the reconstruction of the delivery of health services continues to unfold in the United States, nursing must continue to argue convincingly for its beneficial and cost-effective role, using outcomes-based research as an essential point in this quest for quality care. Nursing must remain faithful to its historical and most fundamental mission—to advocate the best care for patients and families in all health care settings. Only then can components of care articulated in this chapter be practiced by all providers and offered with satisfaction and confidence to every older American.

REFERENCES AND BIBLIOGRAPHY

American Academy of Nursing. (1993). *Managed care and national health care reform: Nurses can make it work.* Washington, DC: American Academy of Nursing.

American Nurses' Association. (1995). *Standards and scope of gerontological nursing practice.* Kansas City, MO: American Nurses Association.

Applegate, W. B., Miller, S. T., Graney, M. J., Elam, J. T., Burns, R., & Akins, D. E. (1990). A randomized controlled trial of a geriatric assessment unit in a community rehabilitation hospital. *New England Journal of Medicine, 322*(22), 1572–1578.

Barker, W. H. (1987). *Adding life to years: Organized geriatrics services in Great Britain and implications for the United States.* Baltimore: Johns Hopkins University Press.

Brush, B. L., & Capezuti, E. A. (1996). Revisiting "A nurse for all settings": The nurse practitioner movement, 1965–1995. *Journal of the American Academy of Nurse Practitioners, 8*(1), 5–11.

Buchanan, J. L., Bell, R. M., Arnold, S. B., Witsberger, C., Kane, R. L., & Garrard, J. (1990). Assessing cost effects of nursing-home based geriatric nurse practitioners. *Health Care Financing Review, 11*(3), 67–78.

Bureau of the Census. (1995). Sixty-five plus in the United States. *Statistical Brief,* Issued May 1995 by the U.S. Dept. of Commerce.

Burns-Tisdale, S., & Goff, W. F. (1989). The geriatric nurse practitioner in home care. *Nursing Clinics of North America, 24*(3), 809–817.

Consensus Development Panel. (1988). National Institutes of Health Consensus Development Conference Statement: Geriatric assessment methods for clinical decision making. *Journal of the American Geriatrics Society, 36*(4), 342–347.

Coughlin, T. A., Liu, K., & McBride, T. D. (1992). Severely disabled persons with financially catastrophic health care expenses: Sources and determinants. *The Gerontologist, 32,* 391–403.

Daley, G. M., & Mitchell, R. D. (1996). Case management in the community setting. *Nursing Clinics of North America, 31* (3), 527–534.

Duffy, M., & MacDonald, E. (1990). Determinants of functional health of older persons. *The Gerontologist, 30*(4), 503–509.

Eccard, W. T., & Gainor, E. E. (1993). Legal ramifications for expanded practice. In M. D. Mezey & D. O. McGivern (Eds.), *Nurses, nurse practitioners: Evolution to advanced practice* (2nd ed.). New York: Springer Publishing.

Editorial. Care of the aged. (1925). *American Journal of Nursing, 25*(5), 394.

Epstein, A., Hall, J., Fretwell, M., Feldstein, M., DiCiantis, M., Tognetti, J., Cutler, C., Constantine, M., Besdine, R., Rowe, J., & McNeil, B. (1990). Consultative geriatric assessment for ambulatory patients. *Journal of the American Medical Association, 263*(4), 538–544.

Evans, L. K., Yurkow, J., & Seigler, E. L. (1995). The CARE program: A nurse-managed collaborative outpatient program to improve function of frail older people. *Journal of the American Geriatrics Society, 43*(10), 1155–1160.

Evans, L. K., Strumpf, N. E., Allen-Taylor, S. L., Capezuti, E., Maislin, G., & Jacobsen, B. (1997). A clinical trial to reduce restraints in nursing homes. *Journal of the American Geriatrics Society, 45*(6), 675–681.

Fanale, J. E., Kennan, J. M., Hepburn, K. W., & Von Sternberg, T. (1991). Care management. *Journal of the American Geriatrics Society, 39*(4), 431–437.

Fulmer, T., & Mezey, M. (1993). *Report of hospital outcomes project for the elderly.* New York, NY: The John Hartford Foundation.

Germain, M., Knoeffel, F., Wieland, D., & Rubenstein, L. Z. (1995). A geriatric assessment and intervention team for hospital inpatients awaiting transfer to a geriatric unit: A randomized trial. *Aging, 7*(1), 55–60.

Green, L. W. (1980). *Health education planning: A diagnostic approach.* Palo Alto, CA: Mayfield.

Haber, D. (1994). *Health promotion and aging.* New York: Springer Publishing.

Health Care Financing Administration. (1995). *Preliminary Annual Summary Controls.* Baltimore, MD: U.S. Government Web Site.

Hogan, D. B., & Fox, R. A. (1990). A prospective controlled trial of a geriatric consultation team in an acute care hospital. *Age and Ageing, 19*(2), 107–113.

Inouye, S., Armapora, D., Miller, R., Fulmer, T., Hurst, L., & Cooney, L., (1993). The Yale Geriatric Care Program: A model of care to prevent functional decline in hospitalized elderly patients. *Journal of the American Geriatrics Society, 41*(12), 1345–1352.

Institute of Medicine Committee on the Future of Primary Care. (1994). *Defining primary care: An interim report.* Washington, DC: National Academy Press.

Kanda, K., & Mezey, M. (1991). Registered nurse staffing in Pennsylvania nursing homes: Comparison before and after implementation of Medicare's prospective payment system. *The Gerontologist, 31*(3), 318–324.

Kane, R. A., Kane, R. L., Arnold, S., Garrard, J., McDermott, S., & Kepferle, L. (1988). Geriatric nurse practitioners as nursing home employees: Implementing the role. *The Gerontologist, 28*(4), 469–477.

Kane, R. L., Garrard, J., Buchanan, J. L., Rosenfeld, A., Skay, C., & McDermott, S. (1991). Improving primary care in nursing homes. *Journal of the American Geriatrics Society, 39*(4), 359–367.

Kane, R. L., Garrard, J., Skay, C., Radosevich, D. M., Buchanan, J. L., McDermott, S. M., Arnold, S. B., & Kepferle, L. (1989). Effects of a geriatric nurse practitioner on process and outcome of nursing home care. *American Journal of Public Health, 79*(9), 1271–1277.

Kramer, A. M., Fox, P. D., & Morgenstern, N. (1992). Geriatric care approaches in health maintenance organizations. *The Journal of the American Geriatrics Society, 40,* 1055–1067.

Lauzon, R. J. (1977). An epidemiological approach to health promotion. *Canadian Journal of Public Health, 68*(4), 311–317.

Liu, K., Perozek, M., & Manton, K. G. (1993). Catastrophic acute and long-term care costs: Risks faced by disabled elderly persons. *The Gerontologist, 33,* 299–307.

Margitic, M., Inouye, S., Thomas, J., Cassel, C., Regenstreif, D., & Kowal, J. (1993). Hospital outcomes project for the elderly (HOPE): Rationale and design for a prospective pooled analysis. *Journal of the American Geriatrics Society, 41*(3), 258–267.

McVey, L. J., Becker, P. M., Saltz, C. C., Feussner, J. R., & Cohen, H. J. (1989). Effect of a geriatric consultation team on functional status of elderly hospitalized patients. *Annals of Internal Medicine, 110*(1), 79–84.

Mezey, M. (1990). GNPs on staff. *Geriatric Nursing, 11*(3), 145–147.

Mezey, M., & Fulmer, T. (1991). The future of nursing home care. *New England Journal of Medicine, 325*(5), 360.

Mezey, M., & Lynaugh, J. (1991). Teaching nursing home program: A lesson in quality. *Geriatric Nursing, 12*(2), 76–77.

Minkler, M., & Pasick, R. J. (1986). Health promotion and the elderly: A critical perspective on the past and future. In K. Dychtwald (Ed.), *Wellness and health promotion for the elderly.* Rockville, MD: Aspen.

National Academy on Aging. (1995, October). Medicare hospital insurance and supplementary insurance. *Gerontology News.*

Naylor, M., Brooten, D., Jones, R., Lavizzo-Mourey, R., Mezey, M., & Pauley, M. (1994). Comprehensive discharge planning for the hospitalized elderly. A randomized clinical trial. *Annals of Internal Medicine, 120*(12), 999–1006.

Newton, K. (1950). *Geriatric nursing.* St. Louis, MO: Mosby.

New York Times. (1996, Sept. 26). *Aging world new wrinkles.* Nicholas D. Kristoff.

Nurses Improving Care to the Hospitalized Elderly (NICHE) Project Faculty. (1994). Geriatric models of care: Which one's right for your institution? *American Journal of Nursing, 94*(7), 21–23.

Omenn, G. S. (1990). Prevention and the elderly. *Health Affairs, 9*(2), 80–93.

Pew Health Professions Commission. (1995, August). *Health professions education and managed care: Challenges and necessary responses* (pp. 1–34). San Francisco, CA: Pew Health Professions Commission.

Provider. (1997, May). *The world of home care* (pp. 33–48).

Rubenstein, L. Z., Bernabel, R., & Wieland, D. (1994). Comprehensive geriatric assessment into the breach. *Aging, 6*(1), 1–3.

Rubenstein, L., Z., Josephson, K., R., Harker, J. O., Miller, D., K., & Weiland, D. (1995). The Sepulveda GEU study revisited: Long-term outcomes, use of services, and costs. *Aging, 7*(3), 212–217.

Ruiz, B. A., Tabloski, P. A., & Frazier, S. M. (1995). The role of gerontological advanced practice nurses in geriatric care. *Journal of the American Geriatrics Society, 43*(9), 1061–1064.

Shaughnessy, P. W., Kramer, A. M., Hittle, D. F., & Steiner, J. F. (1995). Quality of Care in Teaching Nursing Homes: Findings and Implications. *Health Care Financing Review, 16*(4), 55–83.

Sheitel, S. M., Fleming, K. C., Chutka, D. S., & Evans, J. M. (1996). Geriatric health maintenance. *Mayo Clinic Proceedings, 71*(3), 289–302.

Storfjell, J. L., & Cruise, P. A. (1984). A model of community-focused nursing. *Public Health Nursing, 1*(2), 85–96.

Strumpf, N. E. (1994). Innovative gerontological practices as models for health care delivery. *Nursing and Health Care, 15*(10), 522–527.

Stuck, A. E., Siu, A. L., Wieland, G. D., Adams, J., & Rubenstein, L. Z. (1993). Comprehensive geriatric assessment: A meta-analysis of controlled trials. *Lancet, 342*(8878), 1032–1036.

Sullivan, D. H. (1995). Impact of nutritional status on health outcomes of nursing home residents. *Journal of the American Geriatrics Society, 43*(4), 195–196.

U.S. Department of Health, Education, and Welfare. (1979). *Healthy People.* Washington, DC: U.S. Government Printing Office. (DHEW (PHS) Publication No. 79-55071.

U.S. Preventive Task Force Services. (1989). *Guide to clinical preventive services: An assessment of the effectiveness of 169 interventions.* Baltimore, MD: Williams and Wilkins.

U.S. Department of Health and Human Services. (1990). *Healthy People 2000: National health promotion and disease prevention objectives.* Washington, DC: U.S. Government Printing Office.

U.S. Senate Special Committee on Aging. (1986). *Developments in aging.* Washington, DC: U.S. Government Printing Office.

Vaneslow, N. A., Donaldson, M. S., & Yurdy, K. D. (1995). From the Institute of Medicine. *Journal of the American Medical Association, 273*(3), 8192.

Waite, L. J. (1996). The demographic face of America's elderly. *Inquiry, 33*, 220–224.

Wanich, C., Sullivan-Marx, E., Gottlieb, G., & Johnson, J. (1992). Functional status outcomes of a nursing intervention in hospitalized elderly. *Image: Journal of Nursing Scholarship*, *24*(3), 201–207.

Weiland, D., Rubenstein, L. Z., & Ouslander, J. G. (1986). Organizing an academic nursing home. Impacts on institutionalized elderly. *Journal of the American Medical Association*, *255*(19), 2622–2627.

Weiner, J. M., & Illiston, L. H. (1994). Health care reform in the 1990s: Where does long-term care fit in? *The Gerontologist*, *34*(3), 402–408.

Wilensky, G. R. (1987, Feb. 24). Statement before the U.S. Senate Finance Committee, Subcommittee on Health Hearing.

Chapter 17

PRIMARY CARE CONCEPTS IN ADVANCED PRACTICE PSYCHIATRIC-MENTAL HEALTH NURSING

Madeline A. Naegle

IN recognition of the complexity of human and environmental systems, nursing practice has traditionally addressed a broad spectrum of health care needs of clients and their families. This view underlies the biopsychosocial perspective that shapes the current practice of psychiatric-mental health nursing. "Biopsychosocial" connotes that psychiatric-mental health nursing theory derives from biological, cultural, environmental, psychological, and sociological sciences as well as nursing science.

Although psychiatric-mental health nursing was not formally practiced until the early 20th century, Nightingale noted the importance of the human psychological realm by linking anxiety and its control through coping mechanisms. She observed that patients' participation to their maximum potential in activities of daily living decreases apprehension, uncertainty, waiting, expectation, and fear of surprise (Nightingale, 1895). Since the earliest days of psychiatric nursing, nursing care has been directed toward preventing uncomfortable feeling states, dysfunctions, and mental illness and delivering care directed toward alleviating psychic pain and its disabling accompanying behaviors.

The 1996 Institute of Medicine Committee on the Future of Primary Care defines primary care as: "the provision of integrated, accessible health care services by clinicians who are accountable for addressing the majority of personal health care needs, developing a sustained partnership with patients, and practicing in the context of family and community (IOM, 1996). Primary mental health needs, while not specified, can be interpreted as part of personal health care needs. However, key components of this definition seen in early and ongoing nursing models of contractual agreements between the independently practicing nurse and the client and/ or client's family include: (1) *a sustained partnership*, including the assumption of primary and long-term responsibility for the patient regardless of the presence or absence of disease; (2) *the community context* acknowledged in the formation and coordination of networks of resources and care providers within the health care system and/or the community; and (3) *accessibility and consistent contact with other health care providers.*

Today, the mental health-primary care components come together in the primary mental health nurse's role as currently defined by Haber and Billings (1995). By identifying the primary care components of the mental health specialty, the role expands the extent to which the nurse addresses the majority of personal health care needs through direct care provision and referral.

Haber and Billings (1995) note that while psychiatric-mental health nursing has been a specialized area of nursing practice employing theories of human behavior and purposeful use of self as its art, the primary care components of the role have been less frequently emphasized. Primary mental health care in this definition includes all services necessary for the promotion of mental health. Continuous and comprehensive, it includes the *prevention* and *treatment* of mental illness, *health maintenance*, and *rehabilitation*. It begins at or before the first point of contact with the mental health care delivery system (Bellak, 1976) and targets well populations, populations at-risk, and individuals with disorders along the continuum of mental illness.

Primary mental health care interventions fall within the scope of practice of both generalist nurses and mental health nurse specialists. Universal preventive measures, felt to be desirable for everybody in a given population, are implemented to enhance functioning and mental health (Mrazek & Haggerty, 1994). These include culturally congruent activities in parenting education and promotion of self-esteem. Selective preventive interventions are also used for populations at-risk and include activities like elder support groups, respite for caregivers, and bereavement counseling. While this role has only recently been implemented, Leininger identified the lowering of the incidence of mental disorders as a primary care activity in 1973, and Jennings (1977) noted that teaching about stress and mental health risks constitutes mental health nursing.

Advanced practice psychiatric nurses' roles have gained further support with the renewed emphasis on the biological science links to mental health. Not only has recent research elucidated new biological factors which influence mental-emotional illness, but consumer groups have demanded clear definitions of psychiatric illnesses as brain disorders. Neuroscience research that supports brain dysfunction as central to both the diagnosis and treatment of psychiatric disorders is now widely acknowledged by psychiatric nurses. Psychiatric nurse leaders have stressed that neurological and psychiatric mental health knowledge must be integrated if the nurse is to be effective (McBride, 1996) and urged the expansion of the biologic bases for practice (McEnany, 1991).

Today, advanced practice roles in psychiatric-mental health nursing include the psychiatric-mental health clinical nurse specialist and psychiatric-mental health nurse practitioner. While some continue to hold that the scope of practice for these two roles differs, Moller and Haber (1996) present a strong argument for blending the two roles under the title, advanced practice psychiatric-mental health nurse. In the past the *clinical nurse specialist* was recognized for the use of expert psychiatric-mental health nursing knowledge to deliver direct care to acutely ill patients/ clients, families, and groups. Nurses in this role also provide education, consultation, and research perspectives on care provision for colleagues, consumers, and organizations. The *psychiatric nurse practitioner* shares this expert knowledge about mental health and illness, is prepared for the same professional education, consultation, and research responsibilities, but has, to date, been associated with more primary care activities.

In response to the needs of the health care delivery system and the advancement of neurological research related to psychiatric illness, the education and role performance of the mental-health nurse clinical specialist and psychiatric nurse practitioner nurse are increasingly similar. The master's degree is now the accepted requirement for both, and educational programs are preparing students for a role which blends the core component of these original roles. With contemporary changes and role overlap, students preparing for these roles supplement core expert knowledge with additional components and concentrate effort on the direct provider aspects of the role as well as professional activities related to consultation, research, and education. Increasingly, both roles require a master's-degree level of knowledge about basic health problems, and add depth on specific primary care functions of the generalist role.

Master's degree preparation is essential for greater understanding of the biological components of commonly occurring health problems in psychological and physical realms. Such an approach supports the ability of the nurse to ascertain the client's basic health needs, as well as assessing and treating mental health needs. When there are significant medical symptoms, both the clinical nurse specialist and the nurse practitioner make appropriate referrals to a nurse practitioner or physician specialist. The nursing approach of master's degree and generalist levels continues to represent a marked shift away from the medical model, placing heavy emphasis on a comprehensive, sociopsychological assessment of client and family (Aiken, 1978). Increasingly however, advanced practice preparation enables the nurse to work with more autonomy and greater knowledge of the client's health, and that shift has made primary care its center (Aiken & Sage, 1993).

Talley and Caverly (1994) provide excellent examples of primary mental health care services which these nurses are prepared to address. These services include: (1) maintenance of the medical health care record in the mental health treatment record; (2) provision of selected lifetime health screening and health education in mental health settings (e.g., blood pressure and cholesterol screening, weight checks, and education about mammography, family planning, PAP smears, HIV-AIDS), and evaluation of health care risks and problems secondary to psychiatric illnesses or psychopharmacologic interventions (e.g., Diabetes Insipidus, agranulocytosis, tardive dyskinesia, or hypothyroidism), and monitoring before drug treatment, during treatment, and drug discontinuation as well as monitoring of the laboratory and medical procedures needed to ensure safe psychopharmacological interventions.

The forerunner of the primary mental health care model was demonstrated in the 1970s in community mental health centers. Mandated to provide basic services to people with a wide scope of mental health needs, these centers provided community-based inpatient and outpatient care, day care, 24-hour crisis intervention, and consultation and education. The psychiatric-mental health clinical nurse specialists who implemented new roles in these centers (1) worked primarily in ambulatory care; (2) were highly autonomous; (3) delivered treatment in modalities traditionally reserved for psychiatrists, social workers, and others; and (4) provided mental health teaching, education, and consultation to schools, social agencies, and service centers. The nurse was often the client's first contact with the health care delivery system and assumed responsibility for continuing care. This care necessarily included identification, management, and referral of health problems coexisting with acute or chronic mental illness, and required the utilization of knowledge germane to the generalist and specialist preparation of the nurse.

The contemporary role functions of psychiatric mental health nurses continue to include these elements as well as: (1) client advocacy; (2) accountability; and (3) collaborative activities with nurses and members of other disciplines. In addition, nurses implement interventions and professional role responsibilities congruent with *A Statement on Psychiatric Mental Health Clinical Nursing Practice* (ANA, 1994). The direct intervention embedded in psychiatric-mental health nursing at basic and advanced practice levels includes counseling, crisis intervention, health teaching, milieu therapy, case management, and psychobiological interventions including biologic assessment such as laboratory tests. While psychobiologic interventions at the basic level include interpretation and implementation of prescriptions, at the advanced level the nurse may have prescribing privileges in accord with state legal nurse practitioner statutes and collaborative physician and institutional agreements.

Although nurses at both the basic and advanced practice levels function as patient advocates, are involved in professional organizations, and take community level action based on health policy, it is the advanced practice nurse who most clearly embodies the change agent role and assumes leadership responsibility in collaboration with intra- and interdisciplinary colleagues (Chambers, Dangel, Tripodi, & Jaeger, 1987). Nurses at generalist and advanced practice levels must utilize education in culturally diverse traditions, and must acknowledge variation among racial and ethnic groups in manifestations of health and illness and differences in sexual preference and lifestyles to individualize patterns of care delivery. Advanced practice psychiatric-mental health nursing practice of the future must integrate a level of primary care into mental health care to provide a more holistic model of care for clients whose ability to attend to their own physical and mental health needs is compromised (Talley & Caverly, 1994).

ROLES AND PRACTICE SETTINGS FOR THE CONTEMPORARY PSYCHIATRIC NURSE

Professional trends emphasizing quality care, consumer advocacy and accountability all support greater independence of practice in the psychiatric nursing role. Mechanic has noted that combined generalist-specialist preparation, with its capability for complex decision making offers the potential for cost-effective health care delivery (1982). Trends have moved psychiatric nursing away from institution-based interventions, with its focus on pathology, to nursing roles addressing mental health needs along a continuum. Roles that include those of *direct care provider, case manager, consultant and collaborator, and interdisciplinary team member* are implemented in settings that include hospitals, but now increasingly include community agencies, clinics, and long-term residences. Independent practice, an option utilized in the past in psychiatric nursing, is becoming a more frequent choice. Roles in psychiatric-liaison consultation present unique institution-based options to utilize primary care and specialist knowledge bases.

Direct Care Provider

In the climate of managed care, psychiatric hospitalization is reserved for individuals experiencing acute illness states, those with complex diagnostic profiles, and those requiring pharmacologic management, as well as individuals who are of danger to themselves and/or others. Most clients/patients in need of secondary and tertiary psychiatric care live in the community in group homes, halfway houses, with families, in therapeutic communities, or in single-room occupancies. Depending on the region, many are homeless and seek care sporadically in general and psychiatric settings. Many can be maintained in these settings through crises and require hospitalization only during acute exacerbations of illness. These individuals manifest acute psychiatric illness, including dual diagnoses of substance abuse and exacerbations of severe and persistent mental illness and require ongoing management of multiple diagnoses such as substance abuse, HIV, and associated psychiatric illness, as well as management of other coexisting medical conditions.

The advanced practice psychiatric-mental health nurse implements the role of direct care provider for individuals, groups, and families manifesting complex problems in the community. At present, nursing functions are differentiated by the titles of clinical specialist and psychiatric nurse practitioner. The differences in scope of practice are determined primarily by the differences in state statutes. Legislation by state may grant prescriptive authority which is (1) complementary, in which the nurse must have a collaborating physician and/or supervisory mechanism; or (2) substitutive, wherein the nurse may prescribe medication without physician supervision (Talley & Brooke, 1992). Most states grant complementary authority and require written protocols that serve as standards for nurse-physician collaboration.

The scope of practice includes mental and basic health assessments, nursing diagnoses, treatment interventions, including medication prescription and monitoring, counseling and psychotherapy as well as psychoeducational activities. The nurse is accountable for a caseload of clients/patients (case management) in collaboration with members of other disciplines and is responsible for evaluating treatment outcomes. Some examples of treatment settings currently employing mental health nurses in the direct provider role include psychiatric emergency rooms, social agencies that provide mental health care, mental health and substance abuse agencies that are expanding mental health services to include primary care, group homes for the severely and persistently mentally ill and developmentally disabled, day care settings, and centers for vocational rehabilitation counseling and client services.

Case Manager

The case manager role may include elements of the direct provider role or may be limited to case management functions. Case management focuses on meeting treatment outcomes related to an illness episode, in a given period of time. As a case manager, the psychiatric-mental health nurse is responsible for coordinating care delivered to an assigned group of patients or to clients/patients in his or her own caseload. Care is provided according to guidelines for diagnostic groups and standard-based protocols developed between the nurse and a collaborating physician or nurse colleague. It includes some health teaching and health maintenance activities (Cohen & Cesta, 1994). As a direct provider, the nurse focuses on stabilizing acute problems, seeking diagnostic clarification, establishing nursing diagnoses, and monitoring the initiation of treatment. In addition, the nurse oversees the utilization of resources by determining the eligibility and reimbursement potential for a client in a specific program. The nurse case manager also engages in follow-up and review of the case and the client's progress. Psychiatric nurses are increasingly being employed in this role in drug and alcohol treatment facilities, by managed-care companies, and by acute-care psychiatric facilities.

Consultant

The role of the psychiatric nurse as consultant is well described in the *ANA Standards of Psychiatric-Mental Health Nursing Practice* (1994). With nurse practitioner preparation the consultant utilizes knowledge about theories, relationships, and role responsibilities shared with the psychiatric-mental health clinical specialist, but includes a broader base of biologic knowledge. Some excellent examples are the use of psychiatric-mental health nurse practitioners in community-based clinics that treat individuals in the correctional system. Men and women arraigned in the community and evaluated for alternatives to incarceration have a high prevalence of substance-related and/or mental health problems. Onsite, the nurse can implement assessment and screening that considers both the basic health problems of the clients along with the plan of action ordered by the court, i.e., detoxification, community service with mental health follow-up, or psychiatric hospitalization. A comprehensive plan of action by the advanced practice psychiatric nurse involves collaboration with adult health nurse practitioners and/or physicians and/or with social worker or counselor coworkers. In primary care settings where individuals with mental health problems are often seen but undiagnosed or misdiagnosed, the nurse provides consultation for the provision of effective and appropriate mental health care.

Psychiatric-Consultation Liaison Nurse

The psychiatric-consultation liaison nurse seeks to improve mental health services for patients/clients served in settings not specific to mental health or substance abuse. In this advanced practice role the nurse makes psychiatric and psychosocial diagnoses and provides interventions ranging from health promotion to illness rehabilitation. These nurses frequently function as consultants from psychiatric settings and substance abuse treatment centers to general hospital units, primary care clinics, and emergency rooms. The advanced nurse in this role may be specialized by population, i.e., children and adolescents.

Interdisciplinary Team Member

The psychiatric-mental health advanced practice nurse is uniquely prepared to function as a member of multidisciplinary and interdisciplinary teams in all health care settings. Expert knowledge and skills in communication, conflict resolution, leadership, and groups dynamics, as well as interpersonal skills increase the efficiency of teams in their goals to improve organizational functions and provide optimal patient care (McGivern, 1993). Knowledge of human behavior and experience in solving problems related to mental health and human behavior equip the nurse with skills for collaboration, maintenance of a positive work environment, and tolerance for ambiguity and role diffusion which often characterize team development.

Roles in Education and Research

The advanced practice psychiatric-mental health nurse, whether clinical nurse specialist or psychiatric nurse practitioner, functions as educator and researcher. At the basic level the nurse meets the ANA Code requirements by participating in education, obtaining certification, and teaching clients and families. At the advanced practice level, the nurse continues his or her own education and participates in educating others. The psychiatric nurse with basic education uses research findings to improve clinical care and identifies clinical problems for research. At the advanced practice level, the nurse engages and collaborates with others in the research process (ANA, 1994).

With the emergence of newer models of care and an emphasis on primary mental health care, psychiatric-mental health nurses are increasingly developing the role dimension of psycho-education. Teaching skills are honed to address the needs of clients and families for information about preventing mental illness, maximizing well-being, and integrating health-related activities with medical regimens. Behavioral change is the desired outcome of psychoeducation but requires the development of life skills and coping strategies that must be presented, learned, and integrated into behavior. Nurses must be educated in understanding motivation for change, stages of change, and goal setting that results in outcomes of mastery for the client. With a renewed emphasis on empowering clients and families for self-care and disease prevention, this role presents new challenges for the nurse.

Similarly, the advanced practice nurse uses knowledge of research in formulating research-based interventions, evaluating outcomes of care, and formulating questions for further investigation. The need for formulating effective interventions with measurable outcomes has become central to achieving cost-effective use of resources. The nurse integrates research knowledge with the choice and application of interventions with demonstrable outcomes recognized by care providers and the consumer. These often take the form of protocols developed in keeping with standards of psychiatric nursing care and standardized mental health approaches. The implementation and evaluation of protocols serve to shape the directions for new modes of care delivery and new nursing role functions.

PRIMARY CARE AND PSYCHIATRIC-MENTAL HEALTH NURSING CARE

The model which includes primary care enables the nurse to deliver broad-based care while addressing psychotherapeutic needs. Its value in the health care delivery system is best highlighted in the nursing management of illnesses which involve complex psychophysiologic relationships but is not limited to them. Such disturbances are manifested in both dysfunctional behavior and physiologic changes; sensory deprivation dysfunction and alcoholism are examples. Early on others suggested the integration of primary care concepts into specialty services for drug abuse (Klerman, 1980), and geriatric psychiatry (Ebersole, 1989). The traditional psychotherapeutic relationship is enhanced when nursing goals incorporate elements of primary care. To achieve this, the role must change at different stages of therapy, and must be flexible enough to include *primary care delivery, coordination of care providers, and advocacy behaviors* for the client within a variety of community and health care delivery systems.

Three levels of primary mental health care frame the role functions of the advanced practice psychiatric-mental health nurse:

(1) primary mental health activities that focus on "at-risk" groups and are proposed to enhance function and mental health; prevention activities are included in this category;

(2) primary mental health services that address management and treatment interventions. These identify mental health problems as early as possible, reduce the time mental health problems exist, and halt the progression of severity and coexistence of other mental health problems; and

(3) primary mental health interventions that decrease the likelihood of relapse (Haber & Billings, 1995). A final level is added by Murphy and Moller (1993):

(4) maintenance interventions that have as their overriding goal a decrease in disability, the prevention of relapse, and the promotion of optimal functional status and quality of life.

The ways in which the primary mental health care role of the psychiatric-mental health nurse is "analogous" to that of the primary care provider (Haber & Billings, 1995) are easily demonstrated in the care of the depressed elderly client and the alcoholic client. Both depression and alcoholism are multidimensional disorders that are highly prevalent in the population at large. Individuals with these disorders rarely receive comprehensive care, that is, primary care and care of specific psychiatric syndromes. In addition, other disorders such as anxiety disorders, depression and substance abuse are commonly misdiagnosed categories in primary care practice (National Institutes of Health Consensus Development Panel, 1992). Eating disorders and narcotic dependence are equally suited to nursing care delivered in the primary mental health model.

Components of the primary care definition provide a framework for discussion of the broad-based primary mental health nursing functions. These components are: (1) addressing the majority of personal health needs; (2) developing a sustained partnership; and (3) practicing one's role in the context of family and community (IOM, 1996).

The Depressed Elderly Client

Addressing the Majority of Health Care Needs

Depression, in mild to severe forms, occurs in approximately 15% of community residents over age 65. The rates of major and minor depression among elderly people range from 5% in primary care clinics to 15%–25% in nursing homes (NIH Consensus Development Panel, 1992). Most older persons consider themselves in good mental and physical health and are reluctant to acknowledge or admit to psychological difficulty (Jenike, 1996). Many elders are hesitant to talk about feelings of depression, apathy, or discouragement and tend not to seek psychological interventions even when feeling sad and/or dejected (Blumenthal, 1980).

Psychotherapeutic interactions with the elderly can be subsumed under three goals: amelioration of symptoms, restoration of functioning, and enhancement of the perceived quality of life (Lazarus, 1988). The primary mental health nursing orientation is toward total health and the formulation of goals which reflect the client's overall concerns, such as increasing isolation and declining quality of life, as well as evaluating basic health and psychiatric problems. Since these clients tend to place greater emphasis on meeting basic survival needs rather than on mental health needs or may report somatic symptoms and avoid discussing feelings, the nurse works to develop an overall plan that encompasses all concerns. While recognizing that depression may be masked by physical complaints she or he acknowledges the client's priorities which may only indirectly deal with mental health.

The comprehensive approach of *direct care provision* also addresses problems associated with diagnosing depression in the elderly. Depression is often unrecognized in elders because of concurrent medical problems and medications taken for them, like antihypertensives and analgesics which of themselves induce depression. Often the provider associates depression with the aging process. The client may seek treatment for physical complaints such as fatigue, headache, and insomnia, while experiencing concurrent symptoms of dysphoric affect, and feelings of help-lessness, hopelessness, and worthlessness. A broad-based assessment helps to identify possible physical illnesses contributing to depression and to rule out secondary effects of infection, cerebral trauma, malnutrition, misuse of prescribed drugs, and alcohol intoxication, all of which can produce acute brain syndrome (Jenike, 1996; Naegle, 1983). At times, depression is manifested as pseudo dementia and a detailed history from client and family are key to differential diagnosis.

Chronic diseases and disabilities such as cancer, cardiovascular illness, and neurological disorders are often linked with depression. The reasons for this may be psychosocial or biologic. From a biologic perspective, decreased organ system reserve, slowed immunologic response, and changes in metabolism may impact mood (NIH Consensus Conference, 1992). Of prescriptions written in the United States, the largest number are written for persons over 65 (Solomon, Manepalli, Ireland, & Mahon, 1993). Drug properties may produce mood changes, drug interactions may change pharmacotherapeutic outcomes, and side effects of drugs may cause undesirable outcomes in the emotional, sexual, and digestive systems (AHCPR Guidelines, 1993).

A comprehensive history and obtaining or accessing findings of a physical assessment provide data from which the advanced practice mental health nurse can interpret the etiology and significance of depressive symptomatology. For the elder individual where medical problems and depression are often hard to differentiate, laboratory tests that (1) screen for underlying medical causes, and (2) identify biologic abnormalities characteristic of depression, should be ordered (ACHPR, 1993). In conjunction with a mental status exam, signs of depression as an independent versus co-occurring phenomenon may also be revealed. The mental health assessment is conducted with special attention to age-specific themes often associated with depression; selected screening instruments such as the Mini Mental Status Exam and the Geriatric Depression Scale are utilized. Themes include multiple complaints and demands, hypochondriasis and anxiety, multiple losses, disappointment with one's life, a sense of futility, and anticipation of one's own demise and should be evaluated for their links to depressive symptoms. Suicidal ideation and self-destructive thoughts are exacerbated by poor health and limited, unsatisfactory support systems.

Cognitive changes, diminished sensory and learning capacities, and social losses make older individuals especially vulnerable to the confusion caused by fragmentation in the health care delivery system and brief, superficial contacts with a wide variety and number of health care personnel (Bellak, 1976). Whether the depression is mild or severe, the nurse should treat the client with the goals of achieving optimal health not only as a result of treating the depression, but by addressing all contributing psychobiological factors.

A Sustained Partnership with Patients

A trusting therapeutic nurse-patient relationship is the framework within which the primary mental health nurse plans and delivers care. When the single health care professional who is both therapist and primary care provider assumes multiple role functions, the client's security is enhanced. For depressed individuals, primary mental health care activities encompass efforts to prevent depression in the elderly as well as strategies to decrease the severity of depression, shorten its duration, and decrease the likelihood of relapse.

Prevention takes the form of maintaining optimal physical health, dealing with stressful situations early in their onset, avoiding heavy alcohol consumption and overreliance on prescription drugs, and utilizing coping strategies to deal with hassles and problems with a sense of mastery. The nurse focuses on all aspects of the patient's functioning and takes into consideration the elder's preoccupations whether they be with emotional matters, economic security, social relationships, or social conditions. A full awareness of the client's environment, social network, and support systems as well as the willingness to make suggestions to assist the client's optimal manipulation of social and environmental conditions are important provider strategies basic to health promotion and maintenance. In fact, the prognosis will depend heavily on the social context (Jenike, 1996).

For the elderly depressed client, strategies by the nurse psychotherapist include (1) establishing networks supportive to the provision of primary care, including health education and screening; (2) psychotherapeutic work to identify and manage feelings of depression; and (3) planning and coordination of multidisciplinary services essential to the client's support in daily functioning. Because the elderly client needs multiple services, often from private and public agencies, *collaborative* and *coordinating* functions by the therapist may become primary. Information sharing and interpretation of client needs, collaboration with social workers, clergy, public health nurses and/or agency volunteers are necessary to restore and maintain whatever functional level is possible for the client. Such an approach extends the therapeutic activity beyond the one-to-one relationship.

Motivating change and supporting efforts to improve the quality of life will not be appreciated unless the elder trusts the nurse and finds him or her a credible counselor and psychotherapist. The care provider must engage in outreach and invest time and patience in building a trusting relationship. Chronic illness and depressive episodes may necessitate hospitalizations and contact with numerous agencies and/or providers. For trust to continue, a relationship of *continuity* must be maintained between patient and nurse over time and through many communication channels. Continuity in contacts with client and family is essential to offset fears of abandonment and loss in the life of the elderly client. By assuming a central coordinating role, communication, interpretation of the plan for care, and emotional and psychological support are provided by one familiar and trusted care provider. Maintaining a primary relationship and consolidating the emotional investment in one caregiver provides further security that counteracts ongoing fears of desertion, loss, and of death experienced by the elderly (Lazarus, 1988; Levin, 1967). Because of feeling devalued, angry, and lonely, the elderly depressed individual withdraws even further from investing in relationships. In addition, the client's increasing dependence, evident to nurse and patient, needs to be addressed in discussions and through nonverbal support. Most elders have an awareness of increasing dependence and a limited capacity to manipulate the environment which creates feelings of being trapped and helpless in changing environmental circumstances.

Interventions that address decreasing social and physical mobility include efforts to increase community involvement. Theses can prevent a client's feeling increasingly isolated and/or confined and facilitate reconnecting following a depressive episode. Explore the client's involvement and potential participation in community resources such as a nearby synagogue or church, senior center, or volunteer program. When the nurse is at ease with dependency and familiar with systems to decrease it by involvement with the community, greater activity is promoted. *Outreach* efforts, essential in the delivery of broad-based care, are evident in a readiness to visit the client at home and/or assess factors such as family or caretaker interaction with the client, and the safety and stability of the home and community.

Addressing Contexts of Family and Community

For the advanced practice mental health nurse, direct primary care interventions include family and community as well as the individual. The elder's family system is often diminished in size and spirit by death and other losses and separations. Protective, supportive relationships are few in number, and their positive effects such as maintaining self-esteem through others' shared positive feedback may be limited. Expanding and strengthening meager support systems should be major initiatives with this population. "Family" may consist of friends, neighbors, or former business associates because the client is estranged from, or without kin. Knowledge of families, the dynamics of family relationships, and the interrelationships of family members form the basis for interventions. Individuals who provide emotional and practical resources for the client are included in health teaching.

The advanced practice nurse intervenes with family counseling and/or psychotherapy to facilitate problem solving and decision making. These modalities are recommended for the depressed elderly client whose usual need for a supportive family/social network is magnified by the biologic and behavioral manifestations of the illness. In the ongoing relationship, the therapist offers opportunities for the client to have increasing participation in health maintenance activities. Simultaneously, client and therapist can evaluate the effectiveness of implemented plans and modify care plans as treatment progresses. Interested other individuals, including family and other care providers, may be included in this process as necessary. The nurse may include family members in the initial assessment to acknowledge the importance of family structure and members as sources of data and support for the development and implementation of a care plan. In addition, the emotional needs of families can be addressed in support groups to address feelings about the many care-related issues faced by family members (Ebersole, 1989).

Primary mental health nursing role functions include relationships with the professional community and networks for collaborative approaches to patient problems. A well-established network of care providers is most beneficial as a resource for referral and collaborative care. Opportunities to collaborate within an interdisciplinary care team, while they may be limited, should be utilized wherever possible. Depression in the elderly client is a complex phenomenon and depending on the client's age, extenuating medical problems, and the availability of support services, care provision is time-intensive. Components of a database as a foundation for the care plan can be obtained by specialty consultation with a variety of care providers, such as neuropsychologists, psychiatrists, physical therapists, social workers, and others.

The primary care provider must be skilled in identifying needs and making appropriate referrals to other providers. Frequently needed services include short-term hospitalization, psychopharmacologic evaluation, physical and occupational therapy, and diagnostic testing. An excellent example of the nurse's use of referral and interdisciplinary collaboration emerges in differentiating between depression and the affective changes that accompany dementia. Since the blunted affect of dementia resembles the sadness and detachment of depression, a detailed history is essential.

Depression and the tendency for a rapid onset of symptoms suggest that memory impairments are related to emotional dysfunction and constitute pseudo dementia rather than dementia (Franzen & Rasmussen, 1990). A referral for neuro-psychiatric evaluation is indicated in these cases.

Direct Care Provision for the Client with Alcohol Problems

Addressing the Majority of Health Care Needs

As many as 6 million individuals meet DMS-IV criteria for alcohol dependence (SAMSHA, 1995) and another 11 million are heavy drinkers (SAMSHA, 1997). Most persons with these problems are not treated because signs are not recognized by primary care providers and because symptoms of fatigue, headaches, and low-back pain are presented as only physical. In addition, excessive consumption is often denied by the client.

Alcohol-related problems occur on a continuum from early problem drinking to alcoholism. Nursing interventions along the continuum take into consideration the beginning level of severity, intermediate stages, and progression in an entrenched pattern of alcoholism in which the client experiences varying degrees of health and illness. The nurse who understands primary care and its links to illness in acute and chronic stages is able to assist the client during phases of sobriety as well as during preliminary stages of recovery and periods of relapse.

Primary prevention and basic health care are supported by a drug-free lifestyle, and health education is utilized to promote physical and mental well-being. The advanced practice nurse emphasizes health promotion as a premise at all stages of the illness although the signs and symptoms of alcohol-related problems change over time. Health promotion is central to developing a positive attitude about self-care and promoting hope in the early and acute stages. For the chronically ill individual, basic health care can be an essential cornerstone of continuing struggles to achieve sobriety. As a *direct provider* the nurse develops a comprehensive self-care plan with the client. Usually alcohol and other drug use has persisted for long periods, and clients have often neglected self-care like exercise, dental hygiene, and good nutrition. The nurse not only imparts important information in these areas but interprets their importance in the context of positive self-regard and support for sobriety. This requires that the nurse be knowledgeable about nutrition, exercise physiology, relaxation techniques, and alternative modalities which support spiritual growth and mental well-being.

The biologic components of alcohol abuse and dependence figure prominently among client needs and support a biopsychosocial approach to care. Whether acting as a *consultant, direct care provider,* or *case manager,* the nurse develops a database beginning with a comprehensive history and physical assessment, whether performed by the nurse or obtained from a collaborating nurse practitioner or physician. The alcohol and other drug history, in conjunction with physical signs and laboratory data, are central to the formulation of nursing diagnoses. Heavy drinking patterns are suggested when the client manifests elevated liver enzymes (especially GGT) and anemias (particularly macrocytic anemia) in the absence of other diseases that could account for these conditions. Alcoholism is indicated by (1) physiologic and clinical signs; and (2) behavioral, attitudinal, and psychological characteristics associated with stages of alcoholism (Schuckit, 1989). The basic drug history, a major behavioral indicator, includes the amount and frequency of alcohol, illicit and prescription drug use, tobacco and caffeine use, and over-the-counter (OTC) drug use. The client's defensiveness and denial about excessive drinking may result in underreporting, and other sources of data such as collateral reports from family and friends must be considered in reference to national standards of "sensible" drinking (levels unlikely to result in health problems). These limits are 12–14 drinks a week for men and 7–9 drinks per week for women, with no more than 3 drinks per occasion (WHO, 1996).

Screening tools utilized in primary care and specialty practice help to discern if the individual is experiencing effects of drinking that place him or her at-risk. The two that have been found to be especially sensitive in primary care settings are the CAGE (Ewing, 1984) and the WHO (World Health Organization) Audit (Saunders, Aasland, Babor, de la Fuente, & Grant, 1993). In addition, the nurse reviews the physical examination and laboratory findings for biologic indicators of heavy consumption.

Alcohol is rarely the only drug an individual uses. Exceptions to this are persons over 55 who were less influenced than younger people by the prevalence of illicit drug use in the 1960s and 1970s. The physical examination may suggest that the client may also be using other drugs by injection or inhalation. There is a high correlation between smoking and alcohol abuse or alcoholism. Recent research indicates that many alcoholics are also nicotine dependent (Shiffman & Balabaris, 1996). Comprehensive care will include the assessment for readiness to stop smoking and appropriate support and/or guidance toward smoking cessation.

The mental status exam helps to identify affective and cognitive changes that may be related to alcohol consumption such as anxiety disorders and/or depression. In the alcohol-dependent individual, the effects of the drug will distort the assessment of both cognitive performance and affective responses. Findings suggestive of alcohol abuse or alcoholism should be discussed with the client, and be presented as part of the overall health assessment and consultation. The need for intervention, whether through modification of drinking habits or hospitalization for intensive treatment, should be clearly expressed and supported with examples in a caring, nonpunitive manner. Options available to the client must be clearly spelled out. Should the client choose to enter treatment to reduce consumption or treat addiction, a biopsychosocial approach should be utilized throughout.

The advanced practice nurse will find that primary care components are especially important when a client is alcohol-dependent and requires detoxification on an inpatient or ambulatory basis. The appropriate pharmacologic and nursing management in these circumstances are key to the restoration of health and the client's motivation for dealing with the addiction. Basic assessment, nutritional guidance, nursing care, and counseling skills can be implemented by the generalist nurse, but must be a component of comprehensive nursing care provided by the advanced practice nurse. Following detoxification or in stages of illness which do not require it, the nurse may rely on other pharmacologic supports.

Recent research findings suggest that the use of medications such as Naltrexone and Antabuse (Disulfirum hydrochloride) provide helpful, short-term support when the client demonstrates the ability to greatly modify, or abstain from, drinking. When the ability to control drinking is markedly impaired, when the patient is also opioid dependent or has significant liver pathology, the use of these medications may be contraindicated. These medications can be effectively utilized by the nurse practitioner as a part of the comprehensive care approach. Other pharmacologic options are available when depression or anxiety disorder co-occur with alcohol abuse or alcoholism. When depressive symptomatology persist after 2–4 weeks of abstinence, the use of antidepressants may be considered. The nurse must be thoroughly familiar with the medication options, the prescription and management, and the specific guidelines and limitations for the use of medication with people recovering from drug addiction, deriving from the chemical properties of drugs like tricyclic antidepressants and benzodiazepines; these are detailed in the research literature. Their use should only be initiated, however, following a comprehensive psychiatric assessment and a commitment on the part of the patient to abstain from alcohol.

Partnership with the Patient

Alcoholism is an outcome of multiple interrelated factors and affects many aspects of the client's life and the lives of those with whom he or she lives, works, and interacts. Occupational, legal, and social spheres are arenas within which the disease and its associated behaviors are played out, and its ramifications take on a variety of meanings. Basic education for nurses usually prepares them to be sensitive to the psychological impacts of socially stigmatic attitudes about individuals with drinking problems, to know the long-term effects of heavy alcohol consumption, and be aware of the legal difficulties frequently encountered through driving while intoxicated or other legal infractions, and the threats to professional licensure and/or employment. Such awareness influences the attitudes with which the advanced practice nurse enters the *consultation, direct care provision*, and *case management* of the individual experiencing difficulties with alcohol.

While patients may deny the extent to which they are "overusing" or abusing alcohol, their defensiveness suggests some painful awareness of the stigma associated with alcoholism. Fearing criticism and rejection, they rarely seek help for their drinking but are seen in large numbers in clinics, emergency room settings, and general hospital units. It is estimated that the prevalence of alcohol-related problems among individuals with other than psychiatric or addiction diagnoses ranges from 25%–57% depending on characteristics of the facility and geographic region (Dongier, Hill, Kealey, & Lawrence, 1994), and that as many as 1 in 4–7 persons seeking primary care will have an alcohol problem (Morris, 1995). These data have important implications for the advanced practice mental health nurse in *consultation* and *direct provider roles*. While the number of men who use alcohol is almost twice that of women, national numbers for regular users in both groups are high; 58.9% of men and 43.6% of women surveyed had used alcohol in the past month (SAMSHA, 1996). Of drinkers, approximately 1 in 10 men and 1 in 15 women will develop a problem with in alcohol.

Establishing a partnership with these patients can be challenging because when they do seek treatment, usually at the urging of family members, friends, or employers, they are ambivalent about addressing their alcohol problems. Denial of the severity of the problem is common, and shame about the negative outcomes of drinking emerges as the denial gradually decreases. Social stigma, frequent interpersonal and economic losses, and the continuing and generally unsuccessful struggle to control drinking result in diminished self-regard and feelings of hopelessness. Given the frequency with which other drugs are combined with alcohol, legal and job performance problems may further reenforce feelings of low self-esteem.

The client often anticipates responses from the health professional that parallel those of others with whom interpersonal, financial, or legal problems have ensued. The alcoholic's dilemma between perceived dependence on a substance for survival and a perceived "competition" posed by investments in job, family, and friends, results in numerous and painful losses which become all too apparent with sobriety. The constancy of a primary care-nurse therapist relationship facilitates trust and a working relationship characterized by accessibility and commitment. Since "slips" and relapses occur in all phases of the chronic disease of alcoholism, the nurse must establish a contract with the client about a plan. Depending on the nature of the illness that plan may be for controlled drinking or efforts aimed at abstinence. An open agreement and assurance that the nurse will not abandon the patient should relapse occur, supports honest reporting and diminishes expectations about punishment or rejection. A long-term working relationship, characterized by basic health care and psychological support, increases opportunities to achieve personal growth as well as sobriety.

Context of Family and Community

Because they understand the implications of an individual's illness for the community, and community patterns and resources, nurses are aware of the network of community agencies and care providers, that, by providing guidance and information, are invaluable to the recovering alcoholic. Through coordinating and collaborating functions, the nurse facilitates linkages and supports the client's involvement.

Excessive alcohol use in one or more members of a family has the effect of distorting emotional relationships and ultimately disrupting relationships within the family system and the community. The alcoholic may manifest problems at work, is often involved in legal infractions and problems related to compliance with taxes and other indebtedness, and usually engages in behaviors which result in alienation of the family from the community. Dysfunctional family relationships have implications for day-to-day living as well as for the future of the family and its members. These implications include familial predispositions to alcohol and other drug dependence which is genetic and/or environmental, and learned patterns of relationships which are dysfunctional and compromise the family members' capacities for successful interpersonal interactions (Ells, 1991). Adult children of alcoholics report many life problems, and a significant number of them develop dependencies on alcohol and other drugs. By assessing family systems, the psychiatric-mental health nurse can develop strategies for health education, support, and counseling needs of the family with an alcoholic member.

For many, sobriety is most effectively attained through the use of self-help groups as adjuncts to treatment. Alcoholics Anonymous and other programs developed according to this 12-step model provide structure, support, social aspects of a fellowship, and a program for establishing a drug-free lifestyle. Referring the client to 12-step programs and supporting or even requiring their attendance enhances treatment and provides a means of around-the-clock access to understanding persons when drug cravings and other drug-using-related behaviors emerge. For those individuals who find AA unacceptable for ideological, cultural, or other reasons, groups such as Smart Recovery, Rational Recovery, and Women for Sobriety are options.

Tertiary Prevention consists of relapse counseling and health mainte-nance and requires that the client acquire new learning in the psychothera-peutic relationship. Relapse prevention assists the client to learn strategies for recognizing and dealing with high-risk situations, including skill train-ing for coping, cognitive reframing, and lifestyle balance (Marlatt & Gordon, 1988).

When friends and family members have enabled the client's illness to progress by participating in drug use, and/or supplying the drug in an effort to abort negative behavior by the client, these individuals profit from learning the errors of their ways. Al-Anon provides a group setting in which to understand how efforts to "keep the peace" or "save the client" also serve to support the client's continued drug use and lead to poor mental health for everyone. Approaches useful with nontraditional or traditional family systems, such as family therapy, are strategies for promoting behavioral change. The nurse as direct provider is equipped to practice these, or can refer the family to appropriate agencies and care providers. Goals include behavioral change within the family which can support the recovery of the individual as well as resolving old and dysfunctional behaviors, supporting others, and preventing further drug and alcohol problems.

Optimally, advanced practice nurses who assume the *role of primary care/psychotherapy providers* give direct care to clients. Involvement with the family is relevant, but the roles of coordinator of services, collaborator with family and several care providers, and advocate for client and family are particularly important. Because alcoholism and other drug dependencies have wide ramifications for the lives of client and family, the nurse is key in interpreting the availability and appropriate use of reliable community resources.

The focus of the psychotherapeutic work is the client's drug use and central psychological problems, as well as changing the self-concept. Support and learning opportunities which move the individual toward a new view of self are particularly important. The nurse facilitates appropriate opportunities for change at various stages of recovery through referrals to various legal, vocational, and health agencies, as well as other care providers and self-help groups.

SUMMARY

Major changes in health care delivery support the greater use of psychiatric nurses in advanced practice roles generally, and the primary mental health care provider role in particular. Aided by managed-care approaches, access to third-party payment, and federally funded programs, advanced practice nurses are responding to the growing need for community-based mental health care for individuals and families with HIV, the frail elderly, addicts, the severely and persistently mentally ill, the developmentally disabled, and those housed in correctional facilities. In these settings, primary mental health care nurses are cost-effective because they address health in a comprehensive way, while providing psychiatric care at primary, secondary, and tertiary levels. Moller and Haber (1996) stress the importance of supporting the advanced practice role regardless of the title and suggest that a "blended" role provides the most realistic and marketable of future psychiatric-mental health advanced practice nursing roles. Since psychiatric-mental health clinical nurse specialists and psychiatric nurse practitioners share a scope of practice with the same core components of expert knowledge, including primary mental health skills, similar performance outcomes will be demonstrated. In a growing number of settings, the value of the role to the consumer and profession is being demonstrated effectively with target populations of individuals, groups, and families with multiple health and social problems.

The freedom of nurses to practice with high autonomy must still be negotiated on an ongoing basis in institutions and with other members of the health care team. Whatever the confines of practice boundaries, the ability to function as a colleague is essential. Confidence and supporting credentials of one's professional identity are prerequisites if nurses are to participate as colleagues with other professionals. As well as being skilled and contributing members of interdisciplinary teams, nurses must be ready to articulate their role in relationship to that of other mental health professionals. While issues of territoriality restrict the potential for professionals to function together, clarification of boundaries through communication, exploration of competitive striving, and analysis of functions in relation to patient/client needs can improve intra- and interprofessional relations. Advanced practice preparation helps to limit the artificial division of tasks because the nurse can move easily between activities central to primary care and specialty training.

Primary care as a health care delivery model presents challenging opportunities to advanced practice primary mental health nursing as described by Haber and Billings (1995). The prerequisite focus on collaboration, coordination, and direct care delivery supports the nurse's central role on the interdisciplinary team. Skills in addressing client/family problems, organizing environmental patterns to support treatment approaches, and facilitating circumstances to influence the client's ability to attain optimum wellness while addressing both basic and mental health problems support the potential for a broad range of role functions and responsibilities.

REFERENCES AND BIBLIOGRAPHY

Agency for Health Care Policy and Research. (1993). *Depression in primary care: Volume 1: Detection and diagnosis*. Rockville, MD: U.S. Department of Health and Human Services.

Aiken, L. (1978). Primary care: The challenge for nursing. In N. Chaska (Ed.), *The nursing profession: Views through the mist.* New York: McGraw-Hill.

Aiken, L., & Sage, W. M. (1993). Staffing national health care reform: A role for advanced practice nurses. *Akron Law Review, 26,* 1–30.

American Nurses Association. (1994). *Statement on psychiatric-mental health clinical nursing practice and standards of psychiatric-mental health nursing.* Washington, DC: Author.

American Nurses Association. (1995). *Scope and standards of advanced practice registered nursing.* Washington, DC: Author.

Bellak, L. (1976). Geriatric psychiatry as comprehensive health care. In L. Bellak & T. B. Karasu (Eds.), *Geriatric psychiatry: A handbook for psychiatrists and primary care physicians.* New York: Grune and Stratton.

Beyer, J., & Marshall, J. (1981). The interpersonal dimension of collegiality. *Nursing Outlook, 29,* 662.

Blazer, D. C. (1993). *Depression in later life,* 2nd edition. St. Louis: Mosby.

Blumenthal, M. (1980). Depressive illness in old age: Getting behind the mask. *Geriatrics, 35,* 34.

Chambers, J. K., Dangel, R. B., Tripodi, V., & Jaeger, C. (1987). Clinical nurse specialist collaborative practice: Development of a generic job description and standards of performance. *Clinical Nurse Specialist, 1,* 124–127.

Cohen, E., & Cesta, T. (1994). Case management in the acute care setting: A model for health care reform. *Journal of Case Management, 3,* 3.

Dongier, M., Hill, J. M., Kealey, S., & Lawrence, J. (1994). Screening for alcoholism in general hospitals. *Canadian Journal of Psychiatry, 39*(1), 12–20.

Ebersole, P. (1989). *Caring for the psychogeriatric client.* New York: Springer.

Ells, M. A. W. (1991). Family therapy. In G. E. Bennett & D. Woolf (Eds.), *Substance abuse.* Albany, NY: Delmar Publishers.

Ewing, J. A. (1984). Detecting alcoholism: The CAGE questionnaire. *Journal of the American Medical Association, 252,* 1905–1907.

Franzen, M. D., & Rasmussen, P. R. (1990). Clinical neuropsychology and older populations. In A. M. Horton (Ed.), *Neuropsychology across the lifespan.* New York: Springer.

Haber, J., & Billings, C. (1995). Primary mental health care: A model for psychiatric-mental health nursing. *Journal of the American Psychiatric Nurses Association, 1,* 5.

Institute of Medicine. (1996). *Primary care: America's health in a new era.* Washington, DC: National Academy Press.

Jenike, M. A. (1996). Psychiatric illnesses in the elderly: A review. *Journal of Geriatric Psychiatry and Neurology, 9,* 57.

Jennings, C. (1997, January). Primary care and the question of obsolescence. *Journal of Psychiatric Nursing Mental Health Services,* 9.

Klerman, G. (1980). Klerman outlines goals of ADAMHA programs. *Psychiatry News, 40,* 23.

Lazarus, L. W. (Ed.). (1988). *Essentials of geriatric psychiatry.* New York: Springer.

Leininger, M. (1973). *Contemporary issues in mental health nursing.* Boston: Little, Brown.

Levin, S. (1967). Depression in the aged. In M. Berezin & H. Cath (Eds.), *Geriatric psychiatry: Grief, loss and emotional disorders in the aging process.* New York: International University Press.

Liskow, B., Campbell, J., Nickel, E. J., & Powell, B. J. (1995). Validity of the CAGE Questionnaire in screening for alcohol dependence in a walk-in (triage) clinic. *Journal of Studies on Alcohol, 56*(3), 277–281.

Marlatt, G. A., & Gordon, J. R. (Eds.). (1988). *Relapse prevention: Maintenance strategies in the treatment of addictive behavior.* New York: Guilford Press.

McBride, A. B. (1996). Psychiatric nursing in the Twenty-first century. In *Psychiatric-mental health nursing: Integrating the behavioral and biological sciences.* Philadelphia: W. B. Saunders.

McEnany, G. W. (1991, October). Psychobiology and psychiatric nursing: A philosophical matrix. *Archives of Psychiatric Nursing, V,* 5.

McGivern, D. (1993). The role of the nurse on the interdisciplinary treatment team. In M. A. Naegle (Ed.), *Substance abuse education in nursing, Vol. III.* New York: National League for Nursing.

Mechanic, D. (1982). Nursing and mental health care: Expanding future possibilities for nursing services. In L. Aiken & D. Mechanic (Eds.), *Nursing in the 1980s: Crises, opportunities and challenges.* Philadelphia: Lippincott.

Moller, M. D., & Haber, J. (1996). Advanced practice psychiatric nursing: The need for a blended role. *Online Journal of Issues in Nursing, 14*(41), 16–24.

Morris, J. A. (1995). Alcohol and other drug treatment: A proposal for integration with primary care. *Alcohol Treatment Quarterly, 13,* 45–56.

Murphy, M. F., & Moller, M. D. (1993). Relapse management in neurobiological disorders. The Moller-Murphy Symptom Management Assessment Tool. *Archives of Psychiatric Nursing, 7,* 226–235.

Mrazek, P. J., & Haggerty, R. J. (1994). *Reducing risks for mental disorders.* Washington, DC: National Academy Press.

Naegle, M. (1983). The role of psychotherapist within the primary health care model. In L. Breslauer & M. Haug (Eds.), *Depression and aging.* New York: Springer.

National Institutes of Health Consensus Development Conference Statement. (1992). *Depression in the elderly.*

Nightingale, F. (1859). *Notes on nursing: What it is and what it is not.* London: Harrison and Sons.

Rauckhorst, L., Stokes, S., & Mezey, M. (1992). Community and home assessment. *Health assessment for the older individual,* Second Edition. New York: Springer.

SAMSHA. (1995). *Substance abuse and mental health statistics sourcebook.* B. A. Rouse (Ed.). Rockville, MD: U.S.D.H.H.S.

SAMSHA. (1997). *Preliminary results from the 1996 National Household Survey on Drug Abuse.* Rockville, MD: U.S.D.H.H.S.

Saunders, J. B., Aasland, T. F., Babor, T. F., de la Fuente, C., & Grant, M. (1993). Development of the Alcohol Use disorders Identification Test (AUDIT): WHO collaborative project on early detection of persons with harmful alcohol consumption—II. *Addiction, 88,* 791–804.

Schuckit, M. A. (1989). *Drug and alcohol abuse: A clinical guide to diagnosis and treatment.* New York: Plenum Publishing Company.

Shiffman, S., & Balabaris, M. (1996). Do drinking and smoking go together? *Alcohol, Health and Research World, 20,* 107–110.

Solomon, K., Manepalli, J., Ireland, G. A., & Mahon, G. M. (1993). Alcoholism and prescription drug abuse in the elderly: St. Louis University Grand Rounds. *Journal of the American Geriatrics Society, 41*(1), 57–69.

Talley, S., & Brooke, P. (1992). Prescriptive authority for psychiatric clinical specialists: Framing the issues. *Archives of Psychiatric Nursing, 6*(2), 71–82.

Talley, S., & Caverly, S. (1994). Advanced practice psychiatric nursing and health care reform. *Hospital and Community Psychiatry, 45*(6), 545–547.

Whall, A. L. (1990). Nursing approaches to the mental health of the elderly: A position paper. *Issues in Mental Health Nursing, 11*, 71–77.

World Health Organization Study Group. (1996). A cross-national trial of brief interventions with heavy drinkers. *American Journal of Public Health, 86*(7), 948–955.

Chapter 18

NURSE-MANAGED URINARY INCONTINENCE

Joyce Colling

NURSES have always managed urinary incontinence (U.I.). Their role historically, however, has been limited to "mopping up" after an incontinence event occurred, padding patients to contain incontinence, and placing urinals and other collecting devices at patients' disposal. In the early 1970s, a shift began to occur from containment of incontinence to one in which advanced practice nurses began to assess, diagnose, treat, and cure people with urinary incontinence. This new care model was heavily influenced by pioneers in geriatric medicine and continence nurses in England as well as the development of master's-level advanced practice nursing programs in the U.S.

The focus of this chapter is to document the evolution of continence nursing in the U.S., distinguish the nursing model for continence from that of related disciplines such as medicine and physical therapy, discuss barriers to practice, and speculate on future opportunities for practice and research by advanced practice nurses in continence management.

Because little has been written about this new subspecialty in nursing, most of the source material was obtained by interviewing a number of advanced practice nurse informants who have been instrumental in the evolution of continence nursing. These informants are: Christine Norton (England), Diane Newman, Diane Smith, Barbara Woolner, Thelma Wells, Carol Brink, Patricia Burns, Mary H. Palmer, Joanne McDowell, and Molly Dougherty (U.S.).

EVOLUTION OF NURSING MANAGEMENT OF URINARY INCONTINENCE

In England the impetus for improved management of urinary incontinence came in 1977, when Phyllis Friend, the Chief Nursing Officer of England, called for each health district in the country to set up incontinence resource centers, identify continence in nurses' job descriptions, and establish education mechanisms. In 1981, British nurses held the first formal meeting of the Association of Continence Advisors (renamed in 1991 to Association of Continence Advise). By 1983, there were 17 full-time Continence Nurse Advisors, a 10-day national continence certification program, and a national report, *Action for Incontinence*, published by the Department of Health. Early in the 1980s there was opposition by nurses in the Department of Health to nurse specialists for incontinence; however, by the late 1980s this sentiment had been reversed. In 1991, a second national report, *Agenda for Action on Continence Services* (Sanderson, 1991), was published that further underscored the need for expanded services by Continence Nurse Advisors. In 1992, the Continence Foundation established a help-line, public information and education services, and public awareness events, such as the annual National Continence Day.

Currently, there are 30 continence centers where a 10-day course for incontinence management is taught, and over 420 Continence Advisors throughout the United Kingdom. The typical continence nurse advisor has been trained to do an individual assessment, focused physical examination, including a functional and vaginal examination, a diet and medication history, and an evaluation of environmental barriers and toileting aids. All continence advisors teach Kegel exercises, about 50% by verbal instruction only, and 50% through the use of intravaginal weights, perinometers, and electrical-stimulation. Thus, the development of nurses' involvement in continence care was greatly aided in the United Kingdom by national surveys and reports that reached the highest level of government personnel and that released funds to support Continence Nurse Advisors on a national level.

In the U.S., the motivation for innovative, practical, clinical solutions to manage urinary incontinence originated with nurses' clinical experience with patients and as a result of individual nursing projects. The practice of a few of the American interviewees evolved over time with assistance from psychologists and/or in collaboration with physicians.

Early in the development of continence nursing in America, nurses were assisted by the clinical reports published in British nursing journals. Although not data-based, these reports heightened American nurses' awareness as to other possibilities for incontinence management. Several American nurses attended the annual British Continence Nurse Advisors meetings. One U.S. nurse, Thelma Wells, began her study of geriatrics as the first nursing fellow in the Department of Geriatric Medicine headed by Dr. John Brocklehurst at the University of Manchester in England. She began studying general geriatric nursing, but it soon narrowed to incontinence, and she began writing about incontinence management in American journals (Fielding & Wells, 1975; Wells, 1975; Wells, 1980). In 1982, Dr. Wells opened the first American nurse-managed clinic for urinary incontinence in collaboration with Carol Brink, a nurse practitioner, and Dr. Ananias Diokno, a urologist (Brink, Wells, & Diokno, 1983). Dr. Wells also pioneered as the first nurse to receive funding from the National Institute of Aging (NIA) for research on incontinence and was later re-funded through the National Institute for Nursing Research (NINR) (Nursing Intervention: Urine Control in Older Women, NIA, 1982–87; Nursing Intervention: Exercise for Stress UI, NINR, 1987–1992).

Nationally, incontinence management in the U.S. received intense focus in 1983, with the convening of a workshop sponsored by the National Institute on Aging (NIA) (Hadley et al., 1983). The panel of participants was multidisciplinary and included nursing representation. This conference produced a number of recommendations, among which was a call for proposals to test various strategies for urinary incontinence treatment among the elderly through a cooperative agreement between the National Institute on Aging, and the National Center for Nursing Research (NCNR). One nurse, Dr. Patricia Burns, was among the four projects funded in 1985. A nurse practitioner, Dr. Burns's research grew out of a 1980 collaborative project in which nurse practitioners taught Kegel exercises and biofeedback to women with urinary incontinence (Burns, Marecki, Dittmar, & Bullough, 1985; Burns, Pranikoff, Nochajski, Desotelle, & Harwood, 1990). In October of 1988, The National Institutes of Health sponsored a Consensus Development Conference that summarized current knowledge of the prevalence, etiology, costs, pathophysiology, diagnostic assessments, and treatment modalities. Again nursing was represented on the panel of experts and among the presenters during the conference (NIH, 1990).

News of these pioneering nursing efforts to treat incontinence circulated at national meetings and in nursing journals. For instance, an entire 1980 issue of *Geriatric Nursing* was devoted to assessment and management of urinary incontinence. Also during this time, Palmer wrote her master's project on urinary incontinence (Palmer, 1982) and completed a PhD thesis on risk factors for incontinence among nursing home residents (Palmer, 1990). Dr. Palmer's work on prompted voiding techniques with Dr. Kathleen McCormick, a nurse in the U.S. Public Health Service, and Dr. Bernard Engel in NIA's intramural research program at the gerontology research center, led to her appointment as the first research fellow at NINR, where she continued her work on incontinence management techniques (Palmer, 1985, 1996).

The Continence Consensus Conference, the four NIA-NINR-sponsored research projects, focused on behavioral treatments for incontinence, and the NIA intramural research program on incontinence produced a watershed of information and heightened nurses' interest in nurse-managed UI programs. For instance, in the mid-1980s on the East Coast, Dr. Joanne McDowell began treating UI within a multidisciplinary clinic at the University of Pittsburgh. In New Jersey, Diane Smith, a nurse practitioner, began an incontinence nursing practice for home-bound elderly through contracts with the state of New Jersey and the University of Pennsylvania School of Nursing. A year later she was joined by another nurse practitioner, Diane Newman, and the continence practice was expanded to include the city of Philadelphia (Smith-Baigis, Smith, Rose, & Newman, 1989). In Florida, Dr. Molly Dougherty's work began on measurement of pelvic muscle characteristics and stress urinary incontinence in women (Dougherty, Abrams, & McKey, 1986; Dougherty, Bishop, Mooney, Gimotty, & Williams, 1993), and in Virginia, Dr. Jean Wyman began her seminal work with patients with urge incontinence (Fantl et al., 1991). On the west coast, Dr. Joyce Colling and her colleagues launched a multi-site research project to treat incontinence in nursing home residents (Colling, Ouslander, Hadley, Eisch, & Campbell, 1992; Colling, Owen, & McCreedy, 1994) and care-dependent community elderly (Colling, Hadley, Eisch, Campbell, & Newman, 1995). Barbara Woolner, who became certified in biofeedback, began treating patients both in the community in collaboration with a urologist and in nursing homes in California (Woolner, 1995). Knowledge and skills among these nurses were enhanced through frequent collegial discussions at professional meetings, informal clinical site visits, and exchanges with professional colleagues in medicine and the social sciences who were also contributing to the growing knowledge base about incontinence management. This network not only promoted information exchange but provided support in an environment in which many medical and nursing colleagues were at best apathetic and at worst openly critical and disparaging.

Late in 1991, the first multispecialty incontinence nursing conference was held, and in the spring of 1992, the USPHS Agency for Health Care Research and Education (AHCPR) published *Clinical Practice Guidelines on Urinary Incontinence in Adults* (AHCPR, 1992). These two events were pivotal in extending nurses' knowledge about incontinence management and the central role nursing has in assisting people to become continent. The Multi Specialty Conference is now a biannual event and attracts a growing number of nurses and other professionals. In addition, The Wound, Ostomy, Continence Nurses (WOCN) and The Society of Urologic Nurses and Associates (SUNA) in the U.S.; the Association of Continence Advise (ACA) in the U.K.; and the International Continence Society (ICS) now provide yearly conferences that focus partly or wholly on incontinence. These associations are major forums for networking, which is especially useful for American nurses since, unlike our colleagues in the U.K. and Australia, nurses in the U.S. do not have a separate organization directed exclusively toward incontinence.

SCOPE OF INCONTINENCE PRACTICE FOR ADVANCED PRACTICE NURSES

Practice parameters for advanced practice nurses whose clinical work focuses on urinary incontinence are now fairly well established. In addition to urinary incontinence, some practices also include fecal incontinence and pelvic pain. At first, however, nurses in this new subspecialty drew on their general nursing knowledge, such as anatomy and physiology, physical assessment, dietetics, medications, and teaching/learning skills. They learned new behavioral techniques from psychology and biofeedback experts, and worked closely with urologists, gynecologists, and urogyne cologists. Developing broad assessment skills helped them differentiate between acute and chronic incontinence, identify strategies that would be most effective in treating a diverse group of clients with various types of UI, and understand and use various behavioral techniques such as timed voiding, habit training, bladder retraining, prompted voiding, Kegel exercises—with and without various forms of biofeedback and intravaginal weights, and electrical stimulation. As new incontinence products became available nurses were often involved in testing and evaluating their efficacy. Some advanced practice nurses have also added pessary fitting to assist certain patients in regaining continence.

It is beyond the scope of this chapter to describe the various components of UI evaluation and management used by advanced practices nurses in this subspecialty. The 1996 clinical practice guideline update on urinary incontinence from the Agency for Health Care Practice and Research (Fantl, Newman, & Colling, 1996) provides a succinct composite along with extensive references and is accessible through online retrieval from the National Library of Medicine called HSTAT (Health Services/Technology Assessment Text) or by calling (202) 512-1800. It should be noted that the 1992 and 1996 guideline development panels were cochaired by nurses and had nurses on the interdisciplinary panel as well as on the consultant and technical advisers panels.

Of the over 13 million Americans who suffer with UI, less than 50% have ever even mentioned their UI to a health care provider. Some who have disclosed their incontinence have been told there is nothing but surgery or drugs to treat it. Thus, they may just use pads to contain their problem. In the recent past, UI was a silent problem in the media. All of the pioneer nurses, as well as professionals from other disciplines who began working with UI, have spent countless hours in community education. At first, questions at the end of information sessions were handled by written cards because audience participants were so reluctant to reveal that they may have UI. Since publication of the UI guidelines in 1992, there has been a concerted effort to educate the public and health care providers about the treatability of most UI and about the full range of treatment options available to patients.

Patients are especially responsive to nurses as they ask questions, listen, diagnose, teach, and coach them to regain bladder control. One of the positive aspects of behavioral treatments is that they empower patients to take charge of and overcome their UI. Nurses who treat patients with UI receive great satisfaction in their ability to fully assess patients' incontinence and determine what treatment strategies can best assist them to regain continence. Currently, over 400 nurses of the 2,116 members of SUNA have declared incontinence as their subspecialty/interest area (Society of Urologic Nurses and Associates, 1997). An unknown number of WOCN members have also made UI their practice focus.

A small number of psychologists, physical therapists, and physicians also specialize in continence care and include behavioral treatment as part of their practices. Their approach to patients' UI differs from that of nursing in that physicians tend to concentrate on treating the underlying pathology and are less likely to consider environmental, dietary, functional, or psychological factors involved in UI. Their treatment strategies are typically surgical or pharmacologic despite the recommendation of the AHCPR UI guidelines, which state that behavioral treatments are the first-line treatments (Fantl, Newman, & Colling, 1996). Because behavioral treatments are time-intensive, physicians often delegate these treatments to lesser trained office personnel who, while accurately applying the techniques, lack the teaching skills or the judgment to change the treatment regimen, often a key factor needed in achieving continence. Because of their skill in muscle retraining, biofeedback, and electrical stimulation, physical therapists have recently started to treat pelvic muscle dysfunction which includes patients with UI. Here again physical therapists' lack of breadth of knowledge may limit their ability to accurately diagnose and treat UI effectively. Psychologists are also familiar with biofeedback techniques and skilled in counseling and teaching. A few, such as Drs. Kathryn and Louis Burgio, have conducted pivotal research on the use of biofeedback for UI and have served as mentors for some of the pioneer UI nurses (Burgio, Robinson, & Engel, 1985; Burgio, Stutzman, & Engel, 1989; Burgio et al., 1994). Most psychologists, however, lack the physiological knowledge to fully assess the person with UI.

CURRENT ISSUES AND PROBLEMS IN NURSE MANAGEMENT OF UI

Informants identified several major issues and concerns facing advanced practice nurses caring for patients with UI. A concern unanimously described is the lack of any basic content on UI in advanced practice nurses' educational programs. Further, the many UI workshops now available to practicing nurses vary greatly in the quality of content and length. Both

SUNA and WOCN offer certification in UI, but the eligibility to sit for the examinations is variable and few programs require certification to treat patients with UI. Thus, respondents recommended that UI assessment and simple management techniques be taught in basic nursing programs and that curricula preparing RNs for advanced practice with adults include more detailed content on physical assessment of the pelvic floor muscles, common urological and gynecological problems that interfere with normal micturition, incontinence evaluation, and appropriate use of behavioral interventions in treating UI. Advanced practice nurses should be able to differentiate among the types of urinary incontinence and utilize behavioral treatment options effectively. Furthermore, independent learning modules on behavioral treatments for UI should be developed and available to advanced practice nurses.

While respondents had divergent views as to the usefulness of certification for nurses treating patients with UI, respondents felt that future reimbursement for services might be tied to certification. Clearly, this area needs some study so that nurses will be ready with a coherent plan if reimbursement becomes linked to certification.

Respondents also voiced concern about the effect of managed care on UI treatment by advanced practice nurses, especially in light of the demand of managed care that practitioners see more patients at lower cost. Assessing patients with UI and teaching them behavioral management techniques is labor intensive. Thus, there is a continuing need to refine definitive diagnostic skills and to determine the most efficient ways to help patients achieve continence within the changing health care delivery system.

Finally, respondents agreed that the greatest barrier to the advancement of nurses providing incontinence care is the inability to bill third-party payees independently for services, a situation that will change under recent Medicare rulings enacted in January, 1998. Currently, NP practices are typically linked to a medical clinic or medical director to meet current legal requirements for reimbursement. Most NPs, however, receive a percentage of the revenue they generate rather than a straight salary. Several respondents indicated that because UI is a complex problem, a multidisciplinary approach is the ideal practice model; however, such a model may be too costly in this era of managed care.

URINARY INCONTINENCE TREATMENT IN THE FUTURE

Respondents voiced varying viewpoints about advanced practice nurses' treatment of UI in the future. Most thought nurses should take a central role in UI treatment, but whether this goal is accomplished depends on getting UI content into master's programs, targeting care to specific populations such as home care, assisted living, rehabilitation, prevention in younger populations, and modifying the existing direct reimbursement barriers. One respondent expressed concern that while behavioral treatment was becoming recognized, some nurses were beginning UI management without adequate knowledge and training, especially in the use of biofeedback and electrical stimulation. Another respondent emphasized the need for research about the efficiency of specific treatments as well as the need to compare the effectiveness of UI treatment by advanced practice nurses to that of other disciplines.

Other areas for advanced practice nurses to consider in the future are the invention of devices, development of new treatment protocols and educational modules to assist patients and practitioners. Two nurses have already ventured into the area of inventions (Burns—pressure perineometer, patent # 08668800; Colling—incontinence detection device and analysis system, patent # 5258745 and # 5146469). Nurses' broad educational background, coupled with daily access to patients, puts them in a central position to use their observations to invent devices, develop new treatment protocols, and design educational programs for nurses, patients, and family caregivers.

Finally, there was considerable agreement among respondents that the ideal model is that of collaborative management of UI. The knowledge and skills of other disciplines along with nurses is the ideal means by which to craft the best treatment program for patients with UI.

REFERENCES AND BIBLIOGRAPHY

Agency for Health Care Policy and Research. (1992). *Clinical practice guideline: Urinary incontinence in adults.* USDHHS PHS AHCPR Pub. No. 92-0038. Rockville, MD.

Brink, C., Wells, T., & Diokno, A. (1983). A continence clinic for the aged. *Journal of Gerontological Nursing, 9*(12), 651–655.

Burgio, L. D., Engel, B. T., McCormick, K. A., Hawkins, A. M., & Scheve, A. (1988). Behavioral treatment for UI in elderly inpatients: Initial attempts to modify prompting and toileting procedures. *Behavioral Therapy, 19,* 345–357.

Burgio, L. D., McCormick, K. A., Scheve, A. S., Engel, B. T., Hawkins, A. M., & Leahy, E. (1994). The effects of changing prompted voiding schedules in the treatment of incontinence in nursing home residents. *Journal of the American Geriatrics Society, 42,* 315–320.

Burgio, K. L., Robinson, J. C., & Engel, B. T. (1985). The role of biofeedback in Kegel exercise training for stress urinary incontinence. *American Journal of Obstetrics and Gynecology, 154,* 58–64.

Burgio, K. L., Stutzman, R. E., & Engel, B. T. (1989). Behavioral training for post prostatectomy urinary incontinence. *Journal of Urology, 141,* 303–306.

Burns, P. A., Marecki, M. A., Dittmar, S. S., & Bullough, B. (1985). Kegel's exercises with biofeedback therapy for treatment of stress incontinence. *Nurse Practitioner, 10*(2), 111–118.

Burns, P. A., Pranikoff, K., Nochajski, T., Desotelle, P., & Harwood, M. K. (1990). Treatment of stress incontinence with pelvic floor exercises and biofeedback. *Journal of the American Geriatrics Society, 38*(3), 341–344.

Colling, J. C., Ouslander, J., Hadley, B. J., Eisch, J., & Campbell, E. (1992). The effects of patterned urge response toileting (PURT) on urinary incontinence among nursing home residents. *Journal of the American Geriatrics Society, 40,* 135–141.

Colling, J. C., Owen, T. R., & McCreedy, M. R. (1994). Urine volumes and voiding patterns among incontinent nursing home residents. *Geriatric Nursing, 15*(4), 188–192.

Colling, J. C., Hadley, B. J., Eisch, J., Campbell, E., & Newman, D. (1995). Continence program for care-dependent community elderly. Report submitted to NINR under grant No. NR01554.

Dougherty, M. C., Abrams, R., & McKey, P. L. (1986). An instrument to assess the dynamic characteristics of the circumvaginal musculature. *Nursing Research, 35,* 202–206.

Dougherty, M. C., Bishop, K., Mooney, R., Gimotty, P., & Williams, B. (1993). Graded pelvic muscle exercise: Effect on stress urinary incontinence. *Journal of Reproductive Medicine, 39,* 684–691.

Fantl, J. A., Newman, D. K., Colling, J. C., DeLancey, J. O. L., Keeys, C., Loughery, R., McDowell, B. J., Norton, P., Ouslander, J., Schnelle, J., Staskin, D., Tries, J., Urich, V., Vitousek, S. H., Weiss, B. D., & Whitmore, K. (1996). *Clinical practice guideline update, urinary incontinence in adults: Acute and chronic management.* USSHHS, PHS, AHCPR, Publication No. 96-0682, Rockville, Maryland.

Fantl, J. A., Wyman, J. F., McClish, D. K., Harkins, S. W., Elswick, R. K., Taylor, J. R., et al. (1991). Efficacy of bladder training in older women with urinary incontinence. *Journal of the American Medical Association, 265,* 609–613.

Fielding, P., & Wells, T. J. (1975). Clinical trial of an external female urinary collecting device in a geriatric sample. *Nursing Times, 71,* 136–137.

Hadley, E., Burgio, K., Engel, B. T., Jarvis, G. J., Ory, M., Resnick, N. M., Schucker, B., & William, M. (1983). Bladder training and related therapies for urinary incontinence: Prospects and problems for clinical trials in the elderly. Proceedings of workshop sponsored by the National Institute on Aging, April 26 & 27, Betheseda, MD.

McDowell, J. B., Burgio, K. L., Dombrowski, M., Locher, J. L., & Rodriguez, E. (1992). An interdisciplinary approach to the assessment and behavioral treatment of urinary incontinence in geriatric outpatients. *Journal of the American Geriatrics Society, 40,* 370–374.

NIH Consensus Development Conference. (1990). Urinary incontinence in adults. *Journal of the American Geriatrics Society, 38,* 265.

Palmer, M. H. (1982). Perspective on urinary incontinence in the elderly: Implications for nursing practice. Unpublished seminar paper, University of Maryland School of Nursing, Baltimore.

Palmer, M. H. (1985). *Urinary incontinence.* Thorofare, NJ: Slack Inc.

Palmer, M. H. (1990). Urinary continence status of newly admitted nursing home residents: A longitudinal study over a one-year period. Unpublished dissertation, The Johns Hopkins University School of Hygiene and Public Health, Baltimore, MD.

Palmer, M. H. (1996). *Urinary continence: Assessment and promotion.* Gaithersburg, MD: Aspen Publishers, Inc.

Sanderson, J. (1991). *An agenda for action on continence services.* Community Health Division, ML(91)1, Department of Health, London.

Smith-Baigis, J., Smith, D. A., Rose, M., & Newman, D. K. (1989). Management of UI in community residing elderly persons. *The Gerontologist, 29,* 229–233.

Society of Urologic Nurses and Associates. (1997). SUNA membership directory. Pitman, NJ: Author.

Wells, T. J. (1975). A guide for promoting urinary continence in the hospitalized elderly. *Nursing Times, 78,* 1907–1909.

Wells, T. J. (1980). Promoting urine control in older adults. Scope of the problem. *Geriatric Nursing, 1,* 236–240, 275.

Woolner, B. (1995). A clinical odyssey: Ten years of continence care. *Biofeedback, 23,* 16–20.

Chapter 19

ACADEMIC NURSING PRACTICE: POWER NURSING FOR THE 21ST CENTURY

Lois K. Evans, Melinda Jenkins, and Karen Buhler-Wilkerson

For a practice discipline, the notion that those who generate and disseminate nursing knowledge should also be expert practitioners seems self-evident. Yet, the history of "faculty practice" in nursing academic circles has never had a smooth course. Recent developments in health care organization and financing, in roles for advanced practice nurses, and in the struggle of academic nursing for greater equity with academic medicine have heightened the debate about faculty practice in academic nursing. At the close of the 20th century, several ingredients critical for achieving 'power nursing' are now in place: A richer mix of doctorally prepared faculty with research funding, widespread practice reimbursement finally a reality for advanced practice nurse faculty, and potential for school of nursing control of community-based practice. Some of the same factors that enhance nursing's position, however, are also forcing already powerful and wealthy medical schools to expand their reach beyond hospitals to the community. How this impending collision course is played out will have important implications for nursing in the 21st century.

The challenge for academic nursing as we enter this new era is to amass, demonstrate, and disseminate the scientific evidence that nursing makes an essential difference—both in quality and cost—in health care. The next step for the discipline to sustain its foothold is to move beyond previous conceptions of *faculty practice* to institutionalize *academic nursing practice* where research, education, and clinical care converge and are highly integrated. To begin to map this course, we discuss in this chapter the parallels and inherent conflicts between historically community-based academic nursing and hospital-based academic medicine; critique the current definition of faculty practice as it relates to *academic nursing practice*; identify facilitators in the establishment and maintenance of academic nursing practice; and present an illustrative case example.

ACADEMIC PRACTICE: A HISTORICAL REVIEW

Academic Medicine

A comparison of the development of academic medicine and academic nursing is instructive in understanding the critical implications of the debate on faculty practice in nursing circles. Following a 150-year history of academically based training, early 20th century reforms in American medical education established research as a significant expectation of the faculty and a crucial element in the educational milieu; patient care was already incorporated into medical school activities through ownership of, or strong affiliation arrangements with, hospitals. Thus, the triad of education, research, and patient care came to be viewed as inextricably and vitally bound (Burondess, 1991). Federal training and biomedical research monies flowed into academic medicine post-World War II, while medical faculty served as peer reviewers in the distribution of these research funds from the newly formed National Institutes of Health. Whereas income to schools of medicine has traditionally been derived from sources analogous to each of the three arms of the tripartite mission—state appropriations, endowment, and tuition; research grants and contracts; and patient care revenues—the relative proportions changed during the 1980s. Funds for education and research did not keep pace with inflation, while funds from patient care services continued to rise both in absolute and relative terms (MacLeod & Schwarz, 1986; Turner, 1989). These shifts in funding likewise created shifts in time commitments of medical faculty, with increasing numbers on teaching-practice tracks.

Faculty practice plans that were initiated in schools of medicine in response to the introduction of Medicare and Medicaid in the mid-1960s provided an increasingly important supplemental funding source for medical education. Today, in most public medical schools, practice income covers about 25% to 50% of the total operating budget, and in most private medical schools the proportion is much higher, perhaps the largest source of funding for all medical schools (Krakower, Ganem, & Beran, 1994; MacLeod & Schwarz, 1986; Turner, 1989). In fact, among the currently existing 124 medical schools, the revenue stream from practice increased from $5.2 billion to $10.6 billion over the past 10 years (Greenberg, 1997). The traditional faculty practice plan models are becoming less lucrative, however, as the health care arena rapidly changes from fee-for-service to managed-care reimbursement systems. With graduate medical education funding through Medicare also at risk, academic medical centers have quickly acted to build comprehensive health care systems in order to take advantage of risk models and to continue to generate large revenues for their schools of medicine. At the same time, the reimbursement stream is forcing schools of medicine to rapidly shift their locus of education, practice, and research from the institution to the community.

Academic Nursing

While these shifts have posed challenges and conflicts both within medical schools and between medical schools and their parent academic institutions, they are instructive in examining the parallel historical evolution of academic nursing and in planning for its future. As is well known, nursing came late to the academic setting, with little real presence until after World War II (Reverby, 1987). From the 1940s on, nursing education shifted appreciably from a hospital-based apprenticeship model to institutions of higher education. Thus, nursing faculty and students were separated from direct practice responsibilities and revenue generation (for the hospital).

Federal support for the education of nurses in academic settings dates to 1935 (for public health nurses), 1947 (for psychiatric nurses), and 1956 (administration, education, and supervision in all nursing fields). Changes in the educational preparation of the workforce were, however, slow; by

1954, only 1% of nurses had a master's degree and 7.2% a bachelor's degree (Kalisch & Kalisch, 1986). Despite increasing federal aid, by 1962 only 14% of nurses had graduated from a baccalaureate program. Doctoral education for nursing faculty was even more delayed; only 4% of nursing faculty had an earned doctoral degree in 1962, and even today, less than 0.004% of all nurses are doctorally prepared (Jacox, 1993). The first comprehensive doctoral program in nursing was not initiated until 1964 at UCSF. Thus, at a time when faculty of schools of medicine were benefiting from the influx of federal research dollars, few nursing faculty were eligible to apply. Further, from the first $500,000 allocated in 1956 until the late 1970s, federal dollars for projects in nursing focused on educational issues and studies of nurses and nursing rather than clinical nursing practice. Finally, while medical schools' practice income soared in the 1960s, direct reimbursement for much of nursing practice remained essentially unavailable until the late 1990s.

Reuniting Nursing Education and Practice

Concern over the widening split between education and practice reached a high pitch with the advent of advanced practice roles in the 1960s and 1970s (Walker, 1995). Like academic medicine, academic nursing developed model teaching centers for students, where the best of nursing practice could be observed, learned, and examined. Unlike medicine, nursing's academic origins were community based. The first forays into academia in the early 1920s were for postgraduate study for public health nurses (Kalisch & Kalisch, 1986). O. Marie Henry, Director of the Division of Nursing of the Department of Health and Human Services, Bureau of Health Professions, during the 1970s–1980s, challenged nurse educators to take control of practice by creating centers for the integration of practice, education, and research where new methods of nursing care and delivery could be developed, tested, and demonstrated. She proposed that such centers should be in a variety of settings that nursing can influence, such as nursing homes, rehabilitation centers, and the community, and that are dependent on high-quality nursing care (Henry, 1986). While there was consensus regarding the necessity to create centers where nursing would be the primary focus, debate over these centers' practice agendas mirrored that of nursing in the aggregate (Fehring, Schulte, & Reisch, 1986). Like public health nurses who preceded them and created the first nursing centers (Thwing, 1919; Walsh, 1920), contemporary nurses' early "insider" debates reflect our continued struggle to achieve professional autonomy in practice, to legitimize claims for direct reimbursement for practice, to control practice environments, and to define requirements for entry into advanced practice nursing.

Nursing school faculties began again to establish their own practices in the 1970s. The 1979 American Academy of Nursing resolution supporting faculty practice, followed by a series of symposia cosponsored by the Academy and the Robert Wood Johnson Foundation, served to further escalate the debate on the role of practice in academia and stimulate the evolution of a variety of models, including unification/partnerships, faculty practice plans, and nursing centers. By the early 1980s, 63 schools of nursing were affiliated with or were sponsoring nurse-managed centers, the National League for Nursing had established a Council for Nursing Centers, and the first national conference on nursing centers had been held. Consensus was building that nursing faculty must increase their control of the practice environment in order to influence education, conduct research, and facilitate research-based care. Adequate attention to reimbursement, the revenue-generating business aspects of this integration, however, lagged far behind (Aiken, 1992).

Context of Sociopolitical Forces

As the 1990s draw to a close, an unprecedented window of opportunity exists for academic nursing to achieve a more powerful position by finally integrating its tripartite mission. For the first time there appears to be a critical mass of faculty prepared at the doctoral level and successfully engaged in programs of funded research to compete for research dollars. The National Institute for Nursing Research, as well as other institutes and sources, has provided important support for the development of the science (nearly $65 million federal dollars awarded in FY1996 [NIH, 1997]), as well as opportunities for nurse faculty to define the national nursing research agenda and to participate in peer review.

Further, there are a critical mass of advanced practice nurse (APN) faculty for whom there now exist greater opportunities for practice reimbursement. APNs in most states have prescriptive privileges (Pearson, 1997), and other constraints around the advanced practice of nursing are gradually lifting. Resistance from interdisciplinary quarters to the APN role, while still prevalent, has lessened as the data have consistently demonstrated quality- and cost-effectiveness as well as public acceptance and demand (Brush & Capezuti, 1996). The recent passage by Congress of legislation that opens direct reimbursement to APNs under Medicare and Medicaid is expected to pave the way for other insurers to follow suit. Simultaneously, the rapid escalation of managed care has important positive implications for the practice of APNs.

Thus, we are at one of those rare moments in history when all the forces are right—research dollars, practice dollars, research and practice expertise, educational and societal demand—to permit successful integration of the tripartite mission, enabling nursing to take its place with the other academic health professions. Enter academic medicine: Its escalating movement to the community for practice, education, and research places it on a likely collision course with academic nursing which is already ensconced there. In this environment, embracing the new paradigm of academic nursing practice will not be for the faint at heart. To seize the moment, what remains are the formidable tasks of retaining control of nursing's community practice environments, creating acceptance in academic circles for integrating the practice component of the tripartite mission (Rudy, Anderson, Dudjak, Robert, & Miler, 1995), and finding new ways of partnering that will retain newfound equity and meet mutual goals.

DEFINITIONS AND MODELS OF FACULTY PRACTICE

A critique of the current definition and models of faculty practice is important as we move toward a new paradigm.

Faculty practice includes all aspects of the delivery of health care through the roles of clinician, educator, researcher, consultant and administrator. Faculty practice activities within this framework encompass direct nursing services to individuals and groups, as well as technical assistance and consultation to individuals, families, groups, and communities. In addition to the provision of service, the practice provides opportunities for promotion, tenure, merit, and revenue generation. *A distinguishing characteristic of faculty practice within the School of Nursing is the belief that teaching, research, practice, and service must be closely integrated to achieve excellence. Faculty practice provides the vehicle through which faculty implement these missions.* There is an assumption that student practice and residencies as well as *research opportunities for faculty and students are an established component* of faculty practice (Taylor, 1996, p. 474, as cited in Taylor, 1997; *italics added*).

The notion of integrating the tripartite mission does not frame this definition of faculty practice, rather it is added near the end either as an afterthought, or in acknowledgment of its "assumed" establishment. However, the scant research literature (Walker, 1995) and our own experience dictate that this is hardly the case. Moving beyond this concept of faculty practice to that of *academic nursing practice* will permit greater latitude in implementing the tripartite mission. Academic nursing practice allows for the possibility that faculty may move between and among the three arms of the mission, at any one given time concentrating more heavily on one or two roles rather than being master of all three simultaneously. Academic medicine recognized this necessity long ago, and created a range of roles for faculty, while the problem of role overload resulting from lack of academic and administrative support has been acknowledged in survey after survey as a contributing factor in nurse faculty burnout (Walker, 1995).

Models

Historically, nursing has experimented with a variety of faculty practice models (see Broussard, Delahoussaye, & Poirrier, 1996; Hutelmyer & Donnelly, 1996; Potash & Taylor, 1993). Faculty practice may vary by structural type (nursing centers, unification/partnerships, joint appointments, faculty development), faculty roles (practitioner, consultant educator, or researcher), and economic aspects (volunteer, entrepreneurial, joint practice, collaborative, revenue-generating, contractual), and some overlap will occur in any one faculty practice (Taylor, 1996a). Currently, it is the entrepreneurial model that appears to afford the most flexibility for strength and growth of academic practices within a rapidly changing market. The entrepreneurial model allows for a variety of revenue-generating practice designs that may be wholly or partially owned by the School or by affiliates. Prominent examples include Vanderbilt University School of Nursing (Spitzer et al., 1996), University of Texas-Houston Health Science Center School of Nursing (Mackey & McNiel, 1997), and Columbia University School of Nursing (Auerhahn, 1997). Some schools have a faculty practice plan that delineates how faculty-generated practice is governed and revenues shared (Taylor, 1996b). As a resource for faculties considering academic practice, the National Organization of Nurse Practitioner Faculties' guidebook (Marion, 1997) is available.

Facilitators

A distinguishing feature of *academic nursing practice* is the opportunity for *all* faculty, regardless of their degree of clinical practice activity, to participate in practice-related research within school-owned or affiliated practices. Thus, academic practice becomes the medium for testing innovative models, developing a common language to measure nursing interventions and outcomes, and generating new knowledge and evidence-based practice (Lang, Jenkins, Evans, & Matthews, 1996a; Zachariah & Lundeen, 1997), rather than just another opportunity for faculty to maintain clinical skills, gain personal satisfaction, teach students by serving as a role model, and so on. As in academic medicine, academic practice spawns increased research funding and educational program development resources and can also generate much needed revenues for the educational programs.

For this to happen, however, faculty governance and an infrastructure tuned to the business of practice are essential. Patient care responsibilities that feed the education and research missions are constant and demanding and have a rhythm very different from that of the usual academic calendar; discontinuity and tragic consequences can result unless the business of the practice is well managed. Faculty governance and business infrastructure facilitate stability of practices and development of community trust in their ongoing presence. Other facilitators of the practice mission include flexible faculty scheduling and workload, administrative recognition and support for practice, and a valuing of practice in tenure and promotion criteria (Nugent, Barger, & Bridges, 1993; Potash & Taylor, 1993; Walker, 1995; Taylor, 1996b). In addition, practices that fit third-party reimbursement streams and contracts are most likely to achieve fiscal viability. Facilitators in achieving the teaching mission associated with academic practice are faculty confidence in their own skills and expertise and willingness to reach beyond the traditional academic role. The practice-associated research mission is facilitated by the establishment of common databases through collaboration among several schools of nursing to monitor client data, assess costs, and investigate faculty effectiveness in practice (Iowa Intervention Project, 1997; Lang et al., 1996a). Role integration is enhanced when faculty are able to generate research from their practices.

Institutional support of university and dean is essential. In fact, administrative support is perceived to be the greatest overall facilitator of faculty practice (Barger & Bridges, 1987). In schools where administrative policies support practice as a promotion criterion, the mean number of reported practice hours is nearly twice as high. Schools with doctoral programs and those that were public institutions have higher levels of faculty practice time. However, practice is not a criterion for promotion and tenure in most schools, and neither do many schools have formalized faculty practice plans (Barger, Nugent, & Bridges, 1993). For individual faculty members, workload and time demands must balance with financial and academic promotion incentives. Individual faculty pay a high price in role strain and work overload unless roles are integrated. Institutional commitment to policies supporting implementation of an integrated tripartite mission is critical (Walker, 1995).

Several nursing schools have formal criteria for clinical scholarship within the tenure track or on a separate, parallel "clinician-educator" track (Burns, 1997). Oregon's criteria, for example, mesh with Boyer's (1990) proposal that scholarship include the four domains: discovery, integration, application, and teaching. Currently, higher education emphasizes research and the scholarship of discovery. Universities that house medical schools, however, are likely familiar with promotion criteria honoring practice. Valuing the scholarship of research application, including the development of evidence-based care, through inclusion in nursing promotion and tenure criteria enhances excellence in practice, education, and scholarship for individual faculty members and for the school.

THE UNIVERSITY OF PENNSYLVANIA: A CASE EXAMPLE

An examination of the evolution of academic practice at the University of Pennsylvania School of Nursing may be instructive in understanding the forces that have influenced, and continue to shape, its development. Academic medicine and nursing at Penn will first be compared, then the school's evolving academic practice described to demonstrate Penn's unique window of opportunity to achieve 'power nursing' for the 21st century.

School of Medicine

The School of Medicine at the University of Pennsylvania is ranked among the top U.S. academic medical centers, with just under $200 million in annual federal research and training dollars. Opening in 1765 as the first medical school in America, Penn Med early on gained control of its practice environment through developing in 1874 the first U.S. hospital intimately associated with a medical school (Baltzell, 1996). Not only the Hospital of the University of Pennsylvania (HUP) but also several large surrounding teaching hospitals with close medical school affiliations enabled faculty to educate students, practice medicine, and conduct research relatively unencumbered. Its 22 faculty practice plans (Clinical Practices of the University of Pennsylvania) grew rapidly after the influx of Medicare and Medicaid dollars in the 1960s. Responding to the most recent challenge of health care financing changes in Philadelphia, the Medical Center embarked on a bold strategic plan in 1993 to develop an integrated health system. This initiative has enabled the resultant University of Pennsylvania Health System (UPHS) to expand its influence and strengthen its position for the managed-care market by acquiring, through purchase, merger, or affiliation, multiple community-based sites, including a large number of primary care practices, community hospitals, nursing homes, home care agencies, and rehabilitation centers. Access to a clinically diverse patient population and range of health care delivery settings is deemed necessary to ensure continued achievement of its educational and research goals and maintenance of its financial resource base (Iglehart, 1995). A new Department of Family Medicine heralds the school's emerging emphasis on primary care. In its first major curriculum revision since its inception, Penn Med recently implemented Curriculum 2000 which will emphasize prevention and provide multiple elective and required opportunities for community-based learning experiences.

School of Nursing

The University of Pennsylvania remains the only Ivy League University which prepares nurses at the baccalaureate, master's, and doctoral levels. Its School of Nursing has maintained top rankings (first or second place) in its level of federal research funding, totaling nearly $6 million in total federal dollars in FY1996 (NIH, 1997). Like Medicine, Penn Nursing also has a distinctive history. By 1950 an autonomous School of Nursing had evolved at Penn from earlier programs at the Hospital of the University of Pennsylvania Training School (1886), the School of Education (1935), and the Division of Medical Affairs (1945). Master's study was initiated, first in nursing education (1937) and psychiatric-mental health nursing (1961), then in other clinical areas. Penn's first nurse practitioner program began in 1972. Doctoral study (DNSc in 1978 and PhD in 1984) soon followed. One can only speculate on how much energy was dissipated by the simultaneous and rather lengthy coexistence of three separate nursing education programs within the University structure (the HUP school did not close until 1978), surely a peculiar contextual environment for the incubation of nursing at Penn. While the research emphasis of the University and the academic practice histories of Medicine and the other health science schools (Dentistry, Veterinary Medicine) lent precedent for developing the tripartite mission in the younger but autonomous School of Nursing, there was from the beginning disparity between them in size, educational preparation of faculty, research funding, access to practice incomes, and control over practice environments.

Building the Base for the Tripartite Mission

The numbers of doctorally prepared faculty in the School of Nursing grew through the 1970s, yet even by the end of the decade the level of funded research was modest at best. The recruitment of Dean Claire Fagin and faculty with expertise in clinical research, as well as the external funding for a Center for Nursing Research, helped ensure the growth of the research mission and development of a doctoral program. Advanced practice faculty with doctoral preparation were also recruited during this period, thus enhancing the focus on advanced practice within the educational and research domains.

During the 1980s, a number of collaborative medicine and nursing faculty practice and research activities were implemented, and a partnership plan with the HUP evolved to re-link the two entities (Fagin, 1986). Independent of structural change, the partnership focused on ways that the related but separate goals of the School and the Hospital—clinical excellence, developing a research and scholarly base, and providing excellent educational programs—could best be achieved. The extension in 1984 by the University Faculty Senate to nursing faculty of a clinician-educator standing faculty track facilitated the engagement of faculty in scholarly practice initiatives. Nurse practitioner and clinical nurse specialist faculty practiced within a variety of models, including joint appointments, contracts, and entrepreneurial private practices. Other initiatives that helped create an environment that would embrace the tripartite mission included directing the Robert Wood Johnson Teaching Nursing Home Project that emphasized the critical linkage of schools of nursing and clinical facilities to achieve high-quality care (Mezey, Lynaugh, & Cartier, 1988); serving as a training site for the Robert Wood Johnson Clinical Scholars program that demonstrated faculty practice-research role integration; cultivating a faculty research agenda that was primarily clinically focused (Lang, Sullivan-Marx, & Jenkins, 1996b); developing several intradisciplinary research centers that helped to successfully target the faculty's research efforts (Lang, 1996); and building strong affiliations with community partners such as with the Visiting Nurse Association of Greater Philadelphia (Alliance for Academic Home Care) and the Philadelphia Department of Recreation (Reed, 1997). Thus, the stage was set for integrating the tripartite mission through academic nursing practice, a primary emphasis of Dean Norma Lang (Lang, 1996; Lang et al., 1996a; Lang et al., 1996b).

Academic Nursing Practice: The Penn Nursing Network

The academic nursing practices of the School of Nursing, the Penn Nursing Network (PNN), was initiated in 1994 to facilitate full integration of the tripartite mission (see Figure 19.1). Practice evolved as a major component of the school's strategic plan, initiated by the dean and developed and embraced by the faculty and administration with consultation from the national firm APM. Building on a history of nurse-midwifery and geriatric services, clinician educator appointments, and the partnership with HUP, several practices for which the school is 'at risk' were clustered together under the PNN umbrella (Table 19.1). The strategic plan encompassed three types of practice arrangements (see Figure 19.1) and projected an aggressive growth curve from just under $1/2 million in revenues in FY1993 to $10 million in FY2001. While the practices carry out Henry's (1986) agenda in that they are community-based and focus on populations that are dependent on high-quality nursing, their development within the

PENN NURSING NETWORK

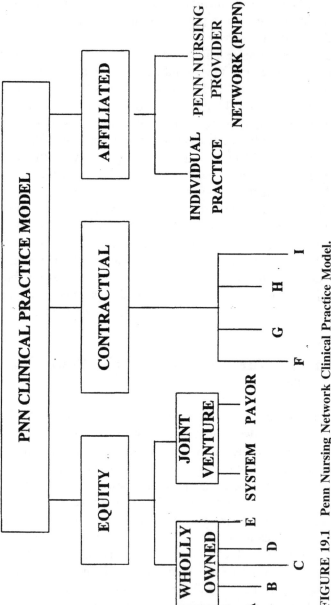

FIGURE 19.1 Penn Nursing Network Clinical Practice Model.

Source: University of Pennsylvania School of Nursing. Printed with permission.

**TABLE 19.1   University of Pennsylvania School of Nursing
Penn Nursing Network**

Overview

Penn Nursing Network (PNN) provides the best practice models of community-based, family-focussed health care services to people of all ages in a variety of settings. Advanced practice nursing services include nurse-midwifery, well-child care, pre-teen and adolescent care, family planning, women's health, primary care for children and adults, continence, gerontologic consultation, comprehensive rehabilitation for older adults, and a capitated acute and long-term care program for frail elders. As the academic practice of a major research school of nursing, the PNN serves uniquely to demonstrate practice fully integrated with education and research.

Brief Descriptions of Each Practice

The Collaborative Assessment and Rehabilitation for Elders (CARE) Program. Functions as a geriatric day hospital, offering comprehensive, intensive nursing and rehabilitation services to very frail older adults with multiple health problems. Operates as a CORF under the Medicare program.

Community Midwifery Services. Provides full-scope obstetric, gynecologic, and family planning services at two community locations, the Myers Health Annex and the Health Corner in the West Philadelphia Community Center.

Continence Program. Provides assessment and nonsurgical treatment for older adults with bowel and bladder incontinence under contract to private physician offices, continuing-care retirement communities, and clinics.

Gerontologic Nursing Consultation Service (GNCS). Provides consultation and education focusing on the care of older adults and the aging process, specifically restraint reduction, consumer education and health promotion, geriatric care models, case management, and expert legal witness services.

The Health Annex at the Myers Recreation Center. A family- and community-centered primary health care practice, integrating physical and mental health services to clients of all ages to promote health and wellness, identifies illness needs, and delivers primary care to a culturally diverse community.

Living Independently for Elders (LIFE). A risk-based program providing integrated acute and long-term care services for the frail elderly who are nursing home certifiable and prefer to live in the community. Based on the On Lok/PACE model in San Francisco, a comprehensive range of health and social services is available on a 24-hour basis, with an adult day health center serving as the focal point.

Neighborhood Midwifery. A full-scope nurse-midwifery, obstetric, and gynecologic practice operated in collaboration with the LaSalle University College of Nursing Neighborhood Nursing Center in Germantown.

Other. The Penn Nursing Network is a licensed home health agency, and also provides women's health services through contracts to agencies in the community.

autonomous School of Nursing, as opposed to the University of Pennsylvania Health System, has not been without challenges (Evans, 1994; Iglehart, 1995).

Governance and Operations

Faculty governance, including review of new practice proposals and business plans, is accomplished through a standing committee of the school's Faculty Senate. Each practice is directly linked to the Standing Faculty through academic directors, each of whom sits on the Practice Committee. The Academic Director closely ties the practices to the academic enterprise of the school by facilitating educational and research opportunities and setting the research agenda. Day-to-day management of each practice is accomplished by a master clinician who serves as clinical director. A Director for Academic Nursing Practices, a tenured member of the standing faculty who reports directly to the Dean, facilitates achievement of operating, fiscal, and quality outcomes within the tripartite mission over the entire network of practices.

Business Infrastructure and Revenues

Infrastructure for practice support is continually evolving, commensurate with overall practice growth. It currently consists of financial, billing, information systems, quality management and support staff; legal services, risk management and insurance, payroll, human resources, purchasing, public relations, development and so on are obtained from the University or school. Members of the School's Board of Overseers with health care interest and experience voluntarily serve in various capacities to advise and assist the practices. Revenue sources include, primarily, patient revenues (fee-for-service, Medicare, Medicaid, private insurers, managed care, and other contracts), and, secondarily, public and private grants and gifts. Excess revenues over expenses generated by any one practice are placed in a 'practice loan pool' to be borrowed by other practices in developmental phases. In addition, a line of credit has been established within the University to permit planned operating shortfall during start-up of new practices. In FY 1997, the six operational practices generated some $2 million in total revenues.

With university and foundation support, an Office for Research in Academic Practice was opened in 1996 to house a repository of clinical, financial, and management data from the School's academic practices. The database contains common data elements across the practices that will facilitate staff, faculty, and student conduct of quality management studies and clinical and health services research (Lang et al., 1996a).

Early Outcomes and the Challenge for the Future

The academic practices have fostered and stimulated new developments in educational, research, and service arenas. Development of new research methods suitable for evaluating practice outcomes in small unique practice settings (Lang et al., 1996a), scholarly leadership in database development within the newly formed regional nursing centers consortium, a graduate-level "Business of Nursing" course, and federal and state policy changes (Jenkins & Torrisi, 1995) have all evolved from the faculty practices at the University of Pennsylvania School of Nursing. Penn is the only School of Nursing in the country to operate a comprehensive outpatient rehabilitation facility (CORF; Evans, Yurkow, & Siegler, 1995) or a Program of All-Inclusive Care for the Elderly (PACE; see Living Independently for Elders in Table 19.1).

Today, 36% of Penn's standing faculty are clinician educators with combined academic and clinical appointments. Six of these faculty are involved in the school's own academic nursing practices, and the others have a variety of roles in affiliated agencies including direct practice, research utilization, leadership, consultation, and so on. The clinician educators have played a vital role in developing the practice mission at Penn, and the school's six research centers are increasingly engaged in developing clinical research proposals that will employ the resources of the academic practices.

At this decisive moment in history, Penn School of Nursing is uniquely poised to be able to move academic nursing forward. A critical mass of seasoned and funded nurse scholars at Penn are producing clinically relevant research findings that are influencing practice on national and international levels. Over 250 advanced practice nurses are graduated each year, along with a substantial number with BSN and PhD degrees and postdoctoral study. Faculty have been instrumental in expanding reimbursement opportunities on a national and state level. And the school controls an increasing number of innovative community-based and -focused clinical settings, demonstrating economic and operational success.

The academic practices of the School of Nursing will increasingly serve as an important vehicle for testing the implementation of clinical findings from nursing faculty research, seeking cost-effective ways to bring innovative practices to market, testing best practices, developing evidence-based care, and preparing students to practice in a new era in health care. Thus, albeit on a much different scale from that of the School of Medicine, the academic practices of the School of Nursing do feed its research and the education mission as well as provide financial resources for the academic programs of the School.

As academic medicine at the University of Pennsylvania moves into the community, the challenge for the School of Nursing will be to maintain control of its practice environments while finding new ways of partnering and collaborating in reaching mutual service, education, and research goals. The LIFE (PACE) program, now in its start-up phase (see Table 19.1), will provide ample opportunities to develop and enhance such partnerships. Now that the School of Nursing has moved toward maturity in its own tripartite mission, it brings a new level of parity to the table. That the *value-added* strengths of the school's academic practices can complement those in the Health System, and vice versa, is increasingly recognized.

We believe that academic nursing practice, in its ability to integrate the tripartite mission, clearly represents a unique power source for nursing in the 21st century. Academic nursing *must* have it to survive and thrive.

The philosophy of the Penn Nursing Network is congruent with that of the School of Nursing. Penn Nursing Network embraces health as a cornerstone for quality of life as defined by the person, the right and responsibility of persons to knowledgeably decide and participate in their own health care, and the belief that nursing has as its primary role the support of persons in their self-care. As the academic nursing practices of the School of Nursing, the mission of Penn Nursing Network is fourfold:

1. To support the education and research missions of the school;
2. To evolve, test, and disseminate best practice models of nursing and integrated health care services;
3. To provide cost-effective, high-quality, community-based health care services to diverse populations; and
4. To provide financial resources to the School.

REFERENCES

Aiken, L. H. (1992). Charting nursing's future. In L. H. Aiken & C. M. Fagin (Eds.), *Charting nursing's future: Agenda for the 1990s* (pp. 3–12). Philadelphia: Lippincott.

Auerhahn, C. (1997). Columbia University School of Nursing faculty practice: A cross-site model. In L. N. Marion (Ed.), *Faculty practice: Applying the models* (pp. 65–72). Washington, DC: National Organization of Nurse Practitioner Faculties.

Baltzell, E. D. (1996). *Puritan Boston & Quaker Philadelphia.* New Brunswick: Transaction Publishers.

Barger, S. E., & Bridges, W. C. (1987). An assessment of academic nursing centers. *Nurse Educator, 15*(2), 31–36.

Barger, S. E., Nugent, K. E., & Bridges, W. C. (1993). Schools with nursing centers: A 5-year follow-up study. *Journal of Professional Nursing, 9*, 7–13.

Boyer, E. (1990). *Scholarship reconsidered: Priorities for the professoriate.* Princeton, NJ: The Carnegie Foundation for the Advancement of Teaching.

Broussard, A. B., Delahoussaye, C. P., & Poirrier, G. P. (1996). The practice role in the academic nursing community. *Journal of Nursing Education, 35*(2), 82–87.

Brush, B. L., & Capezuti, E. A. (1996). Revisiting 'A nurse for all settings': The nurse practitioner movement, 1965–1995. *Journal of the American Academy of Nurse Practitioners, 8*(1), 5–11.

Burns, C. E. (1997). Faculty clinical practice as a tenurable activity. In L. N. Marion (Ed.), *Faculty practice: Applying the models* (pp. 41–48). Washington, DC: National Organization of Nurse Practitioner Faculties.

Burondess, J. (1991). The academic health center and the public agenda: Whose three-legged stool? *Annals of Internal Medicine, 115*, 962.

Evans, L. K. (1994). Overcoming intrainstitutional challenges to collaborative practice. In E. Sieger & F. Whitney (Eds.), *Overcoming barriers to nurse-physician collaboration* (pp. 33–42). New York: Springer Publishing.

Evans, L. K., Yurkow, J., & Siegler, E. (1995). The CARE Program: A nurse-managed collaborative outpatient program to improve function of frail elders. *Journal of the American Geriatric Society, 43*, 1155–1160.

Fagin, C. M. (1986). Institutionalizing faculty practice. *Nursing Outlook, 34*(3), 140–144.

Fehring, R. J., Schulte, J., & Reisch, S. K. (1986). Toward a definition of nurse-managed centers. *Journal of Community Health Nursing, 3*, 59–67.

Greenberg, D. S. (1997, Sept. 9). Med School Millionaires. *The Washington Post,* A-19.

Henry, O. M. (1986). Demonstration centers for nursing practice, education and research. In M. D. Mezey & D. O. McGivern (Eds.), *Nurses, nurse practitioners: The evolution of primary care* (pp. 239–241). Boston: Little Brown & Co.

Hutelmyer, C. M., & Donnelly, G. F. (1996). Joint appointments in practice positions. *Nursing Administration Quarterly, 20*(4), 71–79.

Iglehart, J. K. (1995). Academic medical centers enter the market: The case of Philadelphia. *New England Journal of Medicine, 333*(15), 1019–1023.

Iowa Intervention Project. (1997). Proposal to bring nursing into the information age. *Image: Journal of Nursing Scholarship, 29*(3), 275–281.

Jacox, A. (1993). Estimates of the supply and demand for doctorally prepared nurses. *Nursing Outlook, 41*(1), 43–45.

Jenkins, M., & Torrisi, D. (1995). Nurse practitioners, community nursing centers and contracting for managed care. *Journal of the American Academy of Nurse Practitioners, 7*, 1–6.

Kalisch, P. A., & Kalisch, B. J. (1986). *The advances of American nursing*. Boston: Little, Brown & Co.

Krakower, J., Ganem, J., & Beran, R. L. (1994). Medical school financing: Comparing seven different types of schools. *Academic Medicine, 69*, 72–81.

Lang, N. (1996). Academic nursing practice: A case study of the University of Pennsylvania School of Nursing. In *Penn Nursing: The Publication of the University of Pennsylvania School of Nursing, 1*(1), 17–19, 36.

Lang, N. M., Jenkins, M., Evans, L. K., & Matthews, D. (1996a). Administrative, financial, and clinical data for an academic nursing practice: A case study of the University of Pennsylvania School of Nursing. In *The power of faculty practice* (pp. 79–100), American Association of Colleges of Nursing. Washington, DC: Author.

Lang, N. M., Sullivan-Marx, E. M., & Jenkins, M. (1996b). Advanced practice nurses and success of organized delivery systems. *American Journal of Managed Care, 11*(2), 129–135.

Mackey, T. A., & McNeil, N. O. (1997). Negotiating private sector partnerships with academic nursing centers. *Nursing Economics, 15*(1), 52–55.

MacLeod, G. K., & Schwarz, M. R. (1986). Faculty practice plans. *Journal of the American Medical Association, 256*, 58–62.

Marion, L. N., Ed. (1997). *Faculty practice: Applying the models*. Washington, DC: National Organization of Nurse Practitioner Faculties.

Mezey, M., Lynaugh, J., & Cartier, M. (1988). A report card on faculty practice: The Robert Wood Johnson Teaching Nursing Home Program, 1982–87. *Nursing Outlook, 36*, 285–288.

National Institutes of Health. (1997). *FY 1996 Extramural awards to domestic higher education*. Bethesda: NIH Information Systems Management Section.

Nugent, K. E., Barger, S. E., & Bridges, W. C. (1993). Facilitators and inhibitors of practice: A faculty perspective. *Journal of Nursing Education,32*, 293–300.

Pearson, L. J. (1997). Annual update of how each state stands on legislative issues affecting advanced nursing practice. *The Nurse Practitioner, the American Journal of Primary Health Care, 22*(1), 18, 20, 25–26 passim; published erratum appears in *Nurse Practitioner* (1997) 22(6), 216.

Potash, M., & Taylor, D. (1993). *Nursing faculty practice: Models and methods*. Washington, DC: National Organization of Nurse Practitioner Faculties.

Reed, D. (1997). The development of a community-based, nurse managed practice network by the University of Pennsylvania School of nursing. In *The third national primary care conference case studies* (pp. 229–240). Washington, DC: HRSA.

Reverby, S. M. (1987). *Ordered to care: The dilemma of American nursing, 1850–1945*. Cambridge: Cambridge University Press.

Rudy, E. B., Anderson, N. A., Dudjak, L., Robert, S. N., & Miler, R. A. (1995). Faculty practice; creating a new culture. *Journal of Professional Nursing, 11*, 78–83.

Spitzer, R., Bandy, C., Bumbalough, M., Frederiksen, D., Gibson, G., Howard, E., McIntosh, E., Pitts, V. N., & Reeves, G. (1996). Marketing and reimbursement of faculty-based practice. *Nursing & Health Care, 17*, 309–311.

Taylor, D. (1996a). Faculty practice: Uniting advanced nursing practice and nursing education. In A. Hamric, J. Spross, & C. Hanson (Eds.), *Advanced nursing practice: An integrative approach.* Philadelphia: Saunders.

Taylor, D. (1996b). Faculty practice plan or faculty practice groups? In *The power of faculty practice.* Washington, DC: American Association of Colleges of Nursing.

Taylor, D. (1997). Faculty practice: The next steps. In L. N. Marion (Ed.), *Faculty practice; Applying the models.* Washington, DC: National Organization of Nurse Practitioner Faculties.

Thwing, M. D. (1919). The university public health nursing district in Cleveland. *The Public Health Nurse, 11,* 362–365.

Turner, B. (1989). Future role of academic centers. *Health Care Management Review, 14,* 73–77.

Walker, P. H. (1995). Faculty practice: Interest, issues, and impact. In J. Fitzpatrick & J. Stevenson (Eds.), *Annual Review of Nursing Research* (pp. 217–235). New York: Springer.

Walsh, M. S. (1920). A teaching district in St. Louis. *The Public Health Nurse, 13,* 994–996.

Zachariah, R., & Lundeen, S. P. (1997). Research and practice in an academic community nursing center. *Image: The Journal of Nursing Scholarship, 29,* 255–260.

LEGISLATION, LAW, AND REIMBURSEMENT

PART **IV**

LEGISLATION, LAW, AND REIMBURSEMENT

Chapter 20

PAYMENT FOR ADVANCED PRACTICE NURSES: ECONOMIC STRUCTURES AND SYSTEMS

Eileen M. Sullivan-Marx and Connie Mullinix

B OTH as autonomous providers of health care and members of interdisciplinary teams, nurse practitioners (NP) and other advanced practice nurses (APN) make significant contributions in all sectors of health care delivery. Despite abundant research demonstrating quality and efficacy of advanced practice nurses, barriers to payment have impeded utilization of advanced practice nurses in mainstream health care delivery and stifled development of innovative care models (Sezchenski, Sansom, Bazell, Salmon, & Mullan, 1994; Strumpf, 1994). As a result, nurse practitioners have not been widely included in either private or public payment databases, perpetuating the invisibility of advanced practice nurses in health care policy. Recent landmark federal legislation, however, now enables nurse practitioners and clinical nurse specialists to receive direct Medicare reimbursement in all geographic settings. This new Medicare legislation (part of The Balanced Budget Act of 1997, Public Law 105-33 effective January 1, 1998) removed several payment barriers for advanced practice nurses, placing them in a sound position for business negotiation.

Baer (1993, see chapter 5) notes that advanced practice nurses have the knowledge and thus, the authority and autonomy, to practice primary care. Society, however, has struggled with the *recognition* of the advanced practice nurse's authority. *Payment is society's overt recognition* of a professional group's authority to practice. Barriers to payment for advanced practice nurses, therefore, often reflect a struggle over such professional issues as scope of practice, prescriptive authority, educational preparation, professional certification, and economic competition. Consequently, legislative and policy initiatives for reimbursement of nurse practitioners have developed in a piecemeal fashion and vary from state to state (Mittelstadt, 1993, see chapter 13). Nurse practitioners need to be aware that practice and payment are intertwined, requiring ongoing vigilance by nurses to maintain and expand nursing's contribution to health care delivery.

Changes in both health care financing and restructuring of delivery systems over the last decade have curtailed "solo" practice arrangements and emphasized employment and contractual arrangements for most professional providers, such as nurses, physicians, rehabilitation therapists, and psychologists. In the 1990s, Independent Practice Associations (IPA) and Preferred Provider Organizations (PPO) emerged as the predominant physician practice arrangement in managed care while advanced practice nurses were increasingly developing entrepreneurial independent nursing practices and nurse-managed centers (Sullivan, Fields, Kelly, & Whelan, 1993, see chapter 10). Due to the rapid fluctuation in the business of health care, health delivery system mergers, consolidation of health insurance corporations, and managed care, all health professionals have had to become cognizant and skilled in the nuances of the "business" of health care in order to overcome threats to their practices and take advantage of opportunities.

Regardless of existing barriers for payment, these changes in health care have presented opportunities for nurse practitioners. The much-heralded Oxford Health Plan's decision to pay nurse practitioner primary providers the same as primary physician providers is just one example (Nurses take doctor duties, 1997; also see chapter 13 in this book). Vigilance to the economic forces at work in health care and development of business skills are crucial if nurse practitioners are to take full advantage of such opportunities. This chapter will discuss historical and economic trends affecting payment for nurse practitioners, current payment policies for both fee-for-service and managed care, economic strategies to promote utilization of nurse practitioners, legislative initiatives for payment, and business skills for negotiation of payment.

HEALTH CARE FINANCE REFORM

During the last 25 years, costs of health care in the United States rose faster than the gross domestic product (GDP), the general rate of inflation, and the overall consumer price index for goods and services (Lee, Soffel, & Luft, 1994). In 1995, health expenditures represented 14% of the GDP (Physician Payment Review Commission, 1997), more than in any other major industrialized nation, and are projected to rise to 16% of the GNP by the year 2000 (Lee et al., 1994). Between 1991 and 1994, private employers' health insurance costs per employee-hour worked increased by 24% while rising health care prices explained the largest portion of growth in personal health care expenditures (U.S. Department of Health and Human Services, 1996). In the early 1990s, American employers and consumers of health care were increasingly dissatisfied with the U.S. health care system and its cost (Blendon, Edwards, & Hyams, 1992). Increases in cost, which ultimately limited availability of services for 31 million uninsured, and discontent with the hospital-oriented health delivery system, forged a political agenda in the U.S. in the early 1990s to "reform health care." These reform efforts addressed several overlapping issues including: (1) integration of financial and delivery components of health care; (2) managed competition; (3) health insurance for small groups and the self-employed; (4) standardized, regulatory framework for health care; and (5) universal health insurance (Enthoven, 1992). Although no all-encompassing federal legislation was enacted, health care delivery and financial restructuring occurred throughout the U.S. largely driven by private business, market forces, state legislation, and federal regulatory adjustments.

MANAGED CARE

Role of APNs in Managed Care

Health maintenance organizations (HMOs) evolved from a method developed at the Kaiser Steel Company to provide health care for its employees and their families (Iglehart, 1992). This method of providing care over time, focusing on health and minimizing unnecessary procedures, was viewed in the 1970s as a way to contain cost. In order to curtail the increasing proportion of profits that were being lost due to the rise in cost of providing health care benefits to employees, employers embraced the health maintenance organization model.

Managed care today has developed to include many hybrid models that merge characteristics of health care delivery and payment. Such service models are structured so that financial risk and responsibility for patient outcomes range across a continuum. Preferred provider organizations (PPO) incur the lowest financial risk to providers, while group HMO models incur the highest financial risk and greatest responsibility for outcomes. Independent practice associations (IPA), clinician providers who remain independent practitioners and contract with managed-care payers, assume a moderate financial risk.

In addition to such provider models, hospitals and physician groups have merged in the last decade to form Integrated Delivery Systems (IDS) in which all aspects of health care delivery are integrated at the functional, financial, and clinical levels. Advanced practice nurses have increasingly been utilized in IDS and managed-care models to provide prevention services, primary care, coordinating care, and managing the comprehensive care of high-risk and high-need groups. APNs have contributed to cost-effectiveness in managed care by preventing costly care, such as readmissions and emergency department visits, reducing complications and nursing home admissions (Lang, Sullivan-Marx, & Jenkins, 1996). The willingness of APNs to receive lower salaries than physicians for providing primary care and hospital services is a significant consideration for managed care. Negotiations for higher salaries with more equity to physician salaries will need to emphasize the cost savings in preventive services that APNs can provide (see chapter 13).

Consumer Response to Managed Care

Consumers have expressed concern about the access to and quality of care received from managed-care organizations. Aided by physicians who believed their provider role of advocating for patients was being limited, consumers have urged state legislators to regulate managed-care organizations (Woolhandler & Himmelstein, 1995). Such state regulations take the form of providing a process for consumers to appeal the decisions of managed-care organizations, prescribing the availability of care, and requiring managed-care organizations to pay for certain emergency services (Annas, 1997).

Evidence is beginning to emerge that those patients who are most sick switch from managed-care arrangements to fee-for-service plans under Medicare (Morgan, Virnig, DeVito, & Persily, 1997). Policy observers have suggested that the pendulum has swung from the extreme of excessive care in the fee-for-service era toward far too little care in a managed-care era and that the pendulum will soon return to a midpoint of appropriate care (Ginzberg & Ostow, 1997).

Financial Arrangements for APNs

Advanced practice nurses have had a variety of financial arrangements with managed-care organizations ranging from full risk bearing to receiving a fee for the service provided. Likewise, compensation of APNs by the managed-care organization varies from salary arrangements to reimbursement on a per-member per-month basis. In the current environment of health care financial restructuring and managed-care market penetration, there is considerable variation in the interpretation of state legislation regarding payment for APN services. In North Carolina, for example, psychiatric-mental health nurses who wish to provide psychotherapy and bill insurance companies are increasingly being told that they must be associated with group practices and participate in managed-care arrangements for providing care even though the state insurance law requires that APNs be reimbursed. Decisions to include APNs as providers for a "panel" of patients are made at the business corporate level and may not be regulated by state law. Exclusion of APNs on provider panels undermines the intent of state laws originally enacted to provide third-party reimbursement for these professionals.

Increasingly, APNs are finding it necessary to work toward passing legislation on a state-by-state basis to ensure inclusion of their services in managed-care plans (Sharp, 1995). In Texas and Delaware, HMOs are prohibited from discriminating against APN services; New York has legislation stating that nurse practitioners are qualified as primary care gatekeepers; Arkansas has included advanced practice nurses as "any willing provider" in the 1995 Patient Protection Act (Pearson, 1997). The "any willing provider" provision to state insurance laws requires that any provider licensed to provide services under state law must be considered for privileges with the managed-care organization.

MEDICARE REFORM AND APN REIMBURSEMENT

Background

Medicare provides basic health insurance to Americans over the age of 65, and to those persons who are disabled, or who have end-stage renal disease (approximately 38 million Americans). Medicare consists of two parts: Part A, hospitalization insurance, and Part B, insurance for coverage of physician and other provider services. Part A is provided to Medicare beneficiaries (as an entitlement program through a federal payroll tax; Part B is provided by a voluntary supplementary medical insurance paid by Medicare beneficiary premiums. Nursing services provided in a hospital system, skilled nursing facility, home health agency, and hospice are covered under Medicare Part A. Medicare Part B covers services of physicians (MDs, DOs, dentists, podiatrists), and "nonphysician providers" (such as nurse practitioners, clinical nurse specialists, certified nurse-midwives, certified registered nurse anesthetists, physician assistants, chiropractors, clinical psychologists, psychiatric social workers, and physical therapists). In addition, Medicare part B also covers laboratory services, outpatient hospital care, and some home health care and supplies (Physician Payment Review Commission, 1997).

In 1983, federal efforts to address growth in Medicare Part A (hospital) expenditures led to the development of a prospective payment system based on diagnosis-related groups (DRGs). Following prospective payment enactment, hospital lengths of stay shortened and care provided on a short-stay or outpatient basis increased. Some have argued that efforts such as Prospective Payment Systems (PPS) only shift cost of care rather than address core causes of cost inflation (Morgan, Virnig, DeVito, & Persily, 1997). Significant shifts in population growth, cost of labor and supplies, and expansion of technology and specialty services further contributed to health care cost inflation.

The CPT and RBRVS Process

Federal payment reforms to control rapidly escalating costs of Medicare Part B (primarily physician services), in 1989, led to Public Law 101-239, the Omnibus Budget Reconciliation Act of 1989 (OBRA-89) that established the Medicare Fee Schedule (PPRC, 1991). Prior to this law, physician payment was based on "usual and customary" fees established by regional carriers for Medicare. In the Medicare Fee Schedule, fee-for-service payment for physician and other provider services (including advanced practice nurses when they are performing "physician" services) is based on the resource costs used to provide services. Each service is classified according to the Current Procedural Terminology (CPT) coding system developed by the American Medical Association (AMA) in 1966 (AMA, 1997a). There are over 7,000 CPT codes of which the most common are the Evaluation and Management Services such as an office or outpatient visit for a new patient (99201-99205), ranging from low (1) to high (5) in both complexity and time (AMA, 1997a).

To establish payment for a service provided, Medicare develops allowable charges for each CPT code through a mathematical formula that takes into account the relative work value of the service, practice cost, and professional liability insurance, each adjusted for geographic location. Relative work values are simply scaled estimates of the work involved for a specific code that take into account: (1) time; (2) technical skill and physical effort; (3) mental effort and judgment; and (4) psychological stress associated with patient risk (AMA, 1997b). Use of work values to establish quantified payment for physician services is based on the resource-based relative value system (RBRVS), developed in 1988 and mandated by Congress as a method to set (and presumably contain) costs for "physician" services by measuring work (Hsiao, Braun, Yntema, & Becker, 1988).

Relative work values for each CPT-coded service are established by the Health Care Financing Administration (HCFA) in concert with the American Medical Association's Relative Value Update Committee (RUC), CPT Editorial Panel, and associated Health Care Professional Advisory Committees (HCPAC) to the CPT and RUC committees. Medicare Carrier Medical Directors and public comment contribute to the process. In order to establish value for the work component of a CPT code, practicing clinicians are surveyed to rate the value of work using magnitude estimation methodology. CPT and relative work values are used by HCFA (Medicare and Medicaid) and private payer systems to determine fee-for-service payment. The American Nurses Association (ANA) has a representative to the CPT, RUC, and HCPAC committees. In 1995, nurse practitioners, through the American Nurses Association, were part of a consensus group of primary care providers who contributed survey data from nurse practitioners to AMA and HCFA on NP relative work values for evaluation and management codes (e.g., office and nursing home visits).

In addition to CPT codes, services are also billable to Medicare and other payers by using the HCFA Common Procedural Coding System (HCPCS) and the International Classification of Diseases System (ICD). HCPCS codes are generally supportive services and supplies but may have relative work values associated when applicable, such as physician (or practitioner) review of an electrocardiogram with interpretation (G007) (AMA, 1997b). ICD codes are largely diagnostic codes but may include some procedures; they do not have assigned relative work values for Medicare purposes.

These classification systems were developed for reimbursement of physician services but have been used for all providers (e.g., psychologists, physical therapists) who may provide billable services. The nomenclature of these systems, however, is not based in multidiscipline language or in language that describes work of providers other than physicians. There are CPT codes that describe preventive services and counseling; however, they do not specifically describe nursing practice and are not generally reimbursed by payers. One of the criticisms of the CPT codes is their limitation to describe only physician services and not the full range of health services provided by all health professionals (Henry, Holzemer, Randell, Hsieh, & Miller, 1997; U.S. Department of Health and Human Services, 1997). Since 1993, the American Nurses Association has had a representative on the Health Care Professional Advisory Committee (CPT HCPAC) to the CPT Editorial Panel. It is feasible to introduce nursing services into CPT if they are not otherwise described in another CPT code. Individuals or professional organizations can undertake this process by working with the American Nurses Association to the AMA's CPT editorial process.

Discussion regarding such issues has begun among professional nursing organizations but now takes on new urgency in a cost-conscious health environment in which APNs can now bill directly for their services.

Medicare Part B services, coded by CPT, represent an annual budget of $74 billion dollars. It is crucial to the nursing profession's viability that nursing practice be identified and described so that nursing interventions are visible in federal payment systems and ultimately linked with patient outcomes.

Although Medicare has increasingly expanded participation for beneficiaries in capitated payment and managed-care plans, fee-for-service plans (in which the provider of the service is directly reimbursed) continue to be the most common payment mechanism in Medicare, particularly in rural areas and for the sickest beneficiaries (PPRC, 1997). In addition, the resource-based relative values system is increasingly being used by managed-care systems to set fee schedules and analyze value of services provided under capitation (U.S. Department of Health and Human Services, 1997). Thus, the Medicare Fee Schedule will continue to be an important component of the Medicare system and be maintained as an option in private payer systems.

Since 1982, managed-care plans have had the option to enter into a Medicare risk contract to enroll Medicare beneficiaries. Under the Tax Equity and Fiscal Responsibility Act (TEFRA) of 1982, beneficiaries must be offered all Medicare-covered services. Point-of-service and cost-based contracts with Medicare are also available to managed-care plans to enroll Medicare beneficiaries. In order to offer payment flexibility to plans and test beneficiaries' interest in health delivery options, HCFA implemented the Medicare Choices Demonstration Project in 1997. In early 1997, approximately 13% of the 38 million Medicare beneficiaries were currently enrolled in a managed-care plan, with enrollments expected to increase by 80,000 each month. Generally, those who enroll in Medicare managed-care plans are healthier and thus incur lower costs. Cost savings in managed-care plans may be curtailed with enrollment of "sicker" beneficiaries (Morgan, Virnig, DeVito, & Persily, 1997).

Medicare Reimbursement for APNs

Recent amendments to the Social Security Act passed by Congress and signed by President Clinton as part of The Balanced Budget Act of 1997 (Public Law 105-33) now give direct Medicare reimbursement (at 85% of the physician rate) to nurse practitioners, clinical nurse specialists, and physician assistants regardless of geographic setting (Table 20.1). This long sought legislation is an important opportunity for nurse practitioners and clinical nurse specialists to bill for services directly in all geographic settings, removing barriers that had limited coverage of nurse practitioner services to rural areas and skilled nursing facilities.

Prior to this legislation, billing "incident to" physician services was commonly used, but fraught with such limitations as requiring presence of a physician in the "suite" where services were provided. Under "incident to" billing, payment is made to the physician provider at 100% of the prevailing physician rate since "incident to" billing was intended to reimburse physicians for the services of their employees, not to reimburse health professionals practicing autonomously. The new legislation in the Balanced Budget Act of 1997 does not necessarily eliminate "incident to" billing by nurse practitioners under a physician provider number; however, emerging guidelines from the Health Care Financing Administration should clarify the circumstances in which "incident to" vs. direct billing will apply.

Although new legislation reimburses advanced practice nurses at 85% of the prevailing physician rate, having direct reimbursement places nurse practitioners and clinical nurse specialists in the mainstream of health care payment and, ultimately, of inclusion in Medicare databases, rendering nursing practice costs visible for both business and health policy

TABLE 20.1 Federal Reimbursement for Advanced Practice Nurses

	NP	CNS	CRNA	CNM
Medicare B	Yes	Yes	Yes	Yes
Medicaid †	Yes	No	Yes	Yes
CHAMPUS	Yes	Yes	No	Yes
FEHB	Yes	Yes	per Plan	Yes

†May vary with state discretion.
NP = Nurse Practitioner.
CNS = Clinical Nurse Specialist.
CRNA = Certified Registered Nurse Anesthetist.
CNM = Certified Nurse-Midwife.

Note: From *The Reimbursement Manual: How to Get Paid for Your Advanced Practice Services* (p. 7), by American Nurses Association, 1993, Washington, DC: American Nurses Publishing, American Nurses Foundation/American Nurses Association. Copyright 1993 by the author. Reprinted with permission.

purposes. In addition, dependency on the presence of a physician in the practice setting where services were performed is eliminated, supporting autonomous, collaborative practice for nurse practitioners and clinical nurse specialists. Consequently, opportunities now exist to expand Medicare services provided by advanced practice nurses in homes and other community sites, such as senior citizen centers or nurse-managed centers, fulfilling part of *Nursing's Agenda for Health Care Reform* for community-based care (Nursing's Agenda, 1992).

This new Medicare legislation requires nurse practitioners and clinical nurse specialists to collaborate with a physician for reimbursement of services:

> which the nurse practitioner or clinical nurse specialist is legally authorized to perform by the State in which the services are performed. . . . (Social Security Act, secs. 2158, 2160)

Medicare law defines "collaboration" as:

> a process in which a nurse practitioner [read also clinical nurse specialist] works with a physician to deliver health care services within the scope of the practitioner's professional expertise, with medical direction and appropriate supervision as provided for in jointly developed guidelines or other mechanisms as defined by the law of the State in which the services are performed.

A clinical nurse specialist according to Section 1861 (aa) (5) (B) of the Social Security Act is:

> a registered nurse and is licensed to practice nursing in the State in which the clinical nurse specialist services are performed and holds a master's degree in a defined clinical area of nursing from an accredited educational institution. Collaboration with a physician is required for services reimbursed by Medicare even if this is not required by the state in which the service was rendered.

A potential restriction in the new Medicare legislation is a requirement that reimbursement will be covered "only if no facility or other provider charges or is paid any amounts with respect to the furnishing of such services" (Social Security Act, Sec. 1861). The intent of this provision is to ensure that Medicare will pay only once for a particular service provided by a NP or CNS. Some advanced practice nursing services provided in an inpatient hospital setting or an outpatient hospital clinic are "bundled" into the payment that the hospital receives under the Medicare

Prospective Payment System (PPS), based on the Diagnostic Related Groups (DRGs). In order to ensure correct billing procedures, nurse practitioners and clinical nurse specialists will need to be absolutely clear about the source of their salary so that their services are not considered covered under Medicare Part A and also billed under Medicare Part B. Ensuing interpretations of this legislation by the Health Care Financing Administration will need to be closely monitored by organized nursing groups and practitioners.

In addition to these provisions, APNs must "accept assignment" from Medicare. Accepting assignment simply means that APNs must not bill Medicare beneficiaries for amounts greater than Medicare allowable charges for the service provided.

Certified Nurse-Midwives (CNM) and Certified Registered Nurse Anesthetists (CRNA)

Medicare payment to certified nurse-midwives was established by Public Law 100-203. Payment for services is at 65% of the prevailing physician rate and is made directly to the CNM. No supervision is necessary unless required by state authority.

Certified registered nurse anesthetists provide 65% of all anesthesia services in the U.S.; and 85% of anesthesia services in rural areas (National Commission on Nurse Anesthesia Education, 1990). Direct Medicare reimbursement to CRNAs was established by Public Law 99-509 in 1986. Congress authorized different payment rates in 1990 (effective in 1996) depending on whether services were medically directed. In 1996, payment for nonmedically directed anesthesia services provided by a CRNA is paid at the same rate as an anesthesiologist for the same service (ANA, 1996a).

Issues with APNs and Medicare Payment

In the last 10 years, a number of federal legislative successes enabled payment for Medicare reimbursement of advanced practice nurses in limited ways. The ensuing years have seen growth and increased utilization of APN services despite barriers limiting APNs from participation in mainstream health delivery and payment policy. Furthermore, conflicting and confusing interpretations of Medicare regulations for payment led to infringements on the autonomy of advanced nursing practice. Legislation granting direct Medicare reimbursement to nurse practitioners and clinical nurse specialists regardless of geographic setting has now been passed in the U.S. Congress and signed by President Clinton, effective January 1, 1998.

Because most advanced nurse practitioners receive payment for their services as employees, most are unaware of the intricacies of private or public financial structures involved in setting payment for their services. In 1994, the American Nurses Association (ANA) and its affiliate organizations, the National Organization Liaison Forum (NOLF), conducted a survey of nurses and found that most were unaware of how revenues were generated in their practice settings. Advanced practice nurses represented 46.1% of the sample (N = 104), another 22.1% were nurse administrators or managers; multiple specialties were represented. Respondents were asked to identify coding used in their practices based on 600 CPT and 200 HCPCS (HCFA Common Procedural Coding System) codes identified by an expert panel as common to nursing practice. Respondents indicated that 99% of these codes pertained to their practice. Table 20.2 lists the 15 most common codes identified in the survey. Evaluation and management services (office visits) were the most common codes utilized by the sample (ANA, 1994).

One of the first attempts to ascertain the extent of the use of CPT billing codes by otherwise "invisible" nurse specialists found that use of codes ranged from family nurse practitioners who provided 233 CPT codes to school nurses who performed 58 codes (Griffith & Robinson, 1993).

Table 20.3 ranks Medicare payment to nurse practitioners in the 1996 Medicare Fee Schedule by frequency of CPT code. As expected, nurse practitioners are present in the 1996 database for only those codes and services that were directly or indirectly paid to the nurse practitioner at that time. Thus, the most frequent payment to nurse practitioners is for nursing facility visits (paid indirectly with a modifier) and office visits, likely generated in rural-designated areas. Home visits (Medicare Part B for medical services provided in the home) are least frequently represented because these were not able to be billed to Medicare by nurse practitioners except in rural areas.

Payment to advanced practice nurses for home visits to provide primary care services would increase the access to care for those Medicare beneficiaries who are most underserved—home-bound, elderly, urban-dwelling, women, and minorities (PPRC, 1995). With direct Medicare reimburse-

TABLE 20.2   ANA CPT Survey of HCFA 1993 Procedure Codes

Nurse Rank	HCFA Rank	CPT Code	Descriptor†
1	1	99213	Office visit, established patient, level 3
2	6	99212	Office visit, established patient, level 2
3	4	99214	Office visit, established patient, level 4
4	11	99215	Office visit, established patient, level 5
5	5	99231	Subsequent hospital care, level 1
6	21	99238	Hospital discharge
6	27	99244	Office consultation, level 4
7	3	99232	Subsequent hospital care, level 2
8	14	99254	Initial inpatient consultation
9	7	99233	Subsequent hospital care, level 3
9	9	99223	Initial hospital care, level 3
9	22	99222	Initial hospital care, level 2
9	28	99255	Initial inpatient consultation, level 5
10	17	90844	Psychotherapy, 45 minutes
11	25	99285	Emergency department visit, level 5

†Levels range from simple to complex, lower numbers (1) are the most simple visits and higher numbers (3–5) are the most complex visits.

Note: From ANA/NOLF CPT Utilization Survey Summary (Agenda), 1994, Washington, DC: American Nurses Association. Copyright 1994 by the author. Adapted with permission.

TABLE 20.3   Medicare Part B Payment Schedule
for Nurse Practitioners—1996*

Rank	CPT Code	Descriptor	Freq NP Billed	NP Allowed Charges
1	99312	Nursing facility	1.21%	$3,344,108
2	99311	Nursing facility	0.98%	$1,982,660
3	99313	Nursing facility	0.81%	$803,718
4	99332	Rest home visit	0.67%	$89,952
5	99213	Office visit	0.06%	$1,317,990

*Ranked by NP percentage of total allowed frequency.

Source: U.S. Department of Health and Human Services, Health Care Financing Administration. (1996). Part B Medicare Annual Data.

ment, it is expected that ensuing databases will demonstrate greater percentage of services provided by nurse practitioners and clinical specialists for all evaluation and management services, including home visits and nursing facility visits. Since services provided by nurse practitioners were hidden under physician provider numbers or not billed, future databases will more accurately reflect the contributions (financial as well as clinical) of APNs in all sectors of health care delivery.

Direct Medicare billing presents a challenge to individual APNs and nursing organizations alike. Rather than be "unaware of charges" as indicated in the 1994 ANA survey, APNs will now be able to track revenue that they have generated as employees in a practice or as owners of a nurse-managed practice. Professional nursing organizations will need to establish information services and "hotlines" for questions about correct billing procedures. Two new web sites have done so to date: the American College of Nurse Practitioners (http://www.acnp.org) and The American Nurses Association (http://www.nursingworld.org). APNs need to have a working knowledge of CPT and other coding systems as well as determining payment schedules for individual practices. The AMA resources listed in this chapter are a good beginning to increase awareness of Medicare billing and associated fee schedules. Questions that APNs should be able to answer in their practices include:

1. What specific CPT code is used for the specific services provided?
2. What documentation in the patient's record is required for the service that is billed?
3. When is the service provided a billable service? Or is the service already covered by another Medicare payment source, such as Medicare Part A?
4. What resources do I need so that my services are accurately and legally billed?

Stepping into this new era of Medicare billing will require policy, business, and legal skills. For further discussion, see Business Strategies at the end of this chapter.

Other Federally Sponsored Payment Programs

Four federal programs reimburse advanced practice nurses for their services: Medicare, Medicaid, the Federal Employees Health Benefit Plan

(FEHBP), and CHAMPUS. Table 20.1 lists advanced practice nurse payments in each of the federal programs.

Medicare's Community Nursing Organizations (CNOs)

Another venue for Medicare payment for nursing services, the Community Nursing Organization (CNO) Demonstration Project, was established as a 3-year national demonstration (part of the Omnibus Budget Reconciliation Act of 1987) using a capitated approach to fund Medicare services for older adults. Four sites were initially funded in the 1992–1993 Federal budget and include: (1) Carle Clinic in Urbana, Illinois; (2) Carondelet Health Care in Tucson, Arizona; (3) the Visiting Nurse Service in Long Island City, New York; and (4) the Block Nurse Program in St. Paul, Minnesota. In these models, community-based services to older adults are provided under a capitated nurse-managed model at a controlled rate with integration of financial and health delivery structures (ANA, 1996b).

Ongoing analysis has demonstrated that these projects have been successful to date in providing high enrollee satisfaction, overall lower projected costs, shorter duration of Medicare home care, more cost-effective mix of services, and lower equipment costs (ANA, 1996b). The CNO Demonstration Project was reauthorized by U.S. Congress in the 1997 Balanced Budget Act. Wellness models using nurse management with older adults who are at risk for frequent use of costly services can save funds for Medicare (Burns, Lamb, & Wholey, 1996). The CNO model has not incorporated advanced practice nurses but may serve as a prototype for using APNs in specialized high-risk populations (Lang, Sullivan-Marx, & Jenkins, 1996).

MEDICAID

Medicaid is a federally mandated program that guarantees health care services to low-income families with dependent children, low-income aged and disabled. Medicaid funds are provided by the federal government and administered by the states. Prior to 1989, reimbursement of advanced practice nurses varied according to individual state policy and legislation. To ensure access to primary care services for low-income families and children, the U.S. Congress passed the Omnibus Budget Reconciliation

Act of 1989 establishing direct payment for pediatric and family nurse practitioners in the Medicaid program without the need for supervision or association with physicians or other health care providers. Since 1989, some states have expanded the intent of federal law and allow Medicaid reimbursement for all nurse practitioners. Payment for services provided by CNMs is included under separate state laws (Pearson, 1997). In April, 1997, a bill was introduced in the U.S. House of Representatives (H.R. 1354) to amend title XIX of the Social Security Act mandating coverage of services provided by all nurse practitioners and clinical nurse specialists under state Medicaid plans, but it has not yet been passed as legislation.

In efforts to control costs, many states have reorganized their Medicaid programs using managed-care approaches and capitated payment. States may require Medicaid beneficiaries to access care through a designated primary care provider or enroll in a contracted health maintenance organization. In order for states to alter their method of payment, the federal government must provide a "waiver," part of Sections 1115 and 1915 (b) of the Social Security Act, from specific federal requirements. The scope and nature of "waiver" changes vary with each state, requiring political vigilance on the part of nursing to ensure inclusion of payment for services provided by advanced practice nurses in each of these states (ANA, 1996a; White, 1995).

FEDERAL EMPLOYEE HEALTH BENEFIT PLAN (FEHBP)

Federal employees can voluntarily receive health insurance by participating in the Federal Employees Health Benefit Plan (FEHBP). Two laws have mandated FEHBP coverage of services for nurses, first, in 1985, Congress mandated reimbursement to all nonphysician providers, including registered nurses, for services provided under this plan. In 1990, Public Law 101-509 mandated direct payment to nurse practitioners, clinical nurse specialists, and certified nurse-midwives for services provided to federal employees participating in this plan. Collaboration or supervision by any other health care provider is not required.

CIVILIAN HEALTH AND MEDICAL PROGRAM OF THE UNIFORMED SERVICES (CHAMPUS)

There is limited coverage of services provided by advanced practice nurses in this system. In 1979, Public Law 95-457 provided direct payment for certified nurse-midwives and does not require physician supervision. Certified nurse practitioners and psychiatric clinical nurse specialists were covered by Public Law 97-114 in 1982. Physician supervision is not required (Mittelstadt, 1993).

STATE REIMBURSEMENT FOR APNs

Traditional "Indemnity Plan" Reimbursement

Payment for advanced practice nurses through private "indemnity plan" insurance on a fee-for-service basis is regulated at the state level. In the last 20 years, nurse practitioners and other advanced practice nurses have been successful in establishing state legislation supporting reimbursement for their services. Thirty-seven states have legislation that either requires coverage or prohibits discrimination against reimbursement to nurse practitioners, certified nurse-midwives, certified registered nurse anesthetists, or psychiatric nurses for services (Pearson, 1997).

State insurance laws address components of health care coverage that include insurers affected (nonprofit and commercial or for-profit), providers affected, or reimbursable services. State laws will vary by type of insurer and whether the benefit to be covered for advanced practice nurse services is mandatory or a mandatory option. In a mandatory option, consumers of health care must request to have APN services included in their coverage, while in legislation for mandatory coverage, APN services must be included in coverage. In states where no law exists that covers APN services, APNs have negotiated individually with insurance companies for coverage of their services. Rates of reimbursement vary and may be a percentage of the prevailing physician rate (Pearson, 1997).

Medicaid

All states but Ohio (which only recognizes advanced practice nurses in pilot programs) have complied with federal legislation mandating Medicaid coverage of pediatric and family nurse practitioner services in Medicaid programs. A number of states include all nurse practitioners and advanced practice nurses in coverage for their Medicaid programs. Range of payment varies from 70%–100% of the prevailing physician rate. Twenty-one states reimburse advanced practice nurses at 100% of the physician rate (Pearson, 1997).

Introduction of Medicaid 1115 waivers to allow states greater control of federal Medicaid funds can potentially exclude APNs from participation as primary or identified providers in Medicaid programs. In the District of Columbia and West Virginia, Medicaid waiver programs exclude nurse practitioners as primary providers or "gatekeepers." Advanced practice nurses have needed to take political action in many states to ensure their continued inclusion in state Medicaid programs. Such efforts will need to continue as the federal government seeks ways to reduce costs in the Medicaid program.

BUSINESS STRATEGIES AND INNOVATIVE ECONOMIC PRACTICE MODELS

Advanced Practice Nurse Negotiations

To continue to provide care, advanced practice nurses will need to negotiate with managed-care organizations. Financial relationships vary as described previously from being salaried employees to nurse-managed practices that assume risk in capitated arrangements. Components of business negotiations with managed care include such issues as services to be provided, credentialing, compensation, availability, licensing and privileges, standards of care, referrals, prescription drugs, liability insurance, severability, and details involving name/title usage and record-keeping. Contractual arrangements between Oxford Health Plans and APNs are discussed in chapter 13 of this book.

Buppert (1997) notes that when APNs negotiate salaries with prospective employers they need to consider revenues generated, deducting 40% of that amount for overhead expenses, and deducting another percentage for consultation with collaborating physicians (25% for inexperienced practitioners, 10%–15% for experienced nurse practitioners). In addition, employers will want a percentage, often 10%–15%, for profit. Depending on productivity, experienced nurse practitioner salaries may range from $50,000–$70,000, still less than the average primary physician salary ($100,000–$140,000).

Several federally sponsored programs represent efforts to establish and promote innovative models of health care delivery whose purposes are to provide services to underserved groups employing cost-effective financial arrangements. Nurse practitioners have been intricately involved in these programs and increasingly are establishing advanced nursing practice as the prototype provider for patients served in these models.

Federally Qualified Health Centers (FQHC)

In 1992, HCFA established new facilities—federally qualified health centers—to provide health promotion and preventive services and access to primary care services for Medicare beneficiaries (U.S. Department of Health and Human Services, 1992). Federally qualified health centers originated from community health centers and migrant health centers established under the Public Health Service and include any facility receiving funding from the Public Health Service Act or meeting requirements to receive a grant from this act. Clinics or facilities that meet requirements to receive a public health service grant have been deemed FQHC "look-alikes." Services covered in these health centers include health promotion activities usually not covered in the Medicare program, such as annual physical examinations, health screening and diagnostic tests, immunizations, and preventive health education (Federal Register, 1992). Services of "individual practitioners who may be employed in FQHCs, including . . . nurse practitioners, nurse midwives . . . may be covered under Medicare Part B and would be billable separately . . . under Part B" (Federal Register, p. 24965).

Comprehensive Outpatient Rehabilitation Facilities (CORF)

The Collaborative Assessment and Rehabilitation for Elders (C.A.R.E.) Program at the University of Pennsylvania School of Nursing provides short-term outpatient comprehensive rehabilitation for Medicare beneficiaries using a nurse-managed interdisciplinary model, in which advanced practice nurses directly assess and implement care interventions (Evans, Yurkow, & Siegler, 1995). The program is funded as a comprehensive outpatient rehabilitation facility (CORF) under the Medicare program.

Medicare payment to the CORF are prorated annually for both clinical services and operating costs. Some Medicare Part B services provided by nurse practitioners, clinical nurse specialists, or physicians may be billed separately.

Program for All-Inclusive Care for the Elderly (PACE)

The philosophy of the PACE model is to maintain older adults in the community with minimal disruption of their lives. The PACE model is based on the successful On Lok program in San Francisco which provided a comprehensive, multidisciplinary, community-based program for older adults in their homes with capitated Medicare and Medicaid funding. Initial Medicare waivers were granted to 15 sites yearly but legislation since 1995 has authorized increased waivers. Services provided include primary and specialty medical care, adult day care, home care, nursing, social work, rehabilitative services, prescription drugs, and coordination of hospital and nursing home care by PACE staff. Advanced practice nurses have the potential to provide nursing services as well as primary and specialty medical services. The University of Pennsylvania School of Nursing has received approval as a PACE site for an advanced nursing practice model to provide services to frail, older adults in West Philadelphia beginning in 1997.

SUMMARY AND CONCLUSION

Thirty years ago, nurse practitioners and clinical nurse specialists were considered "pioneers" in health care delivery models, forging a place for themselves in primary care and intensive care units of hospitals. Today, inclusion of APNs in health care systems is increasingly standard practice. Consistent growth in numbers and utilization of nurse practitioners and clinical specialists has forged a need to include APNs in mainstream health care payment structures. Both business and governmental models of practice have recognized the advantages of including advanced practice nursing for cost-savings and quality outcomes. Advanced practice nurses, however, have not generally been cognizant of business practices nor of reimbursement strategies relevant to their practices. Current emphasis in linking financial responsibility with provision of care, and the need to address care of underserved and specialized groups in society, have made it inevitable that APNs take an active part in policy and business in order to continue as essential and viable providers of care.

REFERENCES

American Medical Association. (1997a). *Medicare RBRVS: The physician's guide.* Chicago: Author.

American Medical Association. (1997b). *Physician's current procedural terminology.* Chicago: Author.

American Nurses Association. (1994). *American Nurses Association/National Organizational Liaison Forum Current Procedural Terminology (CPT) Utilization Survey.* Washington, DC: Author.

American Nurses Association. (1996a). *Nursing reimbursement under Medicare and Medicaid.* Washington, DC: Author.

American Nurses Association. (1996b, December 11). *Testimony before the Physician Payment Review Commission.* Washington, DC: Author.

Annas, G. J. (1997). Patients' rights in managed care: Exit, voice, and choice. *New England Journal of Medicine, 337*(3), 210–215.

Baer, E. D. (1993). Philosophical and historical bases of primary care nursing. In M. D. Mezey & D. O. McGivern (Eds.), *Nurses, nurse practitioners: Evolution to advanced practice* (pp. 102–116). New York: Springer.

Blendon, R. J., Edwards, J. N., & Hyams, A. L. (1992). Making the critical choices. *Journal of the American Medical Association, 267,* 2509–2520.

Buppert, C. K. (1997, July/August). Negotiating salary. *Nurse Practitioner World News,* 2(4), 4–5.

Burns, L. R., Lamb, G. S., & Wholey, D. R. (1996). Impact of integrated community nursing services on hospital utilization and costs in a Medicare risk plan. *Inquiry, 33,* 30–41.

Enthoven, A. C. (1992). Commentary: Measuring the candidates on health care. *New England Journal of Medicine, 327,* 807–809.

Evans, L. K., Yurkow, J., & Siegler, E. L. (1995). The C.A.R.E. Program: A nurse-managed collaborative outpatient program to improve function of frail older people. *Journal of the American Geriatrics Society, 43,* 1155–1160.

Ginzberg, E., & Ostow, M. (1997). Managed care: A look back and a look ahead. *New England Journal of Medicine, 336,* 1018–1020.

Griffith, H. M., & Robinson, K. R. (1993). Current Procedural Terminology (CPT) coded services provided by nurse specialists. *Image: Journal of Nursing Scholarship, 25,* 178–186.

Health Care Financing Administration, Bureau of Data Management and Strategy. (1996). *Medicare Part B payment schedule for nurse practitioners.* Washington, DC: Government Printing Office.

Henry, S. B., Holzemer, W. L., Randell, C., Hsieh, S.-F., & Miller, T. J. (1997). Comparison of Nursing Interventions Classification and Current Procedural Terminology codes for categorizing nursing activities. *Image: Journal of Nursing Scholarship, 29*, 133–138.

Hsiao, W. C., Braun, P., Yntema, D., & Becker, E. R. (1988). Estimating physicians' work for a resource-based relative value scale. *New England Journal of Medicine, 319*, 835–841.

Iglehart, J. K. (1992). Health policy report: Managed care. *New England Journal of Medicine, 327*, 742–747.

Jensen, G. A., Morrisey, M. A., Gaffney, S., & Liston, D. K. (1997). The new dominance of managed care: Insurance trends in the 1990s. *Health Affairs, 16*, 125–136.

Lang, N. M., Sullivan-Marx, E. M., & Jenkins, M. (1996). Advanced practice nurses and success of organized delivery systems. *American Journal of Managed Care, 2*, 129–135.

Lee, P. R., Soffel, D., & Luft, H. S. (1994). Costs and coverage: Pressures toward health care reform. In P. R. Lee & C. L. Estes (Eds.), *The nation's health* (4th ed., pp. 204–213). Boston: Jones and Bartlett.

Mittelstadt, P. (1993). Third-party reimbursement for services of nurses in advanced practice: Obtaining payment for your services. In M. D. Mezey & D. O. McGivern (Eds.), *Nurses, nurse practitioners: Evolution to advanced practice* (pp. 322–341). New York: Springer.

Morgan, R. O., Virnig, B. A., DeVito, C. A., & Persily, N. A. (1997). The Medicare-HMO revolving door: The healthy go in and the sick go out. *New England Journal of Medicine, 337*, 169–175.

National Commission on Nurse Anesthesia Education. (1990). *The report of the commission on nurse anesthesia education.* Washington, DC: American Association of Nurse Anesthetists.

Nurses to take doctor duties, Oxford says. (1997, February 7). *The Wall Street Journal,* p. A3–4.

Nursing's agenda for health care reform. (1992). Washington, DC: American Nurses Foundation.

Pearson, L. J. (1997). Annual update of how each state stands on legislative issues affecting advanced nursing practice. *Nurse Practitioner, 22*, 18–86.

Physician Payment Review Commission. (1991). *Annual report.* Washington, DC.

Physician Payment Review Commission. (1995). *Annual report.* Washington, DC.

Physician Payment Review Commission. (1997). *Annual report.* Washington, DC.

Roberts, M. J. (1993). *Your money or your life: The health care crisis explained.* New York: Doubleday.

Social Security Act, sec. 1861 (aa)(4); Medicare Carrier Manual, secs., 2158, 2160.

Sekschenski, E. S., Sansom, S., Bazell, C., Salmon, M. E., & Mullan, F. (1994). State practice environments and the supply of physician assistants, nurse practitioners, and certified nurse-midwives. *New England Journal of Medicine, 331*, 1266–1271.

Sharp, N. (1995). Managed care, nurse practitioners and discrimination. *Nursing Management, 26*(9), 90–93.

Strumpf, N. E. (1994). Innovative gerontological practices as models for health care delivery. *Nursing & Health Care, 15*, 522–527.

Sullivan, E., Fields, B., Kelly, J., & Whelan, E.-M. (1993). Nursing centers: The new arena for advanced nursing practice. In M. D. Mezey & D. O. McGivern (Eds.), *Nurses, nurse practitioners: Evolution to advanced practice* (pp. 251–264). New York: Springer.

White, K. M. (1995). The fate of Medicaid waivers. *Nursing Policy Forum, 1*(3), 37–39.

Woolhandler, S., & Himmelstein, D. U. (1995). Extreme risk: The new corporate proposition for physicians. *New England Journal of Medicine, 333*, 1706–1707.

U.S. Department of Health and Human Services. (1992). Medicare program; Payment for federally qualified health center services. *Federal Register, 57*(11C), 24961–24985.

U.S. Department of Health and Human Services. (1996). *Health United States 1995.* Washington, DC: U.S. Government Printing Office.

U.S. Department of Health and Human Services. (1997). Medical classifications systems. In *The national committee on vital and health statistics, 1995.* Washington, DC: U.S. Government Printing Office.

U.S. Department of Health and Human Services, Health Care Financing Administration. (1996). Part B Medicare Annual Data.

Chapter 21

STATE NURSE PRACTICE ACTS

Bonnie Bullough, and revised by Virginia Gillett
and Vern L. Bullough

ONE of the most noticeable trends in nurse practice acts in the past decade has been the continual revision as legislative regulation struggles to keep up with the changing role of nursing, particularly that of the nurse practitioner. Each state responds somewhat differently to the changes, since in the United States, occupational licensure is a responsibility of the states rather than the federal government. Surprisingly, however, since a statute that seems workable in one state is often copied in other states, there is much similarity among state statutes and regulations. Moreover, communications between the state licensing bodies is facilitated by organizations such as The National Council of State Boards of Nursing. Obviously also, members of the same occupation communicate with each other and advise the state governments as to the kind of licensure and regulations to be used to regulate practice. Not all nurses, however, agree on how practice acts should be revised, and opposition in some states is stronger than in others. This is particularly the case with regulation of nurse practitioners who have often found themselves in conflict with the American Nurses Association.

SOME BACKGROUND

Nurses have not always been registered, and in fact licensure in the United States for any occupation only took place in the last part of the 19th century. It was physicians who set the legal precedents, and their experience helped guide the early nursing efforts to be registered not only in the United States but in England and elsewhere. Interestingly, Florence Nightingale opposed nursing licensure, and the British nurses gained their licensing over her objections.

In the United States, physicians began lobbying for legislative licensing in 1847 with the foundation of the American Medical Association (AMA). The reason for their efforts was twofold: a public reason, namely, to raise the level of competence of physicians, and a less public one, to lessen competition from other healers. This is part of the ambivalence that continues to exist about licensing, since it clearly sets minimum uniform standards for professionals but it also limits the numbers who can become professionals by raising standards. Licensing of physicians, for example, was often opposed by other healers, and it was not until 1873 that the AMA succeeded in getting its first licensure act through a legislature, that of Texas (Derbyshire, 1969). In 1881, a somewhat similar statute was enacted in West Virginia, but in this case the right of the state to license professionals was challenged in the courts. Finally in 1888, the U.S. Supreme Court ruled that occupational licensure was a valid exercise of the political powers of the states (United States Reports, 1888). Following this decision, the lobbying of the AMA increased, and by the end of the 19th century all states had enacted medical licensure laws. The fact that medical licensure had come first had important consequences for other health occupations, since physicians by law were regarded as the key guardians of all health care. This meant that licensing for other professions had to come as amendments to the original medical practice acts, and by implication these other professions had greater limitations put on their practice than did medicine (Roemer, 1973; Shyrock, 1967). This has made for a somewhat uneasy relationship between physicians and nurses because each extension of nursing rights has seemed to imply to physicians that their control was becoming more circumscribed.

The history of the state nurse practice acts can be divided into three distinct phases:

1. Passage of the early nurse registration acts, 1903–1938.

2. Definition and scope of nursing practice: 1938–1971.
3. Development of advanced nursing specialties: 1971 to the present (Bullough, 1976, 1980, 1984).

In the first phase, nurses using the model established by medicine sought to use state licensure to raise standards, eliminate competition from untrained nurses, and increase the power and prestige of their profession. The desirability of achieving licensure served as a catalyst for nurses to organize, with the organization which became the National League for Nursing (NLN) being established in 1894, and that which was later named the American Nurses' Association (ANA), in 1896. Both organizations were instrumental in lobbying state legislatures for registration, although, because of its larger membership, most of the day-to-day work was done by the ANA. The task was made more complicated by the fact that women as yet did not have the vote, and thus had to rely more on powers of persuasion than on the power politics available to the AMA. North Carolina, in 1903, became the first state to pass a registration act, followed by New York, New Jersey, and Virginia in that same year. One by one other states followed, until by 1923 all of the states then in the union had a nurse registration act (Lesnik & Anderson, 1947: 310–314). These early laws were clearly nurse registration acts instead of nurse practice acts because they did not define a scope of practice. Rather the term *registered nurse* referred to a person of good character who had completed an acceptable nursing program and passed a state board examination. In some states, the individual was supposed to have additional attributes, such as good health, but none of the statutes spelled out the functions of a registered nurse.

The second phase in the development of nursing licensure started in 1938, when New York State enacted the first mandatory practice act. The law established two levels of nursing, registered professional and the practical nurse. The law defined each level and the nursing functions, which were to be restricted to members of these two groups (Editorial, 1939; Hicks, 1938).

Mandatory licensure had long been a goal for nursing, but it was not until New York's mandatory practice act that it was possible to restrict the title "nurse." Key to achieving mandatory licensure was the development of licensed practical nurses, a second level of nursing, to satisfy the opposition of hospital employers who argued that all nursing functions did not require 3 years of training. Mandatory licensure of two levels of nursing (with 1-year and 3-years training) was accepted by the hospital administrators as a reasonable response to their needs. The New York statute became a model for other states to copy (Jacobsen, 1940; Lesnik & Anderson, 1947: 315–318).

Mandatory licensing on the New York model made it illegal for an unauthorized person to practice nursing. Older laws of the first phase had merely made it illegal for an unauthorized person to use the title *registered nurse*. Since only registered professional nurses or registered practical nurses could engage in nursing, it became necessary to define just exactly what the scope of function of a nurse was (Lesnik & Anderson, 1947: 47).

To assist state nursing organizations in this endeavor, the ANA in 1955 adopted a model definition of nursing. Professional nursing was defined as:

> ... the performance, for compensation, of any act in the observation, care and counsel of the ill, injured or infirm, or in the maintenance of health or prevention of illness in others, or in the supervision and teaching of other personnel, or the administration of medications and treatments prescribed by a licensed physician or dentist, requiring substantial specialized judgment and skill and based on knowledge and application of the principles of biological, physical, and social science. The foregoing shall not be deemed to include acts of diagnosis or prescription of therapeutic or corrective measures. (ANA Board, 1955)

Unfortunately, the inclusion of the disclaimer in the last sentence about diagnosis, treatment, or prescription of therapeutic measures quoted above, was contrary in fact to what was taking place. Nurses were in fact making diagnostic decisions and acting on them in a variety of settings. It might be that the disclaimer was included to make the practice act more palatable to medicine, but there is no historical evidence that such a statement was demanded by them. Rather, in hindsight, it appears to have been a foolish feminine withdrawal before any challenge was made. Nevertheless, by 1957 15 states had incorporated this model language into their state laws and another six states had used the model with only slight modification (Fogotson, Roemer, Newman, & Cook, 1967). This meant that all the advanced specialty nursing roles which began to develop in the 1960s were illegal until the laws could be changed (Bullough, 1980).

THE DEVELOPMENT OF ADVANCED NURSING SPECIALTIES

Postgraduate specialty courses for nurses were popular as early as the first part of the 20th century. These courses essentially used an apprenticeship model, and nurses worked with their instructors for between 8 and 16 weeks (Bullough, 1990), and although they received a certificate, they did not receive collegiate credit. Basic nursing education was in the hospital diploma schools, although by the 1960s about 14% of new nurse graduates had completed a baccalaureate program (American Nurses Association, 1967). These graduates, along with a smaller group who had earned baccalaureate degrees after their diploma training, made up the pool of applicants available for graduate study. Realizing that higher education was a priority need for nurses, the federal government in 1965 began to offer financial support for graduate nursing education, and universities responded by expanding or initiating graduate programs for nurses (Kalisch & Kalisch, 1982). This expansion allowed the preparation of the major nursing specialties to fall totally in a university setting, either for short-term certificate programs or for graduate degrees.

The initial impetus for graduate programs was to prepare clinical specialists who would improve the quality of nursing care (Johnson, Wilcox, & Model, 1967). Most of the content in the curriculum focused on social psychological support rather than on treatment on the theory that the new clinical specialists could supplement the work of physicians rather than compete with them. The only possible competition to medicine was from the psychiatric clinical specialists simply because psychological support was regarded as therapy in psychiatry (Glover, 1967; Rohde, 1968). As a result, clinical specialists other than the psychiatric nurses fared poorly in the clinical job market. Their avoidance of physician territory left hospital and clinical employers puzzled as to their function and unwilling to pay them more than other nurses, and many turned to teaching or administration as an alternative (Elder & Bullough, 1990).

It was in this setting that the first nurse practitioner program appeared, established at the University of Colorado in 1965 as a short-term certificate rather than a degree program. It was different from the earlier postgraduate courses in the hospitals in that it was an intensive educational experience rather than an apprenticeship program. It was, however, outside the mainstream of nursing education because of the hostility of traditional nurse educators to nursing roles overlapping those of medicine. The federal government, however, felt differently and federal funding through the Division of Nursing (U.S. Public Health Service) enabled nurse practitioner programs to gain a foothold in universities. By 1980 the majority of the nurse practitioner programs were university sponsored and awarded masters' degrees (Sultz, Henry, Kinyon, Buck, & Bullough, 1983).

The reason for the growth of the programs was to meet the shortage of primary care physicians caused by a planned underproduction of physicians encouraged by the medical establishment during the first part of the 20th century as well as an unplanned and unanticipated reallocation of physicians away from the general practice role into specialty roles (Fein, 1967). In 1971 physician specialists outnumbered general practitioners three to one (National Center, 1972–73). In recent years, while the overall physician shortage has abated, a shortage of primary care providers persists and medical specialists still outnumber generalists.

Improvements in health care technology provided a further impetus for the development of specialties in nursing. Most notable were the specialized coronary and other intensive care units in hospitals (Dracup & Marsden, 1990). The early clinical specialists who staffed these units were prepared in short-term certificate programs supplemented by on-the-job training. Presently, critical care nurses are the largest group of specialty nurses (Hartshorn, 1988; Rehm, 1987). The membership of the American Association of Critical Care Nurses in 1995 was more than 60,000, with over 25,000 being certified as Critical Care Registered Nurses (CCRN). The numbers have continued to grow, although the majority of this group are not yet equipped with master's degrees. However, as graduate programs focusing on critical care have grown, so have the master's prepared candidates, and like the other nursing specialties the master's degree will become the means of entering the field.

Midwifery, a time-honored profession in much of the world, became associated with nursing late in the 19th century in many countries of the world with the establishment of nurse-midwifery programs. In the United States, however, physician competition delayed such a development for more than a half century. When the first nurse-midwifery training program in this country started in 1932 in connection with the Maternity Center in New York City, the scope of practice of nurse-midwives was limited and their use was mainly confined to poor neighborhoods (Litoff, 1978; Tom, 1982). As late as 1965, nurse-midwives were licensed only in New Mexico, the eastern counties of Kentucky, and New York City (not in the rest of New York) (Fogotson et al., 1967).

The expansion of nurse-midwifery was greatly enhanced by many of the same factors facilitating development of nurse practitioners: federal funding and changes in the nurse practice acts. The women's movement was also instrumental in revising midwifery by educating clients to demand the personal care long associated with midwife deliveries. By 1990, more than 3,000 practicing nurse-midwives, prepared both in certificate and increasingly in master's programs, were certified by the American College of Nurse-Midwives. By 1997, the ACNM had 6,200 members, but some of these were students and some were retired. Organization officials estimate there are somewhere between 4,500 and 5,000 nurse-midwives in actual practice (ACNM, 1997). Quite clearly the numbers are growing.

Lastly, the nurse anesthetist emerged as a master's-level specialty practice. Nurses started administering anesthesia as early as 1889, particularly in Catholic hospitals (Clapesattle, 1943). Using an apprenticeship format, the first formal course in nurse anesthesia was offered in Portland (Oregon) in 1909. At that time, physician anesthesiologists had no formal training; interns or colleagues were often pressed into service, and nurses were welcomed as assistants (Thatcher, 1953). As the specialty of medical anesthesiology developed the climate changed, and two landmark law cases were brought by medical societies against nurse anesthetists. In 1917, a Kentucky judge ruled in favor of a physician employer of a nurse anesthetist. The ruling indicated that licensure laws are written to benefit people rather than the profession, and that people should not be deprived of the services of nurse anesthetists (Frank v. South, 1917). In 1937, a California nurse anesthetist was sued by the medical society which argued that she was practicing medicine. The nurse won her case with a ruling that she was not practicing medicine because she was supervised by the operating surgeon (Thatcher, 1953).

Ignored by the nursing establishment, the American Association of Nurse Anesthetists established its own certification program in 1945, and began an accreditation program in 1952. A baccalaureate degree was mandated for certification in 1987, and as of 1998 a master's degree has been required (Gunn, 1984). In 1990 there were 22,000 Certified Registered Nurse Anesthetists (CRNA) in the United States and approximately half of the anesthesia in this country was being administered by CRNAs working with anesthesiologists. CRNAs working alone administered 20%, and the other 30% of the anesthesia was administered by physician anesthesiologists (American Association of Nurse Anesthetists, 1990). In 1997 these numbers had grown to 27,000 with increasing numbers working alone (American Association of Nurse Anesthetists, 1997).

EXPANDING STATE LAWS TO COVER NURSE PRACTITIONERS

These early nursing specialties, which operated more or less distinctly from the rest of organized nursing, had developed a system of professional certification. Increasingly, however, as graduate nurse education in the specialties developed, it was recognized that certification was not enough, that a separate level of licensure was needed. The early movement for new kinds of licensure developed out of a need to cover nurse practitioners, who were clearly diagnosing and treating patients in violation of disclaimers written into most nurse practice acts after the ANA model of 1955. The first nurse practitioner legislation was enacted by Idaho in 1971. The legislature instructed the Boards of Medicine and Nursing to draw up rules allowing nurse practitioners to practice. The joint boards decided that nurse practitioners should be regulated by policies and procedures (protocols) written at the local level (Idaho, 1971). The boards, however, did not give separate licensure to nurse practitioners, but since Idaho was first in dealing with the issue, its action was widely copied by other states.

A second approach to accommodate nurse practitioner practice was to expand a state's basic definition of all registered professional nurse practice. This was accomplished by either omitting or limiting the disclaimer in state practice acts against diagnosis and treatment by registered nurses, or by rewriting the definition of registered nursing using broader language. New York, in 1972, was the first state to adopt this approach. Amendment of a state practice act was a major step over the Idaho-type legislation because in theory it removed unnecessary barriers to the full use of all registered nurses. In reality, whether or not a nurse actually functions as nurse practitioner under these amended statutes, even with the use of a protocol, turned out to be dependent on other state statutes and regulations. This forced nursing to turn to the courts, as they did in Missouri.

A 1975 Missouri revision of the Nurse Practice Act removed the blanket prohibition to diagnosis and treatment by nurses, but made no mention of nurse practitioners or other advanced specialists (Missouri, 1975). In spite of this some nurse practitioners in the state used written protocols to guide their practices. Physicians working with nurse practitioners in a rural family planning clinic were charged by the Board of Medicine with aiding and abetting the illegal practice of medicine. The Medical Board won its case at the local level but the State Supreme Court overturned the ruling (Greenlaw, 1984). With impetus from the Missouri decision, a combination of a broad definition of nursing practice plus the use of protocols has been adopted by other states as the mechanism for legal coverage of advanced nursing practice.

In a third approach to facilitating nursing practitioner practice, some states opted to give physicians more delegative powers. Even before the current phase in nursing licensure, some state medical acts, including those of Arizona, Colorado, Florida, Kansas, and Oklahoma, gave physicians broad power to delegate medical acts to other workers. South Dakota in 1972, North Carolina in 1973, and Maine in 1974 added language to their practice acts to facilitate nurse practitioner practice. The Maine act permits professional nurses with additional educational preparation to diagnose, prescribe, and treat when those responsibilities are delegated to them by physicians (Maine, 1974). A number of states followed the Maine example. The current pattern of certification for nurse specialties in each state is shown in Table 21.1.

Individual certification of nurse specialists is the best approach to legal coverage because it makes practitioners accountable for their own practice. Passage of laws to permit individual certification is, however, difficult to achieve, especially in the face of a growing physician surplus. New York State nurse practitioners struggled for 8 years before they succeeded in passing such a law in 1988. Passage of the law was impeded both by physicians and the organized opposition of the New York State Nurses' Association. The state nurses association wanted the ANA practice model (ANA, 1980), which opposed state certification but wanted nursing certifying bodies to decide who was or was not an advanced practice nurse. This model followed the example of the American Medical Association. This philosophical stance meant that the ANA has often found itself opposing much of the legislation for advanced practice nurses. Some state nursing organizations, however, broke with the ANA policy.

As indicated earlier, state practice acts have traditionally afforded medicine very expansive practice privileges simply because when such acts were put on the books, the physician was the only medical professional. The physician licensing was all-encompassing, leaving controls on scope of function either to the certifying boards or to the fear of malpractice litigation (something that has only been a major threat for the past 2 decades). Most legislators have been unwilling in recent years to give any profession this much control and, in fact, have attempted to force medicine to be more responsive. This meant that the ANA policy was in effect politically unrealistic, although it would have given the American Nurses Association much more power.

While the emergence of nurse practitioners was the impetus for nurse practice act revisions, state boards and state legislatures quickly realized that amendments should cover all advanced nursing specialties together instead of dealing with each separately. Consequently many states legis-

(text continued on page 385)

TABLE 21.1   Authorization of Advanced Practice Acts

STATE	DATE[1]	CERTIFICATION					COMMENTS
		NP	NM	NA	NS	PSY	
Alabama	1995	X	X	X			Collaborative practice with physician. Protocols approved by BRN and BOM.
Alaska		X	X	X			No physician relationship required.
Arizona	1993	X	X	X	X		Collaborative relationship with physicians for consultation and referral. CNS not allowed to prescribe.
Arkansas	1995	X	X	X			National certification for CNM, CNS, CRNA or NP. Consulting physician required for CNMs only.
California		X	X	X		X	Standardized procedures when performing medical functions. Collaborative development by nursing, medicine, and administration within the agency.
Colorado			X				Broad definition based on individual nurse's knowledge, skills and abilities. Master's degree in specialty area, accredited program and certification by respective certifying body for CNM and CRNA. Recommended that all NP have national certification.
Connecticut		X		X	X		Advises that all APNs be nationally certified.
Delaware	1994	X		X	X		Full academic year post-graduate educational and national certification requirement (if available). If not a master's level preparation. If the nurse operates under protocols, practice is governed by the BON. If the APN practices or prescribes independently then the practice is governed by the JPC.

TABLE 21.1   *(continued)*

STATE	DATE[1]	NP	CERTIFICATION NM	NA	NS	PSY	COMMENTS
Florida		X	X	X	X	X	Develop a protocol describing the delegated medical acts. General supervision by the physician on site not required. Nurses graduating after Oct. 1, 2001 required to have master's preparation to qualify for mutual certification.
Georgia	1994	X	X	X			Protocols required for performance of certain medical acts. In 1999 a master's degree or higher in nursing is required.
Hawaii	1994						APNs defined as having a master's degree in nursing and certification from a national certifying body recognized by the BON.
Idaho		X	X	X			An Idaho-registered physician must supervise APNs. CRNAs have separate registration.
Illinois	1998	X	X		X		By 2001 applicants must have graduate degrees appropriate to national certification. Practice follows collaborative agreements, which may include delegated prescriptive authority.
Indiana							BON required to adopt rules prescribing standards. BON requires graduation from an approved program and certification from a national certifying body.
Kansas		X	X	X			Additional statutory recognition for CRNs.
Kentucky		X	X	X	X		Practice in accordance with established protocols and seek consultation or referral when required. Practice protocols must be reviewed annually.
Louisiana	1996	X		X	X		Master's degree with concentration in the APN specialty. Acts of medical diagnosis or prescription allowed under direction of an MD or DDS and in accordance with a collaborative practice agreement.

(continued)

TABLE 21.1 *(continued)*

STATE	DATE[1]	NP	NM	NA	NS	PSY	COMMENTS
Maine	1996	X	X	X			National certification and consultation with or referral to medical and other health providers when required by health needs of client. An APRN must be under the supervision of a licensed physician for at least 24 months or be employed by a clinic or hospital that has a licensed physician as medical director.
Maryland		X	X	X	X		Must pass a national certification exam and have a written agreement with a collaborative MD. Certified Nurse Specialists in Psychotherapy are certified by the BON.
Massachusetts	1994	X	X	X	X	X	Graduate degree in advanced nursing practice or certificate of an approved educational program. Collaborative Practice with an M.D.
Michigan		X	X	X			Only nurses certified in specialty field allowed to present themselves as nurse specialists. Clinical nurse specialists are titled nurse practitioners. No physician collaboration or supervision is required.
Minnesota		X	X	X	X	X	No separate category of APNs. Certification by professional nursing organization is approved by the BON.
Mississippi	1995	X	X	X			Must be nationally certified as a NP and submit practice documentation of collaborative, consultative relationship with a physician. Practice must be in an approved site and physician must be within 15 miles of this place. Joint supervision by BON and BOM.

TABLE 21.1 *(continued)*

STATE	DATE[1]	NP	NM	NA	NS	PSY	COMMENTS
			CERTIFICATION				
Missouri	1996	X	X	X			Recognized by their specific clinical nursing specialty. Also recognized as specialties are family, adult, oncology, etc. Recognition as an APN must be done through ongoing compliance with the rules. No written collaboration is required when acting consistent with one's skill and training.
Montana	1993	X	X	X			Completion of a recognized course of study and successful completion of a national exam. New graduates must have a master's degree in their NP specialty, plus national certification.
Nebraska		X	X	X			Since 1996 must have a master/doctorate degree to practice except for Women's Health and Neonatal. CRNAs must practice with consultation, collaboration, or consent of a physician. CNMs must have a practice agreement jointly approved by the BON and BOM, and protocols.
Nevada		X	X	X			Psychotherapist must have a master's degree. APNs will be required to have one by 2005. Written protocols at every job site and a collaborative agreement signed by a physician. The BRN audits 5% of the APN practices annually. CRNAs are not considered APNs and do not have a collaborative practice and cannot (since 1988) prescribe. CRNAs required to have a master's degree by 2005.
New Hampshire		X	X	X			Current national certification, 30 CEUs in the area within 2 years prior to application and transcript from an approved NP program. No requirements for a collaborative practice.

(continued)

TABLE 21.1 *(continued)*

STATE	DATE[1]	NP	NM	NA	NS	PSY	COMMENTS
			CERTIFICATION				
New Jersey	1994			X			Certified by the BON to present, call or represent self as a NP or CNS. Master's degree in nursing with pharmacology and professional certification. Family Planning NPs have until May 2, 2002 before a master's is required.
New Mexico	1993	X	X	X			CNP primary care provider can practice independently without physician supervision. CNSs must have master's and national certification. Cannot diagnose or prescribe.
New York		X	X				NPs authorized to diagnose, treat and prescribe in collaboration with a physician with a practice agreement. No license to practice as a midwife is required.
North Carolina	1995	X	X				APNs apply to a joint subcommittee of the BON and BOM to obtain approval to practice. NPs may own their own practice and contract with an MD for supervision of the medical acts (written protocols for drugs, devices, etc. are required. The physician must also review and cosign all medical acts. CRNAs are regulated by the BON while CNMs have their own separate statute and are regulated by the Midwifery Joint Committee.
North Dakota	1995	X		X			APRNs applying for initial licensure must have a graduate degree with a nursing focus. APRNs must maintain national certification. Prescription with a collaborative agreement.

TABLE 21.1 *(continued)*

STATE	DATE[1]	NP	NM	NA	NS	PSY	COMMENTS
Ohio	1996		X	X	X	X	Must have a collaborating physician. Practice agreement (except psych-mental health). CRNAs practice with a supervising physician. Starting in 2008 all APRNs must have a master's degree with the exception of NPs in title X clinics. All NPs, NMs, and NAs must be certified by a national certifying agency. A standard of care arrangement must be signed by the APN and his/her collaborative physician. The law also extends until 2010 three pilot programs utilizing APNs.
Oklahoma		X	X	X			APNs must have completed a formal program of study and be nationally certified.
Oregon		X	X				NPs and CNMs must receive a certificate from the BON. The NP role is broadly defined and requires a master's degree for entry into NP practice. NPs may be granted hospital privileges and only be denied on the same basis as other providers.
Pennsylvania		X	X	X			Physician supervision of CRNPs medical acts either direct or by voice. Requires predetermined plan for emergencies, consultation and chart review. The BOM licenses and regulates CNMs and a written agreement is required. The department of Health grants and defines the scope of clinical privileges to individuals.
Rhode Island		X	X				NP practice is covered under the NPA by a joint-practice committee. No requirements for physician collaboration except in the case of prescriptions.

(continued)

TABLE 21.1   *(continued)*

STATE	DATE[1]	NP	CERTIFICATION				COMMENTS
			NM	NA	NS	PSY	
South Carolina	1995	X	X	X			Must have MD preceptors to practice in the extended role. Provide evidence of certification by a national credentialing organization and evidence of a master's degree in nursing.
South Dakota	1996	X	X	X			May form professional service corporations. Rules for such are to be under the jurisdiction of the BON. Must have a practice agreement with an MD preceptor. MD on site supervision one half day a week. CRNAs must be under the supervision of a MD licensed in the state (on site supervision is not required).
Tennessee							RNs are not prohibited from expanded roles but they must assume personal responsibility for all their acts.
Texas		X	X	X			Nurses in advanced practice are recognized and regulated by the BNE.
Utah	1992	X	X	X	X		Must be nationally certified to obtain licensure as an APRN. Physician collaboration required for prescribing. CNMs are regulated by a separate Practice Act and CNM board.
Vermont	1994	X	X	X	X		The APRN may perform acts of medical diagnosis and prescribe medical, therapeutic or corrective measures. Must have written practice guidelines which include the name of at least one physician in the same specialty area and provide a method of quality assurance.
Virginia		X	X	X			Joint supervision by the BON and BOM. APNs must be nationally certified to apply for state authorizing.
Washington		X	X	X	X	X	Must submit evidence of completing a nurse course preparing nurses for advanced practice roles.

TABLE 21.1   *(continued)*

STATE	DATE[1]	NP	CERTIFICATION NM	NA	NS	PSY	COMMENTS
West Virginia	1991		X	X			The nurse may announce her advanced practice role if she/he has BON-recognized national certification. As of Jan. 1, 1999 the APN must have an MSN. No collaboration is required unless the APN is prescribing.
Wisconsin			X				The practice is designated as a delegated medical act. The RN must follow protocols or written or verbal orders. The RN must consult with the physician where the medical act may harm the patient. The physician need not be present.
Wyoming		X	X	X			The BON may recognize the APNs after demonstrating education or national certification. The NPA statute uses the term "physician collaboration" when referring to the scope of practice act.
Washington, DC		X	X	X			Grants the APN authority to practice without collaborative agreement with a physician.

[1]The date is given for those revisions made in 1993 or later.

lated what are called umbrella advanced specialty acts, while others amended nurse practitioner statutes to include nurse-midwives, nurse anesthetists, and in some cases, clinical nurse specialists and physician assistants. Nurse practitioners, nurse-midwives, and nurse anesthetists came under the specialty umbrella of state practice acts because: (1) their certifying bodies were outside of the American Nurses Association; and (2) they supported state licensure both as a way to legitimate specialist practice and to protect consumers from untrained practitioners. Although the ANA made attempts to certify various levels of advanced practice nursing, including some nurse practitioners, they could not compete with the advanced practice specialty organizations which developed their own certification processes. Although many individual advanced practice nurses belong to the ANA, most do not now do so, in part because of the ANA's ideological stance. Not only has the ANA opposed advanced licensure for nurse specialists, it has also opposed nurses' treating patients and prescribing drugs. The dominant belief system within the ANA is that the ideal role of the nurse is to "care for" rather than cure patients (Stevenson & Tripp-Reimer, 1990). Motivated by competition from already licensed specialists such as social workers and clinical psychologists, some ANA-certified clinical specialists, especially psychiatric or mental health nurses, have sought to be included in a state's advanced practice legislation. As shown in Table 21.1, 14 states now certify clinical specialists.

The American Association of Critical Care Nurses (AACCN), with its huge workforce of Certified Critical Care Registered Nurses, has behaved like a sleeping giant in relationship to state certification and licensure. THE AACCN has taken no ideological stance either for or against licensure and has not sought coverage for its members under advanced practice status. Rather, AACCN has relied on the use of protocols and standing orders. When their practice extends beyond such safeguards, which is not rare, critical nurses assume that physicians will "cover" for them. There is evidence that physicians in fact are willing to back up (and take credit for) nurses' actions which save patients' lives. It is unclear whether physicians are similarly included to cover nurses' actions which result in negative outcomes. As more master's level recruits enter the field, critical care nurses as a group in all likelihood will become more politically active and vocal regarding licensure.

HOW THE ADVANCED PRACTICE NURSE VIEWS HER OWN PRACTICE

With the new nurse practice regulations each nurse must view how the current laws affect her or his practice, including restrictions, expansions, and relationships with clients. With an adversely restrictive nurse practice regulation, individual nurses often find themselves working outside of the state regulations. This may be accomplished by working in close collaboration with a physician who is comfortable and knowledgeable about how an APN functions, as well as maximizing client care to enable the client to achieve satisfactory health care and maximize feelings of well-being. Physicians who have had a satisfactory relationship with nurse practitioners may be willing to engage in this type of practice. It is known that some physicians may take advantage of this type of relationship and take a high percentage of the practice income with very little input into the practice, outside of being named as the owner or co-owner of the practice.

In interviews with various nurse practitioners who have been willing to share their experiences and views of the nurse practice acts in various sections of the United States, it seems that states with the more restrictive practice laws tend to have a significant out-migration of nurse practitioners and other advanced practice nurses (APNs) to states with less restrictive ones. Those APNs who remain try to find a cooperative physician willing to support the practitioner and incorporate her or him into the practice.

It seems clear that APNs in every state have recognized the importance of becoming more political in order to bring about even further changes in the Nurse Practice Acts. For example, APNs in California have banded together to change the laws to allow prescription privileges and to work with HMOs and other allies to campaign to make such privileges more liberal (Gillett, 1997). Currently APNs as a group have been writing their congressional representatives to change the federal laws to allow APNs to collect the same amount of money as physicians when providing care for Medicare and Medicaid recipients.

The following brief summaries are based on interviews with nurse practitioners in the state described, and list the states with some of the best practice acts and those with some of the weakest (Illinois is the worst in the country).

Alaska

Historically Alaska has had liberal nurse practice statuses because of the shortage of adequate health care in outlying areas. Nurse practitioners were, however, slow to act and much of the early laws were for physician assistants. This meant that APNs initially had to petition through that organization. In 1992 APNs received Drug Enforcement Administration (DEA) registration and beginning in 1993 could dispense drugs without any physician being involved. Although APNs feel it advisable to have a physician backup for an emergency, many work in remote areas where they have to be on their own, asking for support and advice through radio or electronic communication, and in an emergency relying on air support to take patients to a hospital. Medicare reimbursements for APNs started in 1992 at 80% of the rate of physicians.

Iowa

Nurses do not need physician coverage and may admit patients to hospitals with local agreements. There are, however, few APNs in practice in the state. Those in practice receive the same reimbursement rate as physicians. The state practice act (July 1, 1996) provides for payment of necessary medical and surgical care and if the care is given by an APN the policy or contract pays for the service. The APN in private practice receives 80% of what a physician would receive.

New Mexico

A 1993 revision of the registration act allowed APNs to practice independently without physician supervision or collaboration. APNs can write prescriptions and have a DEA number. The current regulations about APNs will cease to exist in 2004 unless renewed as there is a sunset law. Currently the APN may not admit patients to the hospital. Nurse-midwives are currently regulated by the State Department of Health. There is a new State School Health Officer who will oversee the school health regulations.

Utah

APNs must be master's prepared, if they were not licensed before July 1992. Prescriptive privileges may be gained if the nurse has completed advanced courses in physical assessment and pharmacology. Controlled medications may be prescribed and the APN may receive a DEA number. APNs, however, do not have hospital privileges nor can they engage in solo practice. Some insurance plans do not reimburse APNs and in those cases the patient must be seen by a physician; this is also true of Medicaid. Other plans state that the physician must see the patient every third visit and the APN cannot practice independently. Certified Nurse-midwives have a separate board and may have a solo practice.

Maryland

APNs have prescriptive authority including controlled substances with the DEA number. In some practice settings the physician must sign. APNs and CNMs may receive pharmacy samples. HMOs can make their own rules as to reimbursement and prescription. Medicaid is directly reimbursed. There is, however, no solo practice, but those working with a physician may do so off-site. APNs must have passed a national certification exam for recognition. Since 1994 APNs may be listed on managed-care panels.

Minnesota

The state nurse practice act does not recognize a separate category for the APN. CNMs have had prescriptive authority since 1988. In 1990 other APNs also received this when delegated to do so under a written agreement with a physician. The agreement must describe categories of drugs and devices allowed. Independent or private practice is not allowed and there must be written protocols at the employment site. In 1995 it became illegal to deny payment for prescriptions written by the APN.

Ohio

As of September 1996, each APN must have a collaborating physician and must develop a written practice agreement. Beginning in 2000 all new APNs must have master's preparation to practice. There are no prescriptive privileges (this provision was removed in order to have the Nurse Practice Act approved). Currently nurses in Ohio need not have the physician present. The nurses use presigned or call-in prescriptions. There is a pilot program of 22 nurses who have prescriptive authority and receive direct reimbursement. The regulations have come a long way since the 1935 Nurse Practice Act which prohibited the nurse from taking a temperature or blood pressure without a written order, activities still illegal as late as the 1960s. The revised Nurse Practice Act not only admits the existence of APNs but gives RNs official authority to do what they had long done unofficially and often illegally.

Illinois

Until recently, Illinois had the most restrictions and nurses felt unable to practice effectively. However, effective July 1, 1998, licensure was established for advanced practice nurses. By 2001 applicants must have graduate preparation appropriate for national certification in a clinical advanced practice nursing specialty. Written collaborative agreements authorize categories of care, treatment or procedures to be performed, and may include delegated prescriptive authority.

SUMMARY AND CONCLUSIONS

Recent activities in the development of nursing licensure have been characterized by efforts to legitimate specialty nurse practice. This has been done in a variety of ways: by rewriting the registered nurse statutes to cover the advanced specialties through protocols or by augmenting physicians' rights to delegate their responsibilities. In other states nurse specialists carry their own license, their title is protected, and they are responsible for their own actions.

State statutes ordinarily recognize the certification of specialists recognized by national certifying organizations. All specialists are registered nurses with additional education. While the amount of additional education varies from short certificate courses to master's preparation, the trend is clearly in the direction of master's level preparation. Only women's health care nurse practitioners and certified critical care nurses are still prepared primarily in the certificate programs. The reason for the first was the opposition of family planning agencies to a requirement for a master's degree, and the reason for the second is the nature of the development of this specialty which preceded the nurse practitioner movement. As educational requirements become longer, more intensive, and more expensive, it seems clear that all specialties will come to require a graduate degree (Bullough, 1995).

With the development of educational programs and state licensure of advanced nursing practice there are now three levels of nursing:

1. Licensed Practical Nurse (Vocational Nurse)
2. Registered Nurse

3. Advanced Practice Registered Nurse
   Nurse Practitioner
   Nurse Anesthetist
   Nurse-Midwife
   Clinical Nurse Specialist.

Titles, however, may vary from state to state, but the three-level pattern is becoming more clearly entrenched. What their emergence has done is make the baccalaureate degree more important than ever to nursing, since it is only by achieving it that the nurse can gain the graduate training essential to become an advanced practice registered nurse. While only two states, Maine and North Dakota, require a baccalaureate for all nurses, those nurses who plan to go into advanced practice would be advised to gain a baccalaureate degree.

REFERENCES

American Association of Nurse Anesthetists. (1990). Executive Summary. *The report of the National Commission on Nurse Anesthesia Education.* Park Ridge, IL: American Association of Nurse Anesthetists:1.

American Association of Nurse Anesthetists. (1997). *Executive summary.* Park Ridge, IL: American Association of Nurse Anesthetists: 1.

American College of Nurse-Midwives. (1997). Personal communication.

American Nurses Association. (1967). *Facts about nursing: A statistical summary.* New York: American Nurses Association.

American Nurses Association. (1980). *Nursing: A social policy statement.* Kansas City, MO: American Nurses Association: 26.

ANA Board Approves a Definition of Nursing Practice. (1955). *American Journal of Nursing, 55,* 1474.

Arizona Revised Statutes (1973). Chapter 32.1601.

Bullough, B. (1976). The law and the expanding nursing role. *American Journal of Public Health, 66*(3), 249–254.

Bullough, B. (1980). The law and the expanding nursing role. *The law and the expanding nursing role,* Second Edition. New York: Appleton-Century Crofts.

Bullough, B. (1984). The current phase in the development of nurse practice acts. *The St. Louis University Law Journal, 28,* 365–395.

Bullough, B. (1990). Advanced specialty practice: Its development and legal authorization. In N. Chaska (Ed.), *The nursing profession: Turning points.* St. Louis: C. V. Mosby.

Bullough, B. (1995). The professionalization of Nurse Practitioners. *Annual Review of Nursing Research, 13,* 239–266.

Clapesattle, H. (1943). *The Doctors Mayo.* New York: Garden City Publishing Company.

Derbyshire, R. C. (1969). *Medical licensure and discipline in United States.* Baltimore: Johns Hopkins Press: 1–8.

Dracup, K., & Marsden, C. (1990). Critical care nursing: Perspectives and challenges. In N. Chaska (Ed.), *The nursing profession turning points.* St. Louis: C. V. Mosby.

Editorial (1939). All those who nurse for hire. *American Journal of Nursing, 39,* 275–277.

Elder, R. G., & Bullough, B. (1990). Nurse practitioners and clinical specialists: Are the roles merging? *Clinical Nurse Specialist, 4,* 78–84.

Fein, R. (1967). *The doctor shortage: An economic analysis.* Washington, DC: The Brookings Institution.

Fogotson, E. H., Roemer, R., Newman, R. W., & Cook, J. L. (1967). Licensure of other medical personnel. *Report of the National Advisory Commission on Health Manpower.* Washington, DC: U.S. Government Printing Office, 2, 407–492.

Frank et al. v. South et al. (1917). Kentucky Rep. 175:416–428.

Greenlaw, J. (1984). Commentary: Sermchief v. Gonzales and the debate over advanced nursing practice legislation. *Law, Medicine, and Health Care, 12,* 30–31.

Gillett, V. (1997). Personal interviews (recorded telephone conversations).

Glover, B. M. (1967). A new nurse therapist. *The American Journal of Nursing, 67,* 1003–1005.

Gunn, I. (1984). Professional territoriality and the anesthesia experience. In B. Bullough, V. Bullough, & M. C. Soucup (Eds.), *Nursing issues and nursing strategies for the eighties* (pp. 155–168). New York: Springer.

Hartshorn, J. (1988). The President's message: Its up to you. *Focus on Critical Care, 14,* 67–69.

Hicks, A. (1938). Crusade for safer nursing: How New York's new Nurse Practice Law was won. *American Journal of Nursing, 38,* 563–566.

Idaho Code (1971). Section 54-1413 (e).

Jacobsen, M. (1940). Nursing laws and what every nurse should know about them. *American Journal of Nursing, 40,* 1221–1226.

Johnson, D. E., Wilcox, J. A., & Model, H. A. (1967). The clinical specialist as a practitioner. *American Journal of Nursing, 67,* 2296–2303.

Kalisch, B. J., & Kalisch, P. A. (1982). *History and politics of nursing.* Philadelphia: J. B. Lippincott.

Lesnik, M. J., & Anderson, B. E. (1947). *Legal aspects of nursing.* Philadelphia: J. B. Lippincott.

Litoff, B. (1978). *American midwives: 1860 to present.* Westport, CT: Greenwood Press.

Maine Revised Statutes. (1974). Title 32, Chapter 31, Section 2102.

Missouri Statutes. (1975). 335.016.

National Center for Health Statistics. (1972–1973). *Health resources statistics: Health manpower and health statistics.* U.S. Public Health Services Publication, No. 1509.

Nevada Revised Statutes (1973). Chapter 632.020.

Oregon Revised Statutes (1973). Chapter 678-410.

Rehm, A. A. (1987). Personal letter to Y. Scherer.

Roemer, R. (1973). Legal systems regulation of health personnel: A comparative analysis. *Milbank Memorial Fund Quarterly, 46* (1968), reprinted in *Politics and Law in Health Care Policy,* Edited by J. McKinley.

Rohde, I. M. (1968). The nurse as a family therapist. *The American Journal of Nursing, 67,* 1003–1005.

Shyrock, R. H. (1967). *Medical licensing in America, 1650–1965.* Baltimore: Johns Hopkins University Press.

Stevenson, J. S., & Tripp-Reimer, T. (Eds.). (1990). *Knowledge about care and caring: State of the art and future developments.* Kansas City, MO: American Academy of Nursing.

Sultz, H. A., Henry, L. M., Kinyon, J., Buck, G. M., & Bullough, B. (1983). Nurse practitioners—A decade of change, program highlights. *Nursing Outlook, 31,* 138–141.

Thatcher, V. S. (1953). *A history of anesthesia: With emphasis on the nurse specialist.* Philadelphia: J. B. Lippincott.

Tom, S. (1982). Nurse-midwifery: A developing profession. *Law, Medicine, and Health Care, 10,* 262–266.

United States Reports. (1888). (*Cases Adjudged in the Supreme Courts*) 129 Dent v. West Virginia, 114–128.

LEGAL ISSUES AND ADVANCED PRACTICE

Winifred Y. Carson

BACKGROUND FOR ADVANCED PRACTICE

A LTHOUGH the federal constitution does not explicitly grant authority to states to license health professions, states have presumed the right to enact health licensing legislation under the federal constitution reserve powers clause. Under this principle, states license health care professionals under the reasonable expectation that the state is responsible for protecting the health and safety of its citizens.[1] Health licensure laws should not discriminate against out-of-state practitioners; and the regulation of health care professionals should not burden interstate commerce.[2, 3] With state legislators delegating authority to boards of licensed professionals to regulate practice, it is intended that the professions would regulate themselves.[4]

Much has occurred in the 20th century. In less than 100 years, nursing has undergone a major transition. The profession has moved from the original debate in the early 1900s about whether state regulation of nursing was necessary, to a debate about the method of regulation that would allow nurses to safely practice across state lines.[5] When the first mandatory state licensure laws for nurses were enacted in 1938 and afterward, the practice of nursing was defined as the performance of certain functions under the supervision of a physician.[6] As noted by Safriet and Hadley, scopes for nursing practice paralleled their medical counterparts and were written to avoid conflict in nursing practice. The scopes were structured to include narrowly defined independent functions and to mandate a dependent or complementary role as states moved toward mandatory licensure.[7]

Although our focus is on nursing practice, we must review physician licensure and regulation to best understand nursing. As the first health care providers to be licensed, physicians attempted to incorporate all aspects of diagnosis and treatment into the definition of medical practice.[8] And, nurses, recognizing that physician-imposed limitations created by early medical practice acts were written without acknowledgment of the interdependence and independence of other health care providers, attempted to cull out an independent scope for nursing practice.

As medical licensure evolved so did legal theory associated with regulation of health professional regulation. As one legal scholar noted:

> "Modern administrative law scholarship has evolved through three historical periods, each of which emphasized a particular aspect of the field [professional regulation]. In the Progressive and New Deal Eras, scientific experts and political bureaucrats fashioned rational, objective public policies . . . "[9]

Lawyers immediately recognized the need for input/participation into the regulatory process and began working in concert with state legislators to develop and fashion laws to address regulation of licensure and activities of professionals. Like society, the profession was male-dominated, bringing with it a male perspective on regulation. At that time, much like today, the debate about regulation was limited to those participating in the "regulatory/legislative" process, predominately men. And, while nursing, largely a female dominated profession, continued its thoughtful and deliberative study and discussions of regulation and licensure, the ideas and recommendations coming out of those sessions received secondhand interpretation by male legislators and lawyers when incorporated into statute. Thus, nursing statutes were initially structured and continue to perpetuate an organized medicine model which confines nurses to a largely complementary role in the provision of health services.[10] However, with time, the nursing profession has tried to expand and redefine nursing practice within this restrictive regulatory model.

Based upon *state* constitutional law concepts, Boards of Nursing have been delegated the administrative authority not only to issue licenses, but also to provide professional interpretations of scope of licensure. While some legal scholars challenge the appropriateness of executive delegation to administrative agencies,[11] virtually everyone tends to agree that legislative delegation of authority to license and regulate health professionals, by an appointed group of health professionals, is appropriate and consistent with state law theories and interpretation.

Under these constitutional health and safety mandates, State Boards of Nursing developed or expanded educational or certification requirements for licensure, reviewed educational curricula for schools of nursing, and determined the boundaries or scopes of nursing practice including advanced practice.[12] In addition to fighting to enact legislation, nurses also used state boards of nursing to authorize advanced nursing practice through advisory opinions, rules and regulations, depending upon state structure.

ADVANCED PRACTICE SCOPE AND FEIN V. PERMANENTE MEDICAL GROUP[13]

Prior to *Fein v. Permanente Medical Group*, advanced practice nurses relied on the independent scope of registered nursing practice to define and cull out an advanced practice scope. However, with time and legal challenges to the activities of advanced practice nurses, a clear line of cases emerged which defined the advanced practice scope and the independence of advanced nursing practice. *Fein v. Permanente Medical Group* 38 Cal. 3d 137, aff'd 474 U.S. 892 (1985) is cited as the lead case in defining the standard of care for nurse practitioners. In this case a nurse practitioner and a physician missed the symptoms of a heart attack and both were sued. The court went directly to state law as evidenced by the legislative report on the practice bill and acknowledged the legislative intent "to recognize the existence of overlapping functions between nurses and physicians and to permit additional sharing of functions within organized health systems which provide collaboration between physicians and registered nurses." Thus, the court noted that:

" . . . the 'examination' or 'diagnosis' of a patient cannot in all circumstances be said—as a matter of law—to be a function reserved to physicians, rather than registered nurses or nurse practitioners"

The court expanded the standard of care for nurse practitioners to require them to meet "the standard of care of a reasonably prudent nurse practitioner in conducting the examination and prescribing treatment . . . " *Fein*, ibid.

This standard has been applied to other cases as well. In the matter of *Kennedy v. U.S.* 750 F.Supp 206 (1990), the court was asked to determine malpractice in a cancer misdiagnosis which involved a nurse practitioner and two physicians acting independently. In this matter, the court did not directly address the nurse practitioner's malpractice. However, in stating the standard of care utilized in this case, the court noted that "Medical testimony unequivocally establishes that the standard of care relevant to the diagnosis and treatment of breast lumps is uniform . . . " Thus, a uniform standard was applied to all health care professionals in this case, including the nurse practitioner, in determining malpractice.

In another case addressing the activities of a nurse anesthetist who worked under a protocol and scope of practice agreement, the court held that the physician she worked with and his corporation were not responsible for her negligence, stating that:

> "The record shows that the nurse anesthetist who administered anesthesia to Gersheeny was acting independently and not under the direct supervision of a physician within the statute. Accordingly, no physician-shareholder could have been held liable for a nurse anesthetist's negligence." See *Gersheeny v. Martin McFall Messenger Anesthesia Professional Association* 539 So.2d 1131 (1989).

A line of state administrative cases specific to nursing reinforces the concept of licensed professionals regulating their scope of practice. These include Arkansas cases which highlight the historical authority granted to nurses under a separate scope of practice. In May 1993, the State Medical Board adopted new regulations for physicians which would have had a significant and adverse impact on registered nurse practitioners (RNPs). The regulations were virtually identical to regulations adopted by the Medical Board in 1980 which were ultimately declared invalid by the Arkansas Supreme Court.[14] However, 1980 regulations included provisions to limit the number of RNPs a physician could employ or supervise to two. The regulations also included provisions which indicated that regulation of more than two would constitute malpractice. In addition, the 1993 regulations required RNPs to work under "direct supervision" of a physician in violation of the Nurse Practice Act.

The 1980 Arkansas Attorney General's opinion addressed basic licensure and delegation issues. Noting that the Nurse Practice Act gave authority to the Board of Nursing, not the Board of Medical Examiners, to regulate the practice of nursing, the Attorney General stated:

> "The State Board of Nursing has formally adopted rules and regulations for Registered Nurse Practitioners. Therefore it is the State Board of Nursing rather than the State Medical Board which is authorized to regulate the practice of nursing by nurse practitioners. ***"[15, 16]

The subsequent court opinion on these rules reflects consistency in legal analysis and clarity about the authority of nursing to regulate nursing practice. Speaking to the regulation which established nurse/physician ratios, the Arkansas court stated:

> "We find the regulation invalid insofar as it restricts the number of RNPs that may be employed by a physician or a group of physicians and declares that a violation of the restriction is malpractice. The legislature has not even attempted to delegate to the State Medical Board the authority to define punishable malpractice. Quite the contrary, the legislature specified in the Medical Practice Act, the sixteen instances of unprofessional conduct for which a physician's license to practice may be revoked or suspended. . . . The matter of hiring too many RNPs does not fall within the malpractice statute by even the most liberal construction of its language. The Medical Board had no authority to create a non-statutory basis for the revocation of a physician's license."[17]

Likewise, the 1993 Arkansas Attorney General's opinion as well as the Supreme Court's decision consistently express support for retention of the case precedent.[18]

Although state law case precedent is not transferable from one jurisdiction to another, there is continued state support for analysis and interpretations which reinforce the ability of nurses to regulate nursing practice. For example, in a number of opinions by the state Attorney General, there seems to be deference for the authority of the legislature to clearly protect the due process rights of differing classes of individuals. In determining the constitutionality of a pretrial screening procedure for medical malpractice cases, which is applicable only to alleged malpractice by licensed health care professionals, the Attorney General reiterated one of the holdings offered in *Hoem,* which states:

> "We cannot condone the legislature's use of the law to protect one class of people from financial difficulties while it dilutes the rights under the constitution of another class of people. Every professional confronts financial distress at some time, and

that does not justify depriving others of the equal protection guaranteed by the constitution."[19]

Boards of Medicine have attempted to circumvent the authority of the Boards of Nursing to regulate advanced nursing practice in other jurisdictions, and while the efforts have ranged in structure and argument, Boards of Nursing seem to overwhelmingly retain jurisdiction, once established by statute.[20]

PRESCRIPTIVE AUTHORITY AND ADVANCED PRACTICE

Even with the statutory authority and regulatory recognition of advanced practice, Boards of Medicine (BOM) have worked aggressively to control the regulation of nursing in the area of advanced practice. With the advent of nurses obtaining prescriptive authority, physicians and others aggressively worked to limit expansion of the nursing scope of practice. Through the use of joint regulation and other mechanisms, medical and other specialty groups have lobbied so effectively that no 2 of the 48 prescriptive authority statutes, regulations, or attorney general opinions are alike. Twenty-two states with joint regulation of advanced practice[21, 22, 23] have statutes that have been structured in the following manner:

- Statutory definitions of collaboration with definitions of the term collaboration varying from "supervision" to collaboration (as known and understood by nurses);
- Language in the statute authorizing the Board of Medicine to participate in the development of and/or review and approve the rulemaking on prescriptive authority/advanced practice; and
- Statutes which limit or require nurses to practice in legislatively mandated ratios with physicians.

These practice statutes and others continue to limit the ability of the advanced practice nurse to provide complete, comprehensive, and competitive care within the full scope of their education, experience, and professional scope of practice.

The biggest philosophical differences in prescriptive authority are statutes which treat prescriptive authority as a privilege where the advanced practice nurses must apply for the privilege above and beyond APN certification (UT, CA, etc.), as compared to state statutes which treat prescriptive authority as a part of the scope of advanced practice, which does not require additional licensure (CT, NJ). This fundamental difference relates the definition of prescriptive authority to the definition of advanced practice. In states where prescriptive authority is treated as an additional privilege, there is a fear that if the Nurse Practice Act is opened and the scope expanded other challenges will arise. When prescriptive authority is treated as a privilege and not part of the scope of practice, the expansion is especially vulnerable to legal challenge because it may be easily amended and the amendment applied to only a small percentage of nurses in the state. Physician groups are acknowledging and using nursing's failure to incorporate all of the AP functions taught into the scope of advanced nursing practice as another method of limiting AP growth and use. Thus, in states where protocols, and/or practice agreements, are mandated to be approved by physicians, the collaborating physician, not the practice act, tends to define the scope of nursing practice and prescriptive authority is treated not as a right, but a privilege.

Alaska and Washington were two of the first states to authorize prescriptive practice by nurse practitioners, and limited their authority to prescribe via formulary. In the early 1980s, Alaska removed all restrictions and now has one of the most effective statutes that provides independent prescriptive authority to nurses in advanced practice. Like Alaska, Washington State amended its regulation and removed the requirement for practice agreements and supervision by physicians. The statute retains a formulary requirement, yet certified nurse practitioners and clinical nurse specialists may both prescribe. Instead of following this lead, other states developed legislation which was not clear in intent, authority, or scope. Although APNs wanted full authority to prescribe controlled and uncontrolled substances without physician supervision, AP groups recommended using a conservative approach to legislation. Even so, nurses met opposition to development of prescriptive authority and compromise language led to the development of statutes which incorporate the "typical" components of prescriptive authority. These include:

- 26 states authorize nurse prescriptive authority through statute, regulation or opinion;
- 18 states authorize nurse prescriptive practice through legislation which makes the authority dependent upon another licensed professional's scope of practice or regulation or delegation of authority to the nurse from another practice act;

- 5 state boards of nursing have legislation or regulations authorizing prescriptive practice which is regulated by other state boards (such as the board of pharmacy or medicine).

While opponents to nurse prescriptive authority would argue that nurses are not capable of prescribing safely, the number of lawsuits which have been directly attributable to nurses with prescriptive authority are few. In 1994, *Nurse Practitioner* magazine collected data from 1,610 advanced practice nurses regarding their most recent experiences with professional liability allegations and malpractice claims.[24] Of those participants, 25 responded that they had had legal claims filed against them. Thirteen cases involved improper treatment practice, including four which were medication-related. It has not been determined if the four cases occurred because advanced practice nurses were negligent related to their authority to prescribe. The survey did not provide demographic data and, in 1994, there were 43 states with some form of prescriptive authority.

The medication-related cases from the survey are summarized as follows:

- A nurse practitioner treated a woman with a sulpha drug that patient stated she was allergic to. The patient was hospitalized for 3 days with a diagnosis of alcoholic induced hepatitis and "a sulpha versus alcoholic induced" pancreatitis. The woman sued because she alleged she got pancreatitis from the sulpha drug.
- A patient sued the nurse practitioner when the patient reacted with allergic symptoms to amoxicillin prescribed by the NP.
- A patient sued a nurse practitioner alleging negligence regarding the topical application of a medicine.
- A patient was given Provera by a nurse practitioner to stop her excessive menstrual bleeding. The patient then drove in a car a long distance and arrived with a sore leg that was subsequently diagnosed by a local physician as a blood clot caused by the Provera. The patient sued the NP for giving a drug that allegedly "caused the blood clot."

From 1990 through March 1997, 290 nursing medication errors have been reported[25] to the National Practitioner Data Bank (NPDB). Of that number, 11 incidents involved advanced practice nurses.

ANA has seen other instances where anticompetitive actions have led to the inability of nurses to provide care. Although no cases have been litigated to date to address these issues, they include the failure of pharmacies to acknowledge and fill nurse prescriptions,[26] when the nurse has the authority to prescribe; the failure of pharmaceutical companies to provide samples to nurses with prescribing authority; and the failure to fill nurse prescriptions by mail order pharmacies. These types of restraints may be considered group boycotts which limit the ability of the nurse to obtain the necessary "tools" of her profession. Under antitrust law, actions are considered "vertical" or "horizonal" arrangements based upon the grouping of the elements required to compete. Instead of horizontal arrangements, which are typically found in boycotts—a grouping of providers of elements required to compete as opposed to providers or others who may compete directly with the affected party—this arrangement may border upon vertical exclusions. Only upon additional study and review of the actual structure of the companies and their activities, may we prove that the arrangement is a horizontal exclusion, designed to keep the nurse from obtaining essential elements of her profession.

There is a disturbing trend of allowing only pharmacists and physicians to oversee and recommend state actions on drug utilization review panels. Established as a result of the Omnibus Budget Reconciliation Act of 1990, State Drug Utilization Review (DUR) programs are designed to educate physicians and pharmacists to identify and reduce the frequency of fraud, abuse, gross overuse, or inappropriate or medically unnecessary care among physicians, pharmacists and patients. The DUR will assess problems associated with specific drugs or groups of drugs, as well as potential and actual severe adverse reactions to drugs, education on therapeutic appropriateness, therapeutic duplication, drug-disease contraindications, etc. As studies have shown that nurse prescribing patterns differ from physician patterns, concerns arise as to whether these panels, which are usually comprised of pharmacists and physicians, can effectively review and evaluate nursing prescribing competency.

Another major legal issue arising when developing prescriptive authority language is the relationship between nurses and physicians as evidenced through collaboration or supervision provisions, often incorporated into advanced practice statutes.

COLLABORATION VERSUS SUPERVISION

Many states with advanced practice laws or regulations include some provisions that mandate a relationship with a physician. While Alaska's practice arrangement provisions are extremely flexible, other states' laws or regulations all too often require some form of supervision. While some states may term the relationship collaborative, more often than not, it is actually supervisory. While the overall definition of collaboration in most states is consistent with nursing's perception of the concept, when other levels of collaboration are created or conditioned using such terms as "indirect" and "immediate," they are actually levels of supervision. Inconsistency in the definitions utilized not only gives organized medicine fuel to challenge more progressive definition; it also impedes the development of standardized federal law and regulations related to APN practice. Without consistency, we see courts and others looking to other sources beyond the practice act to determine APN scope, including:

- legislative histories of the definitions;
- professional testimony; and
- treatises and academic articles on the given subject within the appropriate context.

When Maine amended its nurse practice act, it included more flexible collaboration requirements. However, in doing so, the physicians proposed language to limit liability in lawsuits. The language offered physicians virtual immunity from civil suit, if in a collaborative relationship, as opposed to sharing the responsibility with each party in the relationship. The language also limited physicians' responsibility to written documents developed through protocol or a physician's written response to a request for consultation. Although the bill passed through the legislature with nursing language which apportioned liability based on responsibility, the governor (a MD) vetoed the bill.[27]

State courts cannot review a definition and challenge subsequent interpretations as articulated in regulations, advisory opinions, declaratory judgments, or hospital policy, which may further limit or restrict interpretations of such terms as collaboration and supervision.

ADVANCED PRACTICE AND ANTITRUST

While all barriers may be challenged, those that are statutorily imposed are the toughest to overcome. When barriers are placed in nurse practice acts or other statutes, the courts presume that the barriers were analyzed, discussed, and developed by legislators prior to enactment. Hence, the courts presume that there is a *rational relationship* between the law enacted and its stated purpose. Unless one can prove:

1. A rational relationship does not exist or the purpose and law are inconsistent;
2. The legislation violates substantive due process; or
3. That equal protection has not been afforded under the law;

it is hard to overturn the law. Hence, nursing organizations and boards should be cautious about what is incorporated in law that may create barriers to practice.

Nurse Midwifery Associates v. B.K. Hibbitt 918 F.2d 605 (U.S.C.A., 6th Circuit) is an insidious example of how other health care providers collaborate to limit the ability of the nurse to compete with physicians. In this case, nurse-midwives had been effective care providers at one of the Nashville hospitals and were seeking to provide their services to an expanded private clientele. They joined together, with the assistance of a collaborating obstetrician/gynecologist, and developed a nurse-midwifery practice. The nurses received privileges at some of the hospitals; however, when the medical community found out about this, physicians joined together to:

1. Force the hospital to rescind the initial admitting privileges granted to the group;
2. Compel other physicians to refuse to provide primary care (pediatrics) to children delivered by the nurse-midwife group; and
3. Coerce the malpractice provider to deny coverage to the backup obstetrician/gynecologist who assisted the midwifery group.

These actions, argued the lawyers for the nurses, constituted a group boycott under both state and federal antitrust laws—concerted action to limit and impede the ability of the nurses to practice their profession. Although nurses were unable to prove a group boycott under state antitrust law, the courts deemed it a boycott under the federal statute, McCarran-Ferguson Act; and the nurses were able to prove a pattern and practice of anticompetitive behavior.

In Washington state, nurses have documented the activities of one preferred provider organization whose assessors admit to directing psychiatric cases which need drug therapies to physicians, instead of to psych/ mental health clinical nurse specialists who have prescriptive privileges.[28]

Nurse-midwives and certified registered nurse anesthetists have complained about the use of insurance surcharges to increase malpractice premiums of physicians who collaborate with nurses. Usually these cases are brought by organizations or groups of nurses against private insurers and a settlement is negotiated prior to trial. However, in the only instance where a case was brought before the insurance commissioner for review, an opinion was rendered which stated that the premium increase allegedly imposed for collaboration had no actuarial basis.[29] Likewise, no other insurer has proven that collaboration increases premiums through actuarial data. The case is *In the Matter of National Capital Reciprocal Insurance Company 1991 Rate Filing* (DC, Order 92-7A, February 7, 1992).

Recently we were informed of refusals by physical therapists to execute orders for care written by advanced practice nurses. This activity may be another form of group boycott. Until we have additional information, we cannot discern whether this is anticompetitive behavior which should be addressed through enforcement of antitrust laws.

Too often hospitals develop position descriptions for nursing and other staff which are in direct contradiction with the scope of nursing as defined by state law.[30] Many institutions utilize perfusionists, medical care technicians, and other nonlicensed staff to provide care that comes directly within the scope of nursing practice. For examples, dialysis technicians are being used to place lines in Ohio;[31] patient care aides are being used for IV monitoring in Maine and Massachusetts; and other unlicensed personnel have been authorized to give injections, IV and subcutaneously, in Oregon;[32] with Oregon being the only state BON to actually promulgate regulations to control this unlicensed practice.[33]

All of the activities described above which may affect nursing cannot be considered per se as violations of the Sherman Antitrust Act. As noted in *Oltz v. St. Peter's Community Hospital*, group boycotts or concerted refusals to deal constitute per se category violations. However, the courts have been hesitant to apply the boycott per se rule to an arrangement when the economic impact of the arrangement was not obvious, 861 F.2d 1440, 1445 (9th Cir. 1988). See also *Harkins Amusement Centers, Inc. v. General Cinema Corp.*, 850 F.2d 477, 486 (9th Cir., 1988). Likewise, some health care lawyers have noted that the group boycott "straddles the per se and rule of reason approaches."[34] With the precedent established by *Arizona v. Maricopa County Medical Center*,[35] *Northwest Stationers v. Pacific Stationary*,[36] and *Oltz*,[37] the courts have specifically narrowed the application of the per se rule.

Bobrow, and other legal scholars, however, argue that courts should grant antitrust immunity to state agencies only if they demonstrate that the state has authorized anticompetitive actions. If the agency's structure encourages it to pursue private rather than public goals, then the state must actively supervise anticompetitive conduct.

Boards of Medicine and vicariously, state medical organizations, use limiting, anticompetitive language in state practice acts to impede competition and limit the ability of the nurse, especially the nurse in advanced practice, to obtain financial parity. And nurses continue to promote use of much of this language, unknowingly creating infrastructures which impede nurse practice. In some cases, state agencies closely resemble private entities and they have "expert agencies." These agencies have a stake in the welfare of the groups they regulate because most of their board members are drawn from the ranks of the industries or professions they regulate. The policies and operations of such agencies tend to be insulated from public view and are subject to minimal state regulation and, like many BON and BOM, their fees are used to staff and finance their operations, and these agencies tend to exercise complete discretion with respect to the policies they pursue.

If nurses are going to respond to anticompetitive activities, the profession must develop a strong database to prove that nurses are suffering from disparate treatment. With the statutory purpose of all practice acts being *protection of health and safety of the public*, legislators can impose seemingly anticompetitive imposed conditions, as long as there is a stated public purpose and intent for such legislation. Nurses must affirmatively work to compel legislators to ask questions about these anticompetitive provisions and the harm to not merely the profession, but to the public as well. The provisions limit access to timely, cost-effective nursing services. Until registered nurses compel legislators to address inequities created by statutes designed to protect existing professional status of other professionals, the battle for equity will continue.

CHANGES IN THE REGULATION OF ADVANCED PRACTICE

The ceding of authority to regulate nursing, however, has been occurring for decades. With internal discussion and debate over the pros and cons of regulating nurses and the continued desire of medicine to control advanced practice, medical boards have and continue to attempt to wrest control of advanced practice. Joint regulation of nurse-midwifery, however, evolved in a different manner from regulation of other forms of advanced practice. Through collaboration, physicians and midwives jointly developed a model for practice which vested authority to regulate nursing-midwifery in Boards of Medicine or, alternatively, departments of health.[38] This dichotomy in approach to advanced practice has led to the promulgation of opinions which often treat midwives differently from other advanced practice nursing categories. Since nurse-midwife prescriptive practice is often treated differently from that of a nurse practitioner, contradictory opinions on the practice have been rendered. It is interesting to note that in a 1977 Attorney General's opinion on the activities appropriate for lay- and nurse-midwives, the Attorney General noted that, even with statutes authorizing a nonlicensed person to administer noninjectible medications, they felt that the activity of placing silver nitrate in the eyes of newborns was a procedure requiring application by a physician or nurse and stated that: "No matter how simple the procedure, yet laudable its purpose, it constitutes administering of medicines and cannot be performed by a lay midwife."[39] Likewise, in efforts to foster and protect clinical nurse specialist (CNS) practice, the nursing profession did not make distinctions in the regulation of this master's-prepared group until after hospitals and other institutional policies expanded their role. Now there is a move afoot to recognize the CNS title through statute, and incorporate this specialty into the group considered advanced practice nurses.[40]

Another pervasive barrier impeding advanced nursing practice is use of protocols, collaborative agreements, and practice arrangements. Generally, state practice acts include language which establishes the parameters for these arrangements. Initially nursing believed these arrangements would enhance practice, but they are increasingly *being used to impede nursing practice*.

PRACTICE ARRANGEMENTS WITH STATUTORILY IMPOSED LIMITATIONS

Some nurse practice acts include statutorily imposed ratios or mandated review of the practice arrangements by physicians in an effort to, allegedly, ensure safe practice. Initially, physicians attempted to impose these limitations directly through statute; however, every time the ratios were challenged, they were overturned. To date, the ratios have been challenged in Oregon, Washington, and twice in Arkansas by nursing organizations and groups. In the opinions mentioned earlier, which address the authority of the Board of Nursing to regulate nursing practice, these cases also addressed mandated ratios. Arkansas physicians attempted to impose the ratios through rulemaking in 1980 and 1993. During the 1993 rulemaking, the Arkansas Board of Nursing and the Arkansas Nurses Association challenged the BOM action and the prohibition against NP/MD ratios was reaffirmed because:

- the ratios unreasonably impeded advanced practice;
- the ratios were not based upon any data and reflected a need to impose limitations on practice and the protection of the public; and
- the courts had addressed this issue earlier.

Now, instead of imposing ratios, which organized medicine knows are illegal, a new approach is being developed and provisions are being placed in nurse practice acts or medical practice acts which would:

- require review of protocols by the BOM or an advisory committee of the BOM to approve protocols, or to require restructuring or additional documentation;
- create a cause of action and impose penalties for unsupervised, under-supervised collaboration with APNs; and/or
- limit liability of the physician in a collaborative relationship with a nurse practitioner.

ADVANCED PRACTICE NURSING AND PRIVILEGING

To ensure that APNs can provide services independently, hospitals must allow nurses to have staff privileges. However, hospitals and staff have not been able to determine the best method for incorporating the APN into the privileging process and assuring due process.

The American Nurses Association (ANA) has determined through surveys that APNs have privileges in more than 29 states. The types of privileges vary from full privileges to admitting, consulting, conditional, and clinical privileges based on the nursing specialty. However, the ANA surveys show that nurses with staff privileges are treated inconsistently in the application process.

In 1981, the Joint Commission on Healthcare Organizations (JCAHO) revised its standards to reflect changes in the health care environment such as hospital diversification into new areas of patient service, and an increase in the number and types of practitioners.[41] Later in 1984, JCAHO relaxed the definition of medical staff[42] and broadened scopes of practice rules to include permissive language to allow hospitals to include " . . . other licensed individuals permitted by law and by the hospital to provide patient care services independently in the hospital."[43] Thus nonphysician providers may obtain privileging but cannot serve on hospital medical staffs and participate in the credentialing or medical staff governance process. JCAHO also established a mechanism to monitor a practitioner's preparation and competence to perform advanced functions. The hospital is also charged with the responsibility to establish criteria for clinical privileges and a process for assuring that individuals who provide patient care services are competent.[44] However, even with these mechanisms in place, standards have been included which are inconsistent with state laws and promote limitations on the licensed independent providers' (LIP) scope of practice.

The inconsistent standards and interpretations of existing JCAHO standards reinforce tradition and create additional barriers to the effective use of APNs. For example, in Alaska advanced practice nurses have clinical and admitting privileges, schedule II through V prescriptive authority, and may provide care independently based upon practice agreements entered into with his or her physician partner. Based on the JCAHO Accreditation Manual for Hospitals (AMH) Standards, the nurse practitioner who has scheduled admission of a patient, based upon her health care plan (and appropriate discussion with medical collaborator), could have her patient admission challenged, and/or the hospital could mandate that a physician examine the patient and coordinate the care, although the primary care provider—the nurse practitioner and the collaborating physician—disagree with the hospital's intervention and action. In addition to usurping the provider's judgment, these actions add to the cost of the patient's care. There is a need to restructure the 1996 Standards to accommodate new classes of providers. And during 1998, the JCAHO will be reviewing the standards and making changes, which hopefully will reflect the existing scope of nursing practice and consistency with state licensure laws, and incorporate provisions which allow nurses to serve on medical staff committees to ensure due process for all members of the medical team.[45]

NURSE PATIENT CONFIDENTIALITY

A privileged communication is the confidential discussion which occurs between patient and health provider of the patient's health status treatment options and course of care and one which is intended solely for this purpose.[46] The communication or discussion may also include information relating to the patient's mental and physical health, as well as other aspects of a patient's lifestyle, all of which may be necessary to assess and diagnose the patient's condition. These discussions receive legal protection from discovery and cannot be used as evidence during legal proceedings. The rules governing these communications may prevent the use of medical records and/or bar the testimony of a physician or nurse.[47] In either case, the patient is the one to claim the privilege, which prevents the health care professional from discussing the information with those outside the circle necessary for treatment. The health professional can also claim the privilege, but only on behalf of the patient. The patient can also waive this privilege voluntarily through contract, or at trial by bringing his or her health into issue.[48]

The applications related to nursing vary. From the clear concerns a nurse practitioner may have about providing independent care to his or her patients to the ethical issues surrounding working with youth, we see that the courts are moving toward an omnibus patient-provider privilege for all health care practitioners. However, until we obtain clarity in all state statutes, we must continue to review and assess the case law related to each state to determine the best practices for nurse practitioners.

Problems have arisen when an advanced practice nurse in the course of practice receives information, which under other circumstances (such as the physician-patient relationship) would be considered privileged; however, with the advanced practice nurse-patient transmission, the privilege is denied. At present two thirds of the states have a physician-patient privilege; and only six states specifically include nurse-patient communications. Some states have judicial interpretations of physician-patient statutes that include nurses, while other states extend the privilege only when the nurse assists the physician. This has occurred in part because confidentiality privilege laws were developed without consideration that the advanced practice nurse would work for and attempt to obtain changes in state laws to address confidentiality.

Previously, two Massachusetts cases were considered seminal on the right of nonphysician providers to maintain patient confidentiality. In *Commonwealth v. Bishop*[49] and *Commonwealth v. Stockhammer*,[50] rape crisis centers or rape crisis counselors defied court orders and refused to hand over counseling records for rape victims. In each instance, counseling was provided by a social worker, psychologist, or psychotherapist. In unanimous opinions, the court held that the trial judge should enter all evidence in the counseling record, and then rule on whether any information gleaned should be entered into evidence. In theses cases, the court seemed to give more weight to the right to a fair trial than to the privacy of a rape victim. The most recent challenge to these cases was decided and the crisis center lost, once again compelling them to transmit privileged information. This line of cases and others like it compel nurses to work with other nonphysician providers to strengthen privileging laws.

However, the case of *Jaffe v. Redmond* 1996 Lexis 3879, 64 U.S.L. W. 4490 (June 13, 1996) seems to be a move toward a clear precedent not just to nurse practitioners, but to all allied health professionals.[51] This case, determined by the Supreme Court, involved a civil action filed by the decedent's estate, after Rickey Allen, Sr. was killed by Mary Lu Redmond, an on-duty police officer. The court ordered Redmond's counselor, Karen Beyer, a licensed clinical social worker (Illinois), to give petitioner notes made during counseling sessions. Beyer refused, citing psychotherapist-patient privilege. At trial, the jury awarded damages to the petitioner after being instructed that the refusal to turn over the notes was legally unjustified. The Court of Appeals reversed and remanded, finding that "reason and experience" compelled recognition of a psychotherapist-patient privileged.

The Supreme Court, using a mandate included in the Federal Rules of Evidence to define new privileges by interpreting the principles of the common law, concluded that a psychotherapist-patient confidentiality privilege existed. Further, the Court determined that the privilege was applicable to state cases, through a balancing test, which determined whether the rejection by states would "eviscerate the effectiveness of the privilege by making it impossible for participants to predict whether their confidential conversations would be protected."

While this case did not specifically address nurse-patient confidentiality, it is applicable to registered nursing practice, because the court placed heavy reliance on:

- A state statute which recognizes a nurse-patient confidentiality privilege;[52]
- The court's recognition of the common public protections intended for all patient confidentiality statutes, regardless of the health provider named in the statute;
- The court's analysis of the purpose surrounding the protection of patient confidentiality, which included concerns about providing for effective care and treatment of patients with mental illness, with the court noting:

"Effective psychotherapy depends upon an atmosphere of confidence and trust in which the patient is willing to make a frank and complete disclosure of the sensitive nature of the problems for which individuals consult psychotherapists, disclosure of confidential communications during counseling sessions may cause embarrassment or disgrace. For this reason, the mere possibility of disclosure may impede development of a confidential relationship necessary for successful treatment." *Jaffe* 64 U.S. L.W. 4490.

This opinion dramatically alters the expansiveness of the confidentiality privilege and no longer allows states to apply the privilege solely to those listed in the statute. Instead, courts are mandated to apply the privilege to all who provide mental health counseling and care, which is consistent with a need for a privilege. As long as an individual is licensed to provide mental health care, the privilege seems applicable to that party.

Jaffe was written to address the application of the confidentiality privilege to federal cases. The language included in the opinion does give guidance to future court interpretations, though. Noting that each state recognizes the need for a privilege between physicians and patients, the Supreme Court anticipates a deferral to its interpretation that all patients should have a reasonable expectation of privacy in their treatment process, stating "it is appropriate to treat a consistent body of policy determinations by state legislatures as reflecting both reason and experience." Using this rationale, the court stated that the privilege will serve a "public good" of reinforcing the ability of mental health professionals to diagnose and treat illness and ailments.[53] Again, it should be noted that nurses are included in the definition of psychotherapists under Illinois statute.

A similar nurse-patient privilege has been articulated in New York state case law;[54] however, there is need for additional clarity in all state law. The *Jaffe* case is but one tool in the arsenal to assist nursing with mounting a campaign to obtain clear state and federal precedent for protecting the confidentiality of nurse practitioner communications.

Without clear precedent, nurse practitioners may find their actions limited or alternatively open to review in suits where traditionally the patient has had his or her confidentiality protected. The fear of public exposure of medical records could impede effective communication and dialogue with the patient.[55] Thus, failure of the law to clearly address nurse practitioner-patient confidentiality privilege may be seen as an impediment to advanced practice.[56]

The nurse practitioner-patient privilege varies and expands upon the nurse-patient privilege. It should be developed in a manner consistent with the regulation of nursing practice in one's state. For example, if the state provides for independent practice and scope for nurses, the privilege should also be independent and not tied to the physician-patient privilege. If the practice law (or regulation) ties nurse practitioner practice to the physician scope of practice, then so should the privilege reflect these distinctions. Presently, two thirds of the states have a physician-patient privilege. Six of these states specifically include nurse-patient communications (Arkansas, Minnesota, New York, Oregon, Vermont, and Wisconsin). Many of the other states have judicial interpretations extending the physician-patient privilege to registered nurses. Two states have incorporated into statute a privilege applicable to the nurse practitioner (Iowa and New Hampshire).[57]

CONCLUSION

Nursing has refused to utilize the state constitutional law concept acknowledging the primacy of all health professions to control the regulation of their practice. In many states nursing boards refuse to use the state-created authority to define nursing practice through declaratory orders, advisory opinions or other r/m mechanisms. And, as a matter of "courtesy," the BON refuses to question any other board's activities which may limit or impede nursing practice. Nurses have to rethink this behavior and understand that they are not protecting nursing or their own power to regulate by ceding responsibility or authority. Instead, this action creates a valid basis for developing multidisciplinary boards and/or transferring regulatory authority for licensure to government bureaucrats.

To change things, nursing should:

- Challenge BOM authority over any issue or portion thereof that impacts on nursing practice;
- Require BON support staff to review all care laws and regulations enacted or considered by the state. If they impose on nursing practice, testify or write legislators—make nursing's position known;
- Issue advisory opinions, interpretative orders, advisory letters that provide additional direction on how the nurse practice acts should be read and used to explain nursing practice; and
- Compel state nurses associations and affected nurses to submit formal complaints, which require investigation and action by boards of nursing to address questionable activity.

NOTES

1.   Tim Searching, "Note: The Procedural Due Process Approach to Administrative Discretion: The Courts' Inverted Analysis" 95 Yale L.J. 1017 (April, 1986). The article notes that the right to pursue a chosen profession is also considered fundamental and will invoke due process entitlement to all forms of professional licensing as adjudicated in *Willner v. Committee on Character & Fitness*, 373 U.S. 96 (1963) (due process protects application for bar membership). *Fleming v. U.S. Department of Agriculture*, 713 F.2d 179, 183 (6th Cir., 1983) (treating revocation of horse training license as intrusion on "right to practice a chosen profession").

2.   *Bowland v. Municipal Court* 134 Cal. Rptr. 630 (Cal, 1977) (en banc).

3.   *Williamson v. Lee Optical Co.*, 348 U.S. 483 (1955), *Dent v. West Virginia* 129 U.S. 114 (1889).

4.   See *Feingold v. Commonwealth, State Bd of Chiropractic*, 568 A.2d 1365 (Pa. Cmwlth, 1990) and *Maryland Chapter of the American Massage Therapy Association v. Maryland*, 928 F.2d 399 (4th Cir., 1991)

5.   On December 12, 1997, the National Council of State Boards of Nursing Special Delegate Assembly passed resolutions authorizing the association to move toward implementation of a mutual recognition model of licensure through interstate compact.

6. In 1938, New York became the first state to pass a mandatory licensure law and 2 other states—New Jersey and Virginia—passed registration acts in the same year. In 1903 North Carolina enacted the first nursing registration law; and by 1923 all the states then existing as well as the District of Columbia and Hawaii had enacted nursing licensure laws, which were largely modeled upon New York law.

7. Safriet, ibid.

8. Safriet, Barbara J. "Health Care Dollars and Regulatory Sense: The Role of Advanced Practice Nursing" 9 Yale J on Regulation 417, 9:2 (September, 1992) and Elizabeth Hadley's article on "Nurses and Prescriptive Authority: A Legal and Economic Analysis" Amer. J of Law and Medicine, IV (2-3):245-266 also touches on the concept that organized medicine attempted to confine nurses to a largely complementary and supervised role through the development of all-inclusive medical scopes of practice."

9. Joseph P. Tomain and Sidney Shapiro "Analyzing Government Regulation," Administrative Law Review, 49:2 (Spring 1997).

10. Hadley, ibid.

11. Gellhorn, Ernest, "A Symposium on Administrative Law: The Uneasy Constitutional Status of the Administrative Agencies: Part 1, 36 Am.U.L. Rev. 345 (Winter, 1987) [p. 347, the Constitution provides that [a]ll legislative powers granted shall be vested in a Congress." Statutes that allow admin. to determine what is in the "public interest, convenience or necessity" simply fail as exercises of that power. To legislate is to make normative policy choices, and broad delegations are defective because they leave basic . . . issues unanswered and thus within the realm of the delegate, p. 347–348. "The theoretical foundation of this basic concept of legislative responsibility derives from John Locke's instance that legislators cannot delegate their legislative authority. **insert quote***

12. BON are often fearful to address scope outside of licensure issues.

13. I *Fein v. Permanente Medical Group* 38 Cal. 3d 137, aff'd 474 U.S. 892 (1985) is the lead case defining the standard of care for nurse practitioners.

14. See *Arkansas State Nurses Association v. Arkansas State Medical Board*, 283 Ark. 367, 677 S.W. 2d 293 (1984).

15. 1980 Ark. AG Lexis 49 (September 9, 1980).

16. In a 1987 Attorney General's opinion, the state of Oregon determined a regulatory structure which allowed an advisory committee to make determinations of prescriptive authority unconstitutional, citing the authority of the Board of Nursing to regulate nursing practice. In this

instance, the state attorney general found that the delegation of control over prescription writing to an advisory committee of physicians impermissible because there were no restraints on their activity. In short, they found that the committee's activities were not limited by statute. With concerns about arbitrary and capricious activities, they found the delegation of authority to an advisory committee outside of the Board of Nursing impermissible. See 45 Op. Atty. Gen. 160 (Oregon, 1987).

17.   *Arkansas State Nurses Association v. Arkansas State Medical Board,* 283 Ark. 366, 677 S.W.2d 293 (1984).

18.   1993 Ark. AG Lexis 455.

19.   *Hoem v. State of Wyoming* 756 P.2d 780 (1988).

20.   See *Louisiana State Medical Society v. The Louisiana State Board of Nursing,* 484 So. 2d 903 (1986) where the Louisiana Medical Society filed petitions against the defendant related to Nurse Board rules establishing and defining the position of Primary Nurse Associate (also known as "nurse practitioner"). The Medical Society challenging the administrative rulemaking process, complaining the Nursing Board exceeded its authority, asked the Nursing Board to repeal the rule or amend it to incorporate the concept of physician supervision. The appeal was based upon state administrative procedures, with the Medical Society challenging the Board's response to their declaratory statement. The Board's counter argument was that the statement was not timely filed. The court found that the Nursing Board had not appropriately addressed the issues and that the Society had a valid issue which should be addressed and which was timely filed. Subsequent regulations were enacted by the Nursing Board.

The Nebraska Nurses Association challenged the opinion of the state Attorney General that their regulations exceeded the authority granted by statute. See *Nebraska Nurses Association and Cording v. State of Nebraska Board of Nursing,* 205 Neb. 792, 290 N.W. 2d 453 (1980). In this instance, the nurses association challenged the decision of the Board of Nursing not to go forward with the promulgation of regulations which were jointly developed, but which the Attorney General determined exceeded the authority of the Board (although the Attorney General did not provide a written opinion). The case turned on the fact that no opinion had been rendered and upon state law which prohibited courts from rendering advisory opinions on matters. Subsequently, these regulations were promulgated appropriately.

21.   American Nurses Association Joint Regulation of Advanced Practice (chart), revised April 28, 1997.

22.   L. Pearson, "Annual Update of How Each State Stands on Legislative Issues Affecting Advanced Nursing Practice," *Nurse Practitioner* (21:1) (January, 1996).

23.   Although some states have prescriptive authority authorized through State Attorney General opinions, declaratory rulings, etc., state boards of nursing have had problems implementing these provisions. Thus, states are opting to amend statutes to obtain prescriptive authority. At the time this book is being prepared, Michigan and Illinois are attempting to obtain statutory prescriptive authority.

24.   "Report on the 1994 Readership Survey on NP Experiences With Malpractice Issues." *Nurse Practitioner* (20:3) (March, 1995), 18–30.

25.   A cumulative total of 2,182 adverse nursing incidents have been reported to the National Practitioner Data Bank for the period (1990 through March 1997).

26.   Even more disturbing are legislative trends designed to complement these activities. Some states are issuing opinions authorizing pharmaceutical companies denial of nurse practitioner-signed prescriptions and one state, Michigan, has limited the type of out-of-state prescriptions which can be filled by pharmacists, to those issued by "physician providers." See Mich. H.B. 4149 (Act 153, Public Acts of 1997).

27.   The next year the bill was reconsidered without the immunity language and passed after considerable debate.

28.   1994 phone call inquiry to the American Nurses Association.

29.   The American Association of Nurse Anesthetists and American College of Nurse Midwives have successfully challenged insurance surcharges and in many instances have compelled reduction of surcharges through negotiated settlements.

30.   Some state nursing practice acts specifically exempt hospitals and health care institutions from adherence to the requirements of the statute. See The Law Related to Nursing Care 18.79 RCW (Washington). Section 18.79.40(c) which sets forth exemptions to the state practice act reads in part: " . . . nothing in this subsection affects the authority of a hospital, hospital district, medical clinic, or office, concerning its administration or supervision. . . .

31.   In 1996, the Board of Nursing developed rules on delegation and dialysis care which allow the LPN at the direction of the registered nurse or licensed physician to perform basic nursing as it relates to dialysis care. Ohio Proposed Rules, 4723-13-10 "Delegation of Dialysis" (1995). In 1997 Ohio filed new proposed rules related to delegation which remove

many of the prohibitions related to delegation of IV therapy; and the rules removed the requirement for on-site supervision of LPNs when the RN delegates IV therapy.

32. Oregon, Division 47, Board of Nurse Examines Standards for Registered Nurse Delegation of Nursing Care Tasks To Unlicensed Persons In Settings Where Registered Nurses Are Not Regularly Scheduled (851-47-000).

33. South Carolina considered similar regulations, however, it enacted delegation regulations which limited the type of functions nurses could delegate based upon the unlicensed person's education, skills, experience, and knowledge of the patient. Other factors to be considered include the patient's status, complexity of care needed, and potential for harm, SC Board Position Statement on Delegation (1995). Most states which have promulgated delegation rules usually incorporate these factors.

34. Alex M. Clarke, "Access to Hospitals by Allied Health Practitioners," presented before the NHLA: The Changing Medical Staff Seminar, October 1992 at 11.

35. 457 U.S. 332, 343 (1982).

36. 472 U.S. 284 (1985).

37. Supra.

38. As advanced practice nurses advocated for the regulation of advanced practice, midwifery expressed ambivalence about changing methods of regulation and as advanced practice nurses coalesced to better define this level of practice, divisions occurred between midwifery and other advanced practice designations because one criterion advocated included master preparation. Because the American College of Nurse Midwifery (ACNM) advocates for nurse and lay midwives, they opposed this option. The ACNM has now developed a regulatory model which allows lay midwives to practice in a manner akin to nurse midwives, and there is a new specialty examination for this practice specialty (New York State has a separate board for midwifery and administers the midwifery examination to lay midwives).

39. See 38 Op. Atty Gen. Ore 967 (1977). In 1986, the Utah Attorney General indicated that one could practice midwifery without being licensed as a physician or a certified nurse midwife, however, the midwife cannot act outside of the scope of midwifery and engage in the practice of medicine. No. 86-48 (1996) At the time, midwifery was considered the practice of medicine in that state.

40. Forty-three states now recognize clinical nurse specialists as advanced practice nurses according to American Nurses Association, States

Which Recognize Clinical Nurse Specialists in Advanced Practice (Chart, revised 9/97).

41.   Quigley, Promoting Autonomy and Professional Practice: A Program of Clinical Privileging. *J. Nurs. Qual. Assur.* 5(3), 27–32 (April, 1991).

42.   See Glenn Richards, "Non-physician Practitioners Make Slow Headway on Staff Privileges," *Hospitals* 58(24), (December 1984).

43.   JCAHO at MS. 1.1. These parties known as licensed independent practitioners are "Any individual permitted by law and by the hospital to provide patient care services without direction or supervision, within the scope of his or her license, and in accordance with individually granted clinical privileges." LIPs may include advanced practice nurses, physician assistants, physical therapists and other allied health staff licensed under state law.

44.   Quigley, et al. *supra.* Also please note that JCAHO at MS 2.16.6 requires that "When physicians or other individuals eligible for delineated clinical privileges are engaged by the hospital to provide patient care services pursuant to a contract, their clinical privileges to admit and/or treat patients are defined through medical staff mechanisms."

45.   At this time the JCAHO is considering amendment of the Medical Staff Chapter of its standards, which include the licensed independent provider (LIP) provisions.

46.   The communication must be intended as confidential. *In the Interest of John Doe*, a mother tried to claim the privilege related to her communications with an outreach nurse to address her abusive behavior toward her son; and the court stated that the mandated counseling sessions were never intended "not to be disclosed to third persons other than those present to further the interest of the patient. . . . ", thus the nurse-patient privilege (through agency relationship) was not held applicable to parent's disclosures. 8 Haw. App. 161, 165, 795 P.2d 294 (1994).

47.   Clear authority to utilize this privilege related to conversations with nurses emerged in the 1950s. With cases related to nursing's influence over their patients in testamentary transfers, see *DeMont v. Renzoni*, 132 Cal. App. 2d 720; 282 P.2d 963 (May 4, 1955), *Northwestern University v. Crisp*, 211 Ga. 636, 88 S.E. 2d 26 (1955).

48.   The privilege can be limited or conditioned by state statute. Classic examples of such include the mandated reporting requirements in the event of elder or child abuse or neglect. However, please note that some states strictly limit the applicability of a statutory limitation. In the 1994

Texas Attorney General opinion on whether the records related to the circumstances of a death of a child being held at a nursing home were discoverable, the Attorney General determined they were not. In the 1994 Tex. AG Lexis 384 (April 29, 1994), the Texas Assistant Attorney General determined that a physicians Discharge Summary and a nurse's notes on the child's condition were not discoverable because they were not developed in response to allegations "That the child's death resulted from either abuse or neglect."

Another instance where a statutory limitation on privilege was strictly construed prohibited a school from using confidential information obtained from law enforcement authorities to require students, under threat of expulsion, to participate in group or individual counseling; and prohibited the school using the information to suspend or expel the students. 1987 Wish. AG Lexis 40 (June 12, 1987).

49.   416 Mass 169, 617 N.E. 2d 990 (1993).

50.   409 Mass. 867, 570 N.E. 2d 992 (1991).

51.   There are no state cases which formally address the issue of advanced practice nurse-patient privilege.

52.   In an Arkansas matter, a licensed psychiatric technician nurse, along with a registered nurse, counseled an individual who committed murder and who discussed specifics related to the case. The court found that a confidential communication can fall within the psychotherapist privilege, but that the state rules of evidence do not grant a privilege to all information or communication between the patient and the health provider. *Cavin v. State of Arkansas*, 313 Ark. 238, 855 S.W. 2d 285 (1993).

53.   In another case where a 10-year veteran of the Air Force was tried before a military judge for raping a seven-year-old female child, the convict challenged the experts provided by the Air Force to him to assist in the preparation of his case. The experts included an ob/gyn nurse practitioner, psychiatrist and social worker. The court found that all were competent to serve as experts. See *U.S. v. Tornowski*, 29 M.J. 578; 1989 CMR Lexis 772 (1989).

54.   See *Lynch v. County of Lewis* (1971) 68 Misc. 2d 78, 326 NYS 243, which is one of the few cases to clearly address nurse-patient privileging.

55.   See 1994 Ill. AG Lexis 27(October 25, 1994). Although this state does not recognize advanced practice nurses, the Attorney General held that a privilege was applicable to a relationship with a registered nurse

who had reviewed the records of a patient, but not treated that patient as part of her job of providing mental health services under the Mental Health and Developmental Disabilities Confidentiality Act ("MHDDCA"), 740 ILCS 110/3(a) which covers all " 'Mental health or development disabilities services including examination, diagnosis, evaluation, treatment, training, pharmaceuticals, aftercare, habilitation or rehabilitation." See also a 1990 Illinois court decision related to the use of nursing notes about mental patients. In the case of *House v. Swedish American Hospital*, 206 Ill. App. 3d 437, 564 N.E. 2d 922 (1990), the appellant argues that the notes are not protected by the MHDDCA or physician-patient privilege and the court found the privileged barred introduction of the notes under the physician-patient privilege only.

56.   This article addresses only one aspect of nurse-patient confidentiality. Another and sometimes greater need is to address nurses in diversion and confidentiality issues related to Board of Nursing disciplinary action. One article addressing this issue is Nancy J. Brent, "The Impaired Nurse: Assisting Treatment to Achieve Continued Employment," *Journal of Health and Hospital Law* (24:4), 112–120 (April, 1991).

57.   Iowa House File 693 (bill prior to including in statute) and New Hampshire, R.S.A. 326-B:30 (1996).

LICENSURE, CERTIFICATION, AND CREDENTIALING

Frances K. Porcher

A LL states have statutes relating to nursing that contain at least a definition of nursing, criteria for licensure and endorsement of those nurses who are licensed in other states, and rules and regulations governing licensure processes. Some state statutes contain more specific and often more restrictive regulatory information. It is the definition of nursing, however, that frames the scope of practice. The definition of nursing is especially important for advanced practice nurses (APNs), whose practice combines both medical and nursing components. This chapter examines regulatory aspects of the APN role, including methods of regulation, licensure, certification, and credentialing.

METHODS OF REGULATION

The purpose of legal regulation of nursing practice is the protection of public health, safety, and welfare. Regulatory criteria should reflect

[*]*Note.* From *Advanced Practice Nursing* by J. V. Hickey, Ed., 1996, Philadelphia: Lippincott-Raven. Copyright 1996 by Lippincott-Raven. Reprinted with permission.

minimum requirements for safe and competent nursing practice. Legal regulation of nursing practice is the joint responsibility of state legislators and boards of nursing.

The first and least restrictive level of regulation is designation/recognition (National Council of State Boards of Nursing [NCSBN], 1992). Advanced practice nurses with state-recognized credentials are granted permission from the State Board of Nursing to represent themselves with those specific credentials: NP (nurse practitioner), CNS (clinical nurse specialist), or CNM (certified nurse-midwife). This approach does not involve any inquiry into competence and accordingly offers the least protection in terms of public health, safety, and welfare. The right of any APN to practice is not limited.

The second level of regulation, registration, requires APNs to list their names on an official roster maintained by the State Board of Nursing (NCSBN, 1992). Again, there is no inquiry into competence and usually scope of practice is not defined.

The third level of regulation, certification (NCSBN, 1992), should not be confused with the meaning adopted by nongovernmental agencies or professional associations to recognize professional competence. In the regulatory sense, certification indicates that individuals have met specified requirements and are therefore "certified." These requirements may vary among states. Boards of nursing often use the professional association certification as a substitute for regulatory certification.

The fourth and most restrictive level of regulation is licensure (NCSBN, 1992). Persons having met predetermined qualifications to engage in a particular profession to the exclusion of others may be granted a license by a regulatory agency or body such as the State Board of Nursing. Rules and regulations define the qualifications, scope of practice, and use of title. Unique to this level of regulation is a high level of accountability and intent to protect public health, safety, and welfare.

In 1986, the NCSBN adopted a position paper on advanced clinical nursing practice, concluding that designation/recognition (level 1) was the preferable method of regulating APNs (NCSBN, 1992). Additionally, educational preparation of APNs was to be at least a master's degree in nursing. Significant changes in health care, nursing, and society since the mid-1980s prompted the NCSBN to review this position, resulting in a position paper that recommends licensure (level 4) as the preferred method of regulation for advanced nursing practice (NCSBN, 1992). According to the position paper, care activities of APNs are complex, require specialized knowledge and skill, great proficiency, and independent decision making. The potential harm to the public is great unless there is a high level of accountability such as is expected with licensure. Advanced practice nursing is defined as "practice based on the knowledge and skills acquired in a basic nursing education, through licensure as a registered nurse, and in graduate education and experience, including advanced nursing theory, physical and psycho-social assessment, and treatment of illness" (NCSBN, 1992, p. 6).

LICENSURE

Nurse practice acts have evolved through four distinct phases. In the early 1900s, the first nursing statutes were actually nurse registration acts. A designated board examined the applicant's competency to hold a "certificate of registration," thereby allowing the nurse to use the title "R.N." (registered nurse). The practice of nursing was not defined. North Carolina was the first state to pass a Nurse Registration Act in 1903, followed shortly by New York, New Jersey, and Virginia. By 1923, all states had passed nurse registration acts.

The passage of the mandatory practice act in New York in 1938 marked the start of the second licensure phase. The New York practice act legally defined nursing by defining scope of practice, specifying the education or training necessary for licensure, and prohibiting the practice of nursing without a license (Bullough, 1976). Nursing was narrowly defined to acknowledge dependent care activities pursuant to physician supervision.

This dependent nursing role predominated in nursing practice acts until the American Nurses' Association (ANA) proposed the following model definition of nursing in 1955:

> The practice of professional nursing means the performance for compensation of any act in the observation, care, and counsel of the ill, injured, or infirm, or in the maintenance of health or prevention of illness of others . . . the foregoing shall not be deemed to include acts of diagnosis or prescription of therapeutic or corrective measures. (Kelly, 1974, p. 1314)

Although this definition modified requirements for physician supervision for all nursing functions, nurses were specifically prohibited from diagnosing and prescribing.

A decade of change followed in the 1960s, marked by the birth of Medicaid and Medicare, a growing shortage of primary care physicians, the start of the first formal nurse practitioner and physician assistant programs, the Vietnam War, and the emerging women's movement. All of these events contributed to the growing recognition that nursing practice was significantly restricted by state laws.

In 1971, Idaho became the first state to amend the nurse practice acts to provide recognition for advanced practice nursing (phase 3). Idaho added a qualifying statement to the portion of the nurse practice act that prohibited nurses from diagnosing and treating patients to allow nurses to diagnose and treat as authorized jointly by the Board of Nursing and the Board of Medicine. Although this was a significant step, advanced practice nursing was still defined by both nursing and medicine.

In 1982, the NCSBN published a new model nursing practice act that defined the practice of nursing to include diagnosis, planning, implementation, and evaluation of care and treatment (NCSBN, 1982). Following publication of this definition, several states modified their nurse practice acts to define both advanced practice nursing as well as who holds regulatory responsibility for advanced practice nursing (nursing versus medicine, or a combination of both).

In 1992, the NCSBN recommended that the preferred method of regulation for advanced practice nursing be licensure rather than designation/recognition. That significant change hallmarked phase 4 of licensure. According to the position statement, advanced practice nursing should be based on graduate nursing education, and boards of nursing should regulate advanced nursing practice by licensure because the risk of harm from unsafe or incompetent clinicians at this complex level of care is quite high.

As of 1997, at least 42 states had specific regulations in their nurse practice acts that identified regulation of advanced practice nursing as belonging to the State Board of Nursing. However, 16 of these 42 states required physician collaboration or supervision as part of the scope of practice definition for nurse practitioners. In another 6 states, advanced practice nursing was authorized by both the state board of nursing and the state board of medicine (Pearson, 1998). Only 3 states (IL, MN, TN) continued to define APN function under a broad nurse practice act. Several states are in the process of revising or refining their nurse practice acts to update the definition of advanced practice nursing and the regulatory mechanism of such practice; still others maintain restrictive practice acts for APNs.

Advanced practice nurses have worked very hard in the past 10 years to obtain authority for autonomous practices in various states. In 1997, nurse practitioners in 18 states (AK, AZ, CO, DC, DE, IA, ME, MT, ND, NE, NH, NM, OR, SC, VT, WA, WI, WY) had legal authority to prescribe independent of any required physician involvement in the prescription writing. Nurse practitioners in another 31 states (AL, AR, CA, CT, FL, HI, ID, IN, KS, KY, LA, MA, MD, MI, MN, MO, MS, NC, NJ, NV, NY. OH, OK, PA, RI, SD, TN, TX, UT, VA, WV) could prescribe with "some" degree of physician involvement. Oftentimes this physician involvement referred to either a protocol or consultation and referral plan written and agreed to by the nurse practitioner and a consulting or supervising physician. Slowly, unnecessary barriers are being removed and restraints are being lifted in order that APNs can practice to the full scope of their ability, experience, and educational preparation.

The 1992 model identified an umbrella classification for advanced practice licensure for the purpose of regulation only. The classification is not intended to be used as a title per se. Licensure at this level is designated as Advanced Practice Registered Nurse in one of the following four categories: nurse practitioner, certified registered nurse anesthetist, certified nurse-midwife, or clinical nurse specialist. The NCSBN believes that consistent titling and uniform use of terminology will improve public understanding of the roles, ensure safe advanced nursing practice, and provide a basis for regulating advanced practice.

Not all nurses support the concept of second licensure as a means to differentiate nurse generalists from nurse specialists. Not all nurses believe that differentiation is necessary. The 1992 NCSBN model legislation has been criticized for not addressing issues of clinical competency, mastery of skills, or validation of specific advanced practice knowledge (Hardy Havens, 1992). Rather, some critics believe the law should identify only the generic category of nurses and not specialists or advanced nurses.

Some nurses believe that a rational, comprehensible system of credentialing needs to be established (Styles, 1990). For example, not all APNs are educationally prepared in the same manner. Although the majority of nurse practitioner programs in the United States are now master's-level programs, there is considerable concern about the recent proliferation of educational programs, particularly certificate level and post-master's certificate programs. Graduates of all these programs are credentialed as nurse practitioners; yet clearly there is considerable variance among these educational programs in terms of length of coursework, curricula for nurse practitioner specialty areas of practice, number of required clinical hours, and faculty qualifications. State boards of nursing have experienced major difficulties in credentialing and licensing nurse practitioners due to these variances. As discussed later in this chapter, it is doubtful that national certification by specialty organizations can serve to ensure a rational system of credentialing either.

In August 1997, the National Task Force on Quality Nurse Practitioner Education released a document entitled "Criteria for Evaluation of Nurse Practitioner Programs" in an attempt to provide a model for evaluating the quality of nurse practitioner education (National Task Force on Quality Nurse Practitioner Education, 1997). The document is intended to be used in conjunction with existing documents and criteria such as "The Essentials of Master's Education for Advanced Practice Nursing" (American Association of Colleges of Nursing, 1996), "Philosophy, Conceptual Model, Terminal Competencies for the Education of Pediatric Nurse Practitioners" (Association of Faculties of PNP/A Programs, 1996), accreditation materials from the National League for Nursing, and materials from various specialty and certifying organizations. It is hoped that licensing (including definition of scope of practice) of APNs will become clearer as some of the titling and credentialing issues are addressed through evaluation and monitoring of advanced practice nurse education programs.

The ongoing debate about titling is directly related to licensure issues in that prescriptive authority had traditionally been afforded only to nurse practitioners. As the scope of practice for other APNs such as clinical nurse specialists expands, prescriptive authority becomes an increasingly more important necessity to the role. Nurse practice acts are beginning to change to reflect the need for non-nurse practitioner APNs, such as clinical nurse specialists, to obtain prescriptive authority without having to meet licensure requirements as a nurse practitioner in addition to those for clinical nurse specialist.

There is a growing interest among nurse educators in merging the roles of clinical nurse specialist and nurse practitioner. Titles found in the literature addressing the combined clinical nurse specialist/nurse practitioner role include "advanced nurse practitioner" (Calkin, 1984), "advanced registered nurse practitioner" (Sparacino, Cooper, & Minarik, 1990), and "advanced practice nurse" (Safriet, 1992). Supporters of a merger claim that many similarities already exist in the educational preparation, clinical roles, and practice settings for both types of APN, which are expanding and overlapping. Furthermore, supporters have suggested that professional unity would lead to greater power in activities with legislators, administrators, and consumers. Opponents of a merger assert that the scope of practice is quite different, graduate programs would need to be lengthened, and the legal entanglements outweigh the benefits of a merger (Soehren & Schumann, 1994). Full discussion of this issue is beyond the scope of this chapter.

Phase 4, second licensure for APNs, reflects the many internal and external forces acting on the nursing profession. The health care reform movement of the 1990s forced the nursing profession to increase professional accountability and set national practice standards, particularly at the advanced practice level. Changes in state nurse practice acts, including advanced practice licensure, represent responses by the profession to an increasing public demand for comprehensive, quality health care.

It seems that the fifth licensure phase, interstate licensure, is beginning to emerge or develop reflecting one impact that technology has had on health care. The rapid growth of "telehealth" has stimulated the need to explore alternatives to the current licensing system for nurses. Nursing practices such as providing advice over the telephone which might occur through a managed care organization or telephone triage firm frequently do occur across state lines. The NCSBN has proposed a multistate licensure model entitled "Interstate Compact for Mutual Recognition of Nursing Regulation and Licensure" for RNs/LPNs. Implementation would require legislative activity by each state to address the development of an agreement or compact for knowing the law, rules, and regulations of the state in which the practice would occur. Although the current proposal focuses on RN/LPN practice, it is reasonable to expect that the proposal has significance to APN practice as well. Several liability and legal issues will need to be addressed prior to implementation however.

CERTIFICATION

Certification is a process by which a nongovernmental agency or association attests that an individual licensed to practice a profession has met certain predetermined standards specified by that profession. In response to a proliferation of specialties in nursing and a growing emphasis on quality care in the health professions, the ANA initiated a national certification program in 1974 to recognize excellence in nursing practice. The certification process was voluntary, and initially 191 nurses were certified.

In 1975, the National Certification Board of Pediatric Nurse Practitioners and Nurses (NCBPNP/Ns) began offering pediatric certification examinations, also on a voluntary basis.

In 1978, the purpose of the certification process had expanded to include assurance of quality beyond basic registered nurse licensure, identification of nurses who may be eligible for direct reimbursement for services, and recognition of professional achievement and quality of practice (Hawkins & Thibodeau, 1993). Ten generalist and specialty certification examinations were available from ANA in 1978. Three more specialty examinations were added in 1979. By 1996, more than 130,000 nurses had achieved ANA certification in 24 categories consisting of 21 clinical areas, 2 administrative areas, and 1 staff development area.

In 1980, the Nurses' Association of the American College of Obstetricians and Gynecologists assumed responsibility for certification of obstetric/gynecologic nurse practitioners, neonatal intensive care nurses, and inpatient obstetric nurses. In 1993, the name of the group was changed to National Certification Corporation for the Obstetric, Gynecologic, and Neonatal Nursing Specialties, and five other area-related certification examinations were added.

Although the ANA served as a leader in the development of national certification examinations for nurses, several professional organizations or associations offer APN certification processes. For example, the American College of Nurse Midwives certifies nurse-midwives; the American Association of Nurse Anesthetists certifies nurse anesthetists; and the National Certification Board of Pediatric Nurse Practitioners and Nurses (NCBPNP/N) certifies pediatric nurse practitioners. In 1993, the American Academy of Nurse Practitioners (AANP) began to offer national certification examinations for family and adult nurse practitioners. Reflective of the rapid technological growth in the mid-1990s the NCBPNP/Ns exams became computer-based in 1997 and are offered at specific technology centers throughout the United States.

In response to the growing need for appropriate credentialing of acute care nurse practitioners, ANCC offered the first Acute Care Nurse Practitioner Certification Examination in December 1995. A clear distinction between acute care and primary care nurse practitioners was finally made within the nursing community.

Certification of APNs serves to protect the public by assuring that an individual titled as an APN has mastered a certain body of knowledge and acquired a particular set of specialized skills. Specialists are expected to have expert competence, and certification serves as one means to verify the knowledge and skills of nurses who claim competence at a certain level. Certification of nursing specialists represents a judgment made by the nursing profession about an individual's credentials. Many nurses are certified in more than one area.

Because several specialty groups offer certification, much variability exists in the certification processes. In the past, attempts to standardize certification processes have not been successful for several reasons, one being the intense concern of specialty organizations to maintain control of their specialty practice. For example, in the late 1970s, following 3 years of extensive study, an ANA committee on credentialing recommended that a separate national credentialing center be established (Hawkins & Thibodeau, 1993). The intent was to have one national credentialing center that would be responsible for certification for all nursing specialty groups. Although a national center was never established, the ANA did establish its own credentialing center, which now offers 24 certification exams for nurses. Another attempt to standardize certification processes in nursing was attempted in 1995–1996, perhaps in response to the concern about the proliferation of nurse practitioner programs and the quality of these programs and their graduates. The issue may also have been related to some accreditation process issues that were occurring with the National League for Nursing (NLN). This effort to standardize was unsuccessful as well because specialty organizations again fought to maintain control of their specialty practices.

Specialty designation and national certification also play a central role in both state licensure and reimbursement for specialty nursing services. Several states now require national specialty certification as a requirement for APN licensure. Furthermore, Medicaid reimburses only certified family and pediatric nurse practitioners for their services. These activities mandate that the professional organizations address the certification issue. What does certification mean in the 1990s? Should certification be linked to professional licensure or third-party reimbursement? Who should set the standards for certification?

Of special note is the requirement of state-specific certification for APN licensure by individual states. Currently, three states (CA, FL, NY) require state certification for APN licensure (Pearson, 1998). In addition to providing documentation of formal educational preparation as an APN, applicants must also meet other statutory requirements such as written protocols or supervisory agreements with a physician. The state certification may or may not be designated on the license. Some states recognize national certification in lieu of state certification.

CREDENTIALING

Credentialing refers to the validation of required education, licensure, and certification. Credentialing of APNs is necessary not only to assure the public of safe healthcare provided by qualified individuals but also to assure compliance with federal and state laws relating to nursing practice. Legal regulation provides clear authority for qualified APNs to provide advanced nursing care including certain aspects of healthcare such as diagnosing and prescribing. Credentialing acknowledges the APN's advanced scope of practice. It mandates accountability. Individual APNs must be held accountable for the quality of healthcare they provide as well as their continued professional growth. Credentialing systems must be accountable to the public by providing appropriate avenues for public or individual practice complaints. Credentialing allows the profession to be accountable to the public and its members by enforcing professional standards for practice.

A number of disturbing problems are evident in the nursing profession's current credentialing system for advanced practice nursing. Because the requirements for the various certification examinations very widely, the term "certification" lacks uniform meaning (Hawkins & Thibodeau, 1993). In some states, the scope of advanced practice nursing is so severely restricted that the financial cost and time investment to become appropriately credentialed outweigh the benefits. This is particularly true if the employment situation also fails to recognize the significance of credentialing.

Currently, the issue of titling or name designation is also somewhat controversial. To most nurses, the particular advanced practice designation seems to signify certain professional accomplishments and some political advantages or disadvantages. In this era of healthcare reform, both legislators and the public are confused by nursing's many titles. What exactly is a "nurse practitioner," or a "clinical nurse specialist," or a "certified nurse specialist?" Clarification through simplification of the APN title will foster professional unity and ultimately facilitate and cement the APN role in health care reform.

CONCLUSION

The health care reform movement of the 1990s has provided nursing with an opportunity to reevaluate the regulatory aspects of the APN role. At the state level, there seems to be an increasing trend toward more physician involvement in regulation of advanced practice nursing. Many states require joint regulation of APNs by the board of nursing and the board of medicine. Many require restrictive controls such as protocols or detailed written practice agreements between the APN and physician. Yet other states legally acknowledge the professional contribution of the APN to health care through regulation by the board of nursing only. There is also a trend to specify in state statutes that a master's degree in nursing be the mandatory minimum educational requirement for the APN role and that national certification serve as a requirement for APN licensure.

On the national level, the most significant trend is toward standardization and uniformity. APN licensure is being proposed as the most effective method of self-regulation. It is postulated that second licensure will facilitate mobility among states and increase professional accountability. The proposed interstate compact may serve to address some of the issues that have arisen due to the impact of technology on healthcare. Current trends also include use of national certification as a credentialing mechanism rather than as a voluntary measure of competence. Nationally there is a growing need to set practice standards and monitor APN educational programs relative to these standards. It is definitely an exciting yet challenging time to be an APN.

REFERENCES

American Association of Colleges of Nursing. (1996). *The essentials of master's education for advanced practice nursing.* Washington, DC: American Association of Colleges of Nursing.

Association of Faculties of Pediatric Nurse Practitioner and Associate Programs. (1996). *Philosophy, conceptual model, terminal competencies for the education of pediatric nurse practitioners.* New Jersey: National Association of Pediatric Nurse Associates and Practitioners.

Bullough, B. (1976). Influence on role expansion. *American Journal of Nursing, 76,* 1476–1481.

Calkin, J. D. (1984). A model for advanced nursing practice. *Journal of Nursing Administration, 14*(1), 24–30.

Hardy Havens, D. (1992). Licensure for advanced practice: Be informed, be alert. *Pediatric Nursing, 18,* 540.

Hawkins, J. W., & Thibodeau, J. A. (1993). *The advanced practitioner: Current practice issues* (3rd ed.). New York: Tiresias Press.

Kelly, L. Y. (1974). Nursing practice acts. *American Journal of Nursing, 74,* 1310–1319.

National Council of State Boards of Nursing. (1982). *The model nursing practice act.* Chicago: Author.

National Council of State Boards of Nursing. (1992, May). *National Council of State Boards of Nursing position paper on the licensure of advanced nursing practice.* Chicago: Author.

National Task Force on Quality Nurse Practitioner Education. (1997). *Criteria for evaluation of nurse practitioner programs 1997.* Washington, DC: National Organization of Nurse Practitioner Faculty.

Pearson, L. J. (1998). Annual update of how each state stands on legislative issues affecting advanced nursing practice. *Nurse Practitioner, 23*(1), 14–66.

Safriet, B. J. (1992). Health care dollars and regulatory sense: The role of advanced practice nursing. *Yale Journal on Regulation, 9*(2), 417–487.

Soehren, P. M., & Schumann, L. L. (1994). Enhanced role opportunities available to the CNS/nurse practitioner. *Clinical Nurse Specialist, 8*(3), 123–127.

Sparacino, P. S. A., Cooper, D. M., & Minarik, P. A. (1990). *The clinical nurse specialist: Implementation and impact.* Norwalk, CT: Appleton-Lange.

Styles, M. M. (1990). Nurse practitioners creating new horizons for the 1990s. *Nurse Practitioner, 15*(2), 48–57.

INTERNET RESOURCES FOR NURSE PRACTITIONER STUDENTS

updated regularly on *http://nurseweb.ucsf.edu/www/arwwebpg.htm*

T HIS list appears on the Web site of the School of Nursing, University of California–San Francisco.

Compiled by
Amy Rosenbaum-Welsh

I. Huge Health Information Servers

- *Doctor's Guide to the Internet*
  www.pslgroup.com/DOCGUIDE.HTM
- *Reuters Health Information Services*
  www.reutershealth.com/news/
- *MEDSCAPE*
  www.medscape.com
- *Jim Martindale's Extensive Health-Science Guide '96*
  www-sci.lib.uci.edu/HSG/HSGuide.html
- *Yahoo! Health Page*
  www.yahoo.com/Health

- *Medical Matrix: Guide to Internet Clinical Medicine Resources*
  www.medmatrix.org/index.asp
- *Internet Grateful Med*
  http://igm.nlm.nih.gov

II. Nurse Practitioner/Nursing Resources

- *ANPACC Listserv*
  http://pobox.upenn.edu/~jtv/button8.html
- *Nursing Connection*
  http://home.earthlink.net/~mjsevero
- *"Nurse Practitioner"* online journal
  www.springnet.com/np/npract.htm
- *California Coalition of Nurse Practitioners*
  www.ccnp.org
- *American College of Nurse Practitioners*
  www.nurse.org/acnp
- *American Academy of Nurse Practitioners*
  www.aanp.org
- *Nurse Practitioner Web:* A Primary Care Homepage for Nurse Practitioners
  www.npweb.org
- *Nurse Practitioner Support Services* (includes national job listings)
  www.nurse.net/np/index2.html
- *Virtual Nursing College* (an ftp server in Canada)
  www.langara.bc.ca/vnc
- *Nightingale,* University of Tennessee, Knoxville School of Nursing
  http://nightingale.con.utk.edu/
- *150 Sites for Nurses, Children & Families,* University of Central Florida
  http://pegasus.cc.ucf.edu/~wink/home.html
- *Nurseweek Hotlinks*
  www-nurseweek.webnexus.com
- *Nursing World* (American Nurses Association site)
  www.nursingworld.org

III. Primary Care Resources

- *New England Journal of Medicine* online journal
  www.nejm.org/
- *Diabetes Net*
  www.diabetesnet.com/index.html
- *Arthritis Foundation*
  www.arthritis.org
- *Primary Care Teaching Modules* (a collaborative effort by UCSF and Stanford)
  www-med.stanford.edu/MedSchool/DGIM/Teaching/
- *Primary Care Baseline Project*, University of Florida
  www.med.ufl.edu/medinfo/baseline/
- *Geriatrics Education Project*, University of Florida
  www.med.ufl.edu/medinfo/geri/geri.html
- *VOLC-R Primary Care Resources on the Internet*
  http://griffin.vcu.edu/~dimlist
- *American Family Physician*, online full text journal of AAFP
  www.aafp.org/afp
- *American College of Preventive Medicine*
  www.acpm.org
- *Mental Health Net*
  www.cmhc.com
- *Dr. Rose's Peripheral Brain*
  http://weber.u.washington.edu/~momus/PB/tableofc.htm
- *National Rural Health Association*
  www.nrharural.org/index.html
- *Internal Medicine Notes*, UC Davis
  www-informatics.ucdmc.ucdavis.edu/
  IntMedNotes/IntMedNotesHome.htm
- *University Health Services Home Page*, University of Chicago
  http://uhs.bsd.uchicago.edu/uhs/index.html#homepage
- *AMA Publications Home Page* (JAMA, Archives of Family Medicine, etc)
  www.ama-assn.org/register/welcome.htm
- *Journal of Family Practice*, Wayne State University, Michigan
  www.phymac.med.wayne.edu/jfp/JFP.HTM
- *General Practice On-Line*
  www.priory.com/gp.htm

IV. Government Agency Resources

- *Centers for Disease Control and Prevention* (CDC)
  www.cdc.gov/
- *CDC Morbidity and Mortality Weekly Report*
  www.cdc.gov/epo/mmwr/mmwr.html
- *National Institutes of Health*
  www.nih.gov
- *Agency for Health Care Policy and Research* (AHCPR)
  www.ahcpr.gov
- *Health Resources and Services Administration, Dept. of Health and Human Services, US PHS*
  www.hrsa.dhhs.gov

V. Pharmacology Resources

- *PharmInfoNet*, Pharmaceutical Information Network
  www.pharminfo.com
- *RxList*, The Internet Drug Index
  www.rxlist.com
- *Pediatric Pharmacotherapy Newsletter*
  www.medscape.com/UVA/PedPharm/public/
  index.PedPharm.html

VI. Case Study Resources

- *Med Files*
  www.geocities.com/~fnp
- *Medical Rounds* University of Colorado
  www.uchsc.edu/sm/pmb/medrounds/index.html
- *webRounds* Williams & Wilkins
  www.wwilkins.com/rounds/intro.html
- *The Virtual Hospital*, University of Iowa
  http://vh.radiology.uiowa.edu/Providers/Providers.html
- *The Interactive Patient*, Marshall University School of Medicine, West Virginia
  http://medicus.marshall.edu/medicus.htm

- *Pathophysiology Case Studies*, Cornell University School of Medicine
  http://edcenter.med.cornell.edu/Departments3.html
- *Pediatric Case of the Month*, Baylor College of Medicine
  www.wwilkins.com/rounds/Clerkships/Baylor/toc.html

VII. HIV/AIDS Resources

- *HIV Insite* Gateway to AIDS Knowledge
  http://hivinsite.ucsf.edu
- *The Body*, a multi-media AIDS and HIV information resource
  www.thebody.com/cgi-bin/body.cgi
- *Critical Path AIDS Project*
  www.critpath.org
- *CDC Division of HIV/AIDS Prevention* (DHAP)
  www.cdc.gov/nchstp/hiv_aids/dhap.htm
- *CDC HIV/AIDS Surveillance Report*
  www.cdc.gov/nchstp/hiv_aids/stats/hasrlink.htm
- *Assoc. of Nurses in AIDS Care*
  www.anacnet.org/aids
- *HIV InfoWeb*
  www.infoweb.org
- *Immunet* for AIDS/HIV caregivers; includes archive of AIDS Treatment News
  www.immunet.org
- *JAMA HIV/AIDS Information Center*
  www.ama-assn.org/special/hiv/hivhome.htm
- *AIDS Treatment Data Network*
  www.aidsnyc.org/network/index.html
- *Project Inform*
  www.projinf.org

VIII. Women's Health Resources

- *Alan Guttmacher Institute*
  www.agi-usa.org
- *Women's Health Links*
  http://walden.mo.net/~bmizes/links.html

- *Guide to Women's Health Resources on the Internet*
  www.indra.com/natracare/guide.html
- *Atlanta Reproductive Health Centre*
  www.ivf.com//index.html
- *Women's Health Weekly,* Office of Research on Women's Health, NIH
  www.holonet.net/homepage/1w.htm
- *Online Birth Center*
  www.efn.org/~djz/birth/birthindex.html
- *Female Genital Mutilation Research Home Page*
  www.hollyfeld.org/fgm

IX. Pediatric Resources

- *The Virtual PNP* (a phenomenal, comprehensive PNP link)
  http://home.earthlink.net/~emgoodman/virtualpnp.htm
- *Parents' Place, Health Issues and Your Children*
  www.parentsplace.com/readroom/health.html
- *Pedinfo: A Pediatrics Web Server,* University of Alabama
  www.lhl.uab.edu:80/pedinfo
- *Med Web: Pediatrics,* Emory University
  www.gen.emory.edu/MEDWEB/keyword/pediatrics.html
- *Pediatric Points of Interest,* Johns Hopkins University
  http://medweb.uni~muenster.de/mirror/poi/jobs.html
- *National Parent Information Network*
  http://npin.org
- *American Academy of Pediatrics*
  www.aap.org
- *Pediatrics,* on line full text journal of AAP
  www.pediatrics.org
- *Bright Futures Periodic Childhood Exam Guidelines*
  www.brightfutures.org
- *AMA Adolescent Health On-Line*
  www.ama-assn.org/adolhlth/adolhlth.htm

X. Healing Arts Resources

- *American Association of Colleges of Osteopathic Medicine*
  www.aacom.org

- *Alternative Medicine Homepage*
  www.pitt.edu/~cbw/altm.html
- *Complementary and Alternative Medicine Homepage*
  http://galen.med.virginia.edu/~pjb3s/
  ComplementaryHomePage.html
- *Acupuncture.com*
  http://208.233.90.104

INDEX